Atlas of Procedures in Neonatology

EDITORS

Mary Ann Fletcher

M.D.

Associate Professor of Pediatrics and Obstetrics and Gynecology
George Washington University School of Medicine and Health Sciences
Associate Director of Nurseries
The George Washington University Medical Center
Washington, DC

Mhairi G. MacDonald

M.B.Ch.B., F.R.C.P.(E), D.C.H.

Professor of Pediatrics
George Washington University School of Medicine and Health Sciences
Vice-Chairman, Division of Neonatology
Children's National Medical Center
Washington, DC

With 27 Contributors

ILLUSTRATORS

Judy Guenther   Virginia Schoonover

PHOTOGRAPHY

Audio Visual Departments
The George Washington University Medical Center
Children's National Medical Center

Atlas of Procedures in Neonatology

SECOND EDITION

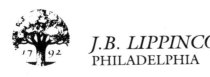
J.B. LIPPINCOTT COMPANY
PHILADELPHIA

Acquisitions Editor: Charles McCormick, Jr.
Assistant Production Manager: Lori J. Bainbridge
Production: Barbara A. Conover, Publications Management
Compositor: The Composing Room of Michigan, Inc.
Printer/Binder: R.R. Donnelley & Sons
Cover Designer: Lou Fuiano Design

6 5 4 3 2

Library of Congress Cataloging-in-Publication Data

Atlas of procedures in neonatology / editors, Mary Ann Fletcher, Mhairi G.
  MacDonald : with 27 contributors : illustrators, Judy Guenther, Virginia
  Schoonover : photography, Audio Visual Department, George Washington
  University Medical Center, — 2nd ed.
      p.   cm.
    Includes bibliographical references and index.
    ISBN 0-397-51195-7
    1. Neonatology. 2. Neonatology—Atlases. 3. Neonatal intensive care.
  4. Neonatal intensive care—Atlases. I. Fletcher, Mary Ann. II. MacDonald,
  Mhairi G.
    [DNLM; 1. Neonatology—atlases. 2. Neonatology—outlines. WS 18
  A881]
  RJ251.A84 1993
  618.92′01—dc20
  DNLM/DLC
  for Library of Congress   92-49106
                                                               CIP

The authors and publisher have exerted every effort to ensure that drug selection and dosage set forth in this text are in accord with current recommendations and practice at the time of publication. However, in view of ongoing research, changes in government regulations, and the constant flow of information relating to drug therapy and drug reactions, the reader is urged to check the package insert for each drug for any change in indications and dosage and for added warnings and precautions. This is particularly important when the recommended agent is a new or infrequently employed drug.

We have attempted to use product names only when the commercial availability of specific items of equipment is relatively restricted. Use of the product name does not imply endorsement of the product.

Contributors

Kathryn D. Anderson, M.D.
Professor of Surgery and Pediatrics
George Washington University School of Medicine
and Health Sciences
Senior Associate, Surgery
Children's National Medical Center
Washington, DC

Garth Asay, M.D.
Fellow in Neonatal/Perinatal Medicine
Clinical Instructor in Pediatrics
George Washington University School of Medicine
and Health Sciences/Children's National
Medical Center
Washington, DC

Kathleen M. Cronin, M.D.
Clinical Assistant Professor of Ophthalmology
Loyola University Medical Center
Stritch School of Medicine
Foster G. McGaw Hospital
Maywood, Illinois

Maureen C. Edwards, M.D., M.P.H.
Associate Professor of Pediatrics and of Obstetrics
and Gynecology
Director of Nurseries
The George Washington University Medical Center
Washington, DC

Martin Raymond Eichelberger, M.D.
Professor of Surgery and of Pediatrics
George Washington University School of Medicine
and Health Sciences
Attending, Pediatric Surgery
Children's National Medical Center
Washington, DC

Ayman A.E. El-Mohandes, M.D., M.P.H.
Assistant Professor of Pediatrics and of Obstetrics
and Gynecology
George Washington University School of Medicine
and Health Sciences
Attending Neonatologist
The George Washington University Medical Center
Washington, DC

Arthur J. Engler, R.N.C., M.S., N.N.P.
Doctoral Candidate
The Catholic University of America
Neonatal Nurse Practitioner
Holy Cross Hospital
Silver Spring, Maryland

Robert J. Fink, M.D.
Associate Professor of Pediatrics
George Washington University School of Medicine
and Health Sciences
Chairman, Department of Pulmonary Medicine
Children's National Medical Center
Washington, DC

Mary Ann Fletcher, M.D.
Associate Professor of Pediatrics and of Obstetrics
and Gynecology
George Washington University School of Medicine
and Health Sciences
Associate Director of Nurseries
The George Washington University Medical Center
Washington, DC

Harold M. Ginzburg, M.D., J.D., M.P.H.
Professor of Psychiatry, Preventive Medicine
and Biometrics
Uniformed Services University of the Health Sciences
School of Medicine
Bethesda, Maryland

Kenneth M. Grundfast, M.D.
Professor of Surgery
George Washington University School of Medicine
and Health Sciences
Chairman, Department of Otolaryngology
Children's National Medical Center
Washington, DC

Robert P. Howard, M.S.
Director, Biomedical Engineering
Children's National Medical Center
Washington, DC

Dorothy S. Hsiao, M.D.
Clinical Assistant Professor of Pediatrics
Georgetown University Medical Center
Associate Neonatologist
Columbia Hospital for Women Medical Center
Washington, DC

Dennis L. Johnson, M.D.
Associate Professor of Neurosurgery and of Pediatrics
George Washington University School of Medicine
and Health Sciences
Associate Neurosurgeon
Children's National Medical Center
Washington, DC

Aileen T. Kelly, M.B., B.Ch., B.A.O.
Former Fellow in Neonatal/Perinatal Medicine
and ECMO
Former Clinical Instructor of Pediatrics
George Washington University School of Medicine
and Health Sciences
Children's National Medical Center
Washington, DC

Gail R. Knight, M.D.
Assistant Professor of Pediatrics
University of California, San Diego
Attending Neonatologist
Children's Hospital San Diego
San Diego, California

Andrea Lotze, M.D.
Assistant Professor of Pediatrics
George Washington University School of Medicine
and Health Sciences
Attending Neonatologist
Children's National Medical Center
Washington, DC

Naomi L.C. Luban, M.D.
Professor of Pediatrics and of Pathology
The George Washington University Medical Center
Director, Blood Bank and Hematology
Children's National Medical Center
Washington, DC

**Mhairi G. MacDonald, M.B. Ch.B.,
F.R.C.P.(E), D.C.H.**
Professor of Pediatrics
George Washington University School of Medicine
and Health Sciences
Vice-Chairman, Department of Neonatology
Children's National Medical Center
Washington, DC

S. Lee Marban, M.D., Ph.D.
Assistant Professor of Pediatrics
George Washington University School of Medicine
and Health Sciences
Associate Neonatologist
Children's National Medical Center
Washington, DC

Kathleen A. Marinelli, M.D.
Assistant Professor of Pediatrics
University of Connecticut School of Medicine
Farmington, Connecticut
Attending Neonatologist
Hartford Hospital
Hartford, Connecticut

Marilea Kay Miller, M.D.
Associate Professor of Pediatrics
George Washington University School of Medicine
and Health Sciences
Medical Director of the Nurseries
Holy Cross Hospital
Silver Spring, Maryland

Claire Bohince Pagano, R.N.
Assistant Director
Neonatal Intensive Care Unit
Children's National Medical Center
Washington, DC

Majid Rasoulpour, M.D.
Associate Professor of Pediatrics
University of Connecticut Health Center, School
of Medicine
Director, Pediatric Nephrology and Hypertension
Hartford Hospital
Hartford, Connecticut

Mary E. Revenis, M.D.
Assistant Professor of Pediatrics
George Washington University School of Medicine
and Health Sciences
Attending Neonatologist
Children's National Medical Center
Washington, DC

Oswaldo Rivera, B.S.
Assistant Director, Biomedical Engineering
Children's National Medical Center
Washington, DC

Lucienne S. Sanchez, M.D.
Associate Neonatologist
University Hospital Nijmegen
Department of Neonatology
Nijmegen, The Netherlands

H. Joel Schmidt, M.D.
Major, Medical Corps, U.S. Army
Teaching Fellow, Department of Pediatrics
F. Edward Herbert School of Medicine
Uniformed Services University of the Health Sciences
Bethesda, Maryland
Senior Fellow
Department of Pulmonary Medicine
Children's National Medical Center
Washington, DC

Billie Lou Short, M.D.
Professor of Pediatrics
George Washington University School of Medicine
and Health Sciences
Director ECMO Services
Children's National Medical Center
Washington, DC

Foreword

Procedures play a critical role in Neonatology. The first edition of *Atlas of Procedures in Neonatology* was designed to delineate the anatomy of the newborn necessary to guide these procedures, to discuss methodology, to point out recorded complications, and to review the literature and supply salient references to the reader. Each chapter was organized in parallel, with major headings for indications, contraindications, equipment, precautions, technique, and complications. The intent was to provide both a practical guide and an understanding of the procedures that were described.

The second edition recognizes the rapid pace of change in Neonatology and the evolution of bedside techniques. New chapters, or considerable amplification, have been directed at central venous catheterization including percutaneous techniques, cannulation for ECMO, flexible fiberoptic bronchoscopy, intraosseous infusions, tapping ventricular reservoirs, cryotherapy for RLF, and dialysis/ultrafiltration. New emphasis is given to physiologic monitoring, including the use of pulmonary function tests. Recognizing current sensitivities, chapters on analgesia and informed consent have been added.

This second edition, like the first, should become a friendly and well-worn companion in the intensive care nursery.

Gordon B. Avery, M.D., Ph.D.

Preface

There is nothing more gratifying to editors than to see their book lying open and dog eared during a bedside visit to another facility. We have been pleased to find the first edition of the *Atlas of Procedures in Neonatology* used not only by trainees and staff in neonatology but also by other members of the neonatal-perinatal health care team, including radiologists and respiratory therapists.

The primary purpose of the *Atlas* is to provide a detailed, step-by-step approach to procedures, most of which are performed by neonatologists, pediatricians, and nurses within the nursery. Some procedures, such as ECMO cannulation, operative tracheotomy, gastrostomy, and cryotherapy, are usually done by surgical specialists, but are included to promote understanding by those who are responsible for the perioperative care of the neonate.

The editors wish to emphasize that following recipes by rote does not replace applying good judgment, should a better method be devised or a patient's condition change. We acknowledge that there are often several acceptable methods of performing the same procedure. While some optional techniques are described, we have not exhaustively included all alternatives, selecting instead those techniques that, in our experience, are most frequently successful and have the fewest complications. Recognizing that techniques are often passed on to trainees more because of personal bias than because of supporting data, we have tried, as much as possible, to base all of our recommendations on sound clinical and scientific data. However, we have not excluded personal experience or preferences when they appeared appropriate.

On the advise of our readers, we have selected a binding that will allow the book to open flat to facilitate bedside use during procedures. The organizational format of the first edition remains. We recommend studying an entire procedure before starting it, not only to review the technique but also to better weigh benefits against risks by understanding the complications and precautions. As in the first edition, we have emphasized the anatomical differences between the neonate and older patients which influence the performance of certain procedures. After every procedure we have attempted to include a comprehensive list of complications, in order to heighten awareness of their potential impact on both morbidity and mortality. The order of listing does not necessarily reflect the frequency or severity of any single complication.

It is sobering to observe that a significant number of complications, some of them not previously recognized, continue to be reported for procedures that have been standard in neonatal nurseries for more than two decades. For example, since the first edition of the *Atlas* was published, reports in the literature on complications of umbilical artery catheterization have approximately tripled. With every new procedure there is a learning curve, but one would expect the incidence of complications to decrease as experience and expertise increase. Clearly, the number of reported complications does not represent their true incidence. An optimistic view might be that increased reporting of complications reflects a more universal respect for the possibility of their occurrence and attempts to find ways of preventing or minimizing them.

When any procedure is applied to smaller and more immature infants, it is not only technically more difficult, but also more likely to be accompanied by side-effects or complications. For all procedures performed in the newborn there is a baseline morbidity; no procedure will be absent complications. For example, placement of a peripheral IV line is a basic procedure essential for the survival of sick newborn babies. There have been significant improvements in the size and quality of intravenous cannulas and pumps specifically to allow for pressure obstruction alarms, low flow rates, etc. However, no matter how good the care of the infant and the

IV, there will always be incidents of infiltration and chemical skin burns. It behooves each clinician to weigh carefully the risks versus the benefits of every procedure before beginning it, while any piece of equipment remains in place, and even in the months and years after completion.

"One cannot possibly practice good medicine and not understand the fundamentals underlying therapy. Few if any rules for therapy are more than 90% correct. If one does not understand the fundamentals, one does more harm in the 10% of instances to which the rules do not apply than one does good in the 90% to which they do apply"—Fuller Albright.

Mary Ann Fletcher, M.D.
Mhairi G. MacDonald, M.B. Ch.B., F.R.C.P.(E), D.C.H.

Preface to the First Edition

The rapid advances in neonatology in the last 15 years have brought with them a welter of special procedures. The tiny premature and the critically ill term neonate are attached to a tangle of intravenous lines, tubes, and monitoring leads. As a result, more and more procedures are done at the bedside in the intensive-care nursery, rather than in a procedure room or operating room. With these technical advances has come the opportunity for more vigorous physiologic support and monitoring. With them also has come a whole new gamut of side-effects and complications. The old dictum to leave the fragile premature undisturbed is largely ignored. It is therefore the responsibility of those who care for sick newborns to understand the complications as well as the benefits of new procedures and to make systematic observations of their impact on both morbidity and mortality. Unfortunately, the literature on outcome and complications of procedures is widely scattered and difficult to access. Manuals that give directions for neonatal procedures are generally deficient in illustrations giving anatomic detail and are often cursory.

We are offering *Atlas of Procedures in Neonatology* to meet some of these needs. A step-by-step, practical approach is taken, with telegraphic prose and outline form. Drawings and photographs are used to illustrate anatomic landmarks and details of the procedures. In several instances, more than one alternative procedure is presented. Discussion of controversial points is included, and copious literature citations are provided to lead the interested reader to source material. A uniform order of presentation has been adhered to wherever appropriate. Thus, most chapters include indications, contraindications, precautions, equipment, technique, and complications, in that order.

The scope of procedures covered includes nearly all those that can be performed at the bedside in an intensive-care nursery. Some are within the traditional province of the neonatologist or even the pediatric house officer. Others, such as gastrostomy and tracheostomy, require the skills of a qualified surgeon. Responsibility for procedures such as placement of chest tubes and performance of vascular cutdowns will vary from nursery to nursery. However, some details of surgical technique are supplied for even the most invasive procedures to promote their understanding by those who are responsible for sick neonates. We hope this will help neonatologists to be more knowledgeable partners in caring for babies and will not be interpreted as a license to perform procedures by those who are not adequately qualified.

The book is organized into major parts (e.g., "Vascular Access," "Tube Placement," "Respiratory Care"), each of which contains several chapters. Most chapters are relatively self-contained and can be referred to when approaching a particular task. However, Part I, "Preparation and Support," is basic to all procedures. Occasional cross referencing has been used to avoid repetitions of the same text material. References appear at the end of each part.

Many persons have contributed to the preparation of this atlas, and we are grateful to them all. Some are listed under Acknowledgments, and others have contributed anonymously out of their generosity and good will. Special thanks is due to Bill Burgower, who first thought of making such an atlas and who has been gracious in his support throughout this project.

If this atlas proves useful to some who care for sick newborns, our efforts will have been well repaid. Neonatology is a taxing field: strenuous, demanding, confusing, heartbreaking, rewarding, stimulating, scientific, personal, philosophical, cooperative, logical, illogical, and always changing. The procedures described in this atlas will eventually be replaced by others, hopefully more effective and less noxious. In the meantime, perhaps the care of some babies will be assisted.

Mary Ann Fletcher, M.D.
Mhairi G. MacDonald, M.B.Ch.B., F.R.C.P.(E), D.C.H.
Gordon B. Avery, M.D., Ph.d.

Acknowledgments

Assembling a book always involves more work than ever anticipated during the euphoria of planning. It has been through the support and encouragement of our coworkers, staff, and families that we have been able to meet our deadlines. We thank the editorial and production staff of J.B. Lippincott for their patience, assistance, and advice. We would like especially to thank John Scanlon, M.D., for reviewing the First Edition in detail and Bob White, M.D., John Sequin, M.D., and David Kushner, M.D., for their helpful suggestions for changes in this edition. We would like to thank again the major contributors to the first edition, as they generously provided pathologic and radiologic case examples: Roma Chandra, M.D., William S. McSweeney, M.D., David S. Rockoff, M.D., and Sylvan Stool, M.D. We especially appreciate the patience and cooperation of our fellow neonatology attendings and office support personnel. Allowing us to add major projects to busy departmental schedules meant sacrifices by our colleagues. For their ever cheerful support, we are grateful. Finally, to our most important supporters, our own spouses, John Hurley, M.D., and Harold Ginzburg, M.D., J.D., M.P.H., we offer our special thank you.

Mary Ann Fletcher, M.D.
Mhairi G. MacDonald, M.B.Ch.B., F.R.C.P.(E), D.C.H.

COLOR FIGURES

A   B

COL. FIG. 11-1
Transillumination. (*A*) Arteries and veins on volar aspect of left wrist. (*B*) Venous arch on dorsum of hand. (*C*) Vessels in right antecubital fossa. (*D*) Left posterior tibial artery.

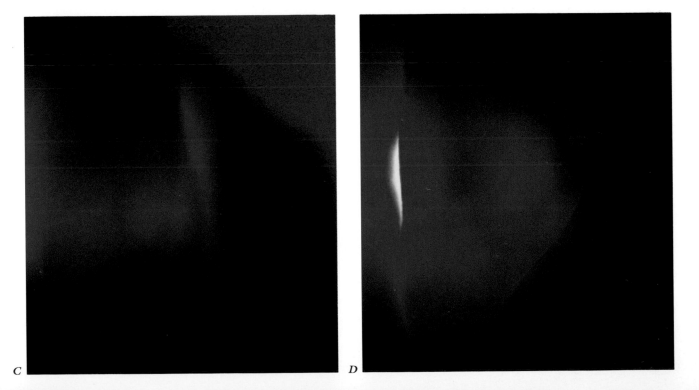

C   D

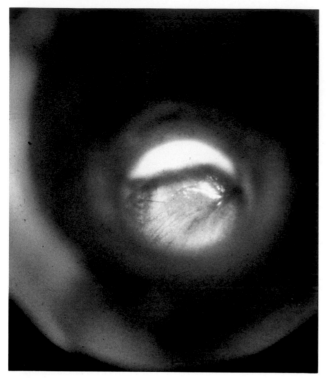

COL. FIG. 20-1
Normal newborn eardrum. View through speculum.

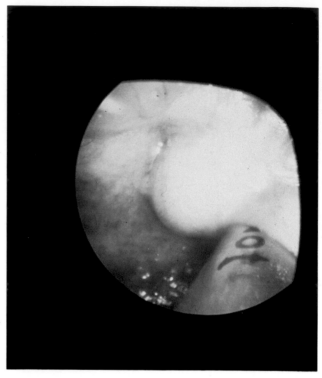

COL. FIG. 32-1
Cyst in aryepiglottic fold causing stridor and proximal airway obstruction. Endotracheal tube passes
beneath cyst.

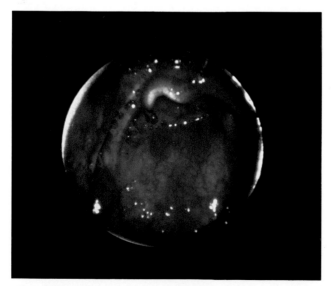

COL. FIG. 32-2

A

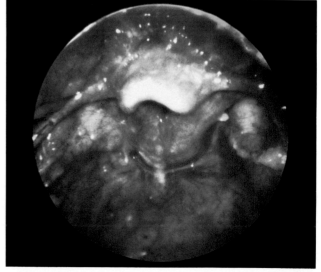

B

(*A*) Normal epiglottis obscuring glottis. Tip of laryngoscope blade in vallecula would lift epiglottis for tracheal
intubation. This amount of clear secretions does not require suctioning for visualization. (*B*) Same airway as in
Col. Fig. 32-1 after surgical removal of cyst. Glottic opening is visible just beneath epiglottis. Gentle tracheal
pressure or decreasing neck extension while lifting tip of laryngoscope blade will improve visibility.

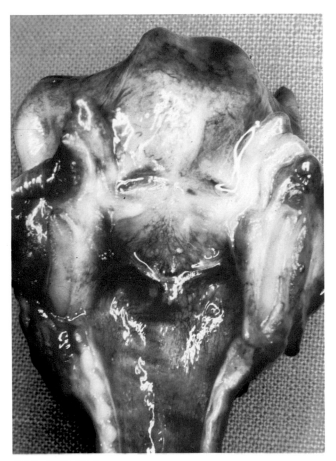

COL. FIG. 32-3
Subglottic erosion and stenosis postintubation.

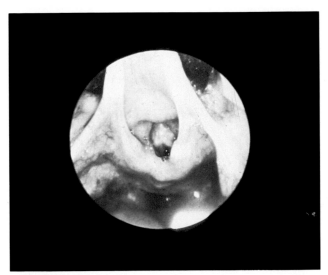

COL. FIG. 32-4
Glottic granuloma postintubation. Epiglottis is manually retracted to reveal granuloma below cords. Esophageal opening is clearly visible beneath airway.

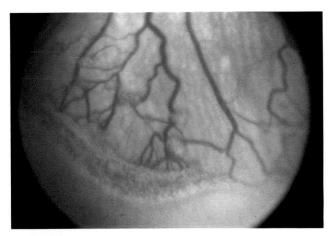

COL. FIG. 48-1
Dilated, tortuous vessels end in vascular shunts at a thickened ridge of fibrovascular tissue. Avascular retina lies anterior to the ridge.

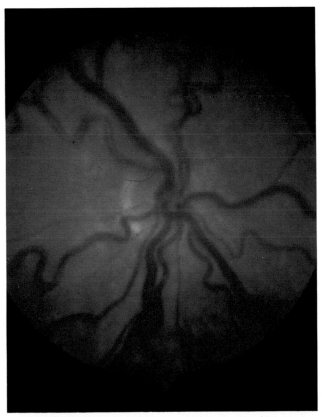

COL. FIG. 48-2
Plus disease as seen by direct ophthalmoscopy. Retinal vessels are dilated and tortuous.

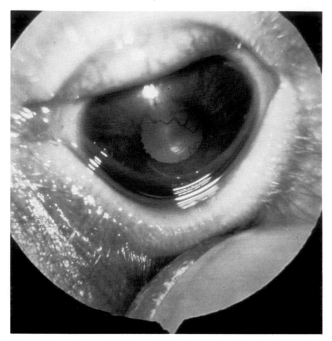

COL. FIG. 48-3
Dilatation and tortuosity of iris vessels may be seen in severe threshold ROP.

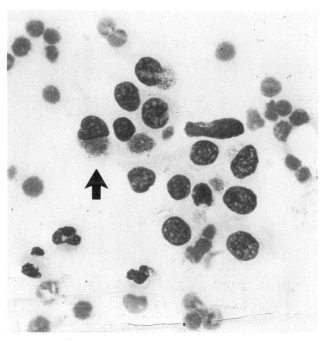

COL. FIG. 50-1
Smear from chlamydial eye infection stained with Gram's stain to show acidophilic cytoplasmic inclusions capping nuclei.

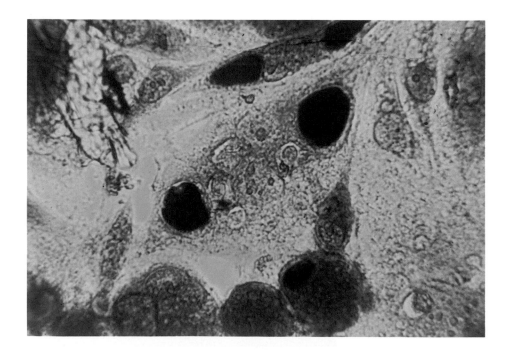

COL. FIG. 50-2
Chlamydial eye infection. Iodine-stained inclusion bodies from tissue-culture specimen.

Contents

Part 1
Preparation and Support

1 Informed Consent for Procedures on Neonates

Harold M. Ginzburg

A. GENERAL COMMENTS

1. Medical care is generally provided by "teams" of medical personnel, including physicians, nurses, therapists, and technicians (e.g., extracorporeal membrane oxygenation, respiratory therapy, dialysis). By medical tradition, the physician and the hospital have been held responsible for the actions of the team members.[1-3] Each team member is also medically and legally responsible for his or her own actions.

2. It is the fundamental duty and responsibility of those providing medical care and treatment to neonates to appropriately inform the parent or guardian and to document that relevant information has been provided, and understood, and that consent has been obtained. Failure to provide informed consent may result in legal liability under either a claim of negligence or a claim of assault and battery (depending on state law).[4-7]

3. The Federal government and the individual states have laws, regulations, guidelines, policies, and practices that directly and indirectly affect the practice of medical care.[8,9] Federal and state reimbursement, licensure, inspection, and enforcement functions may vary and even be in conflict. Therefore, health care providers are encouraged to consult with local legal counsel when potential legal issues arise.

4. "The law does not permit [a health care provider] to substitute his own judgment for that of the patient [or guardian]."[10]

B. CONCEPTUAL BASIS

1. Duty
   a. Legal. A Duty is a legal and ethical responsibility. A breach (violation) of a duty owed to another person may result in legal liability. Duties are a reflection of the moral fiber of a community. Public policies and laws are the vehicle for expressing a community's moral imperatives.
   b. Medical. A health care provider has a duty to conform his or her practice to a reasonable (or, in some instances, usual) standard of care in the particular type of case, and in the particular circumstances in which the care and treatment are being provided. He or she also has a duty only to perform procedures for which, under normal circumstances, appropriate equipment and support are available and which he or she is professionally competent to perform.

2. Health care provider–patient relationship
   a. Health care providers, and hospital care systems, have a fiduciary duty to patients and their parents or guardians. A fiduciary duty is a responsibility that emanates from the trust and confidence placed by the patient/parent/guardian in the health care professional. Health care providers are assumed to have superior medical knowledge; they are expected to warn and to protect their patients from untoward or predictable harm. The relationship is created when a health care provider responds to an expressed or implied request for treatment by the patient, his or her guardian, or a third party (e.g., emergency medical service personnel). The health care provider has a duty to share his or her knowledge about the nature of the illness, its prognosis, treatment options, and associated risks (informed consent) with the parent or guardian.
   b. The health care provider–patient relationship is a contract. A health care provider and a patient (or his parent or guardian) enter into the contract,

either verbal or written, for the performance of medical services. The contract created is based on the fiduciary relationship and not a financial one.

3. Standard of Care
   a. Legal. The health care provider has a duty to conform his or her practice to a reasonable standard of care in the particular type of case, and in the particular circumstances in which the care and treatment are being provided.
   b. Medical. The health care provider must not undertake any procedure that will place the patient at an unreasonably great risk of harm when weighed against the potential benefits. The health care provider must consider the consequences of his or her actions, or inactions, and exercise his or her best judgment.

4. Negligence
   a. General Negligence. Negligence is the failure to do something that a reasonable man or woman, guided upon those considerations that ordinarily regulate the conduct of human affairs, would do, or doing something that a prudent and reasonable man or woman would not do.
   b. Medical Negligence. Medical negligence, or medical malpractice, is a special instance of negligence. A missed operative diagnosis, a therapeutic misadventure, or a failure to inform, warn, or protect the patient, or in some instances, a third party, are special instances of medical negligence. The medical care profession is held to a specific minimum level of performance based on the possession, or claim of possession, of "special knowledge or skills" that have accrued through specialized education and training. A health care provider may be successfully sued only if there was a duty or obligation, recognized by law, that required the defendant to conform to a particular standard of conduct in order to protect others against unreasonable risks of harm and that standard of conduct was violated.

5. Informed Consent
   a. Clinical. Informed consent is educated consent; it is a cornerstone in the provision of medical care.[11] Fundamentally, informed consent is a contract between the physician and the patient, and/or the parent or guardian. Informed consent requires that sound, reasonable, comprehensible, and relevant information be provided by a health care professional to a competent individual (patient) for the purpose of eliciting a voluntary and educated decision, by that patient, about the advisability of permitting one course of clinical action as opposed to another.[12] Thus, it is an understandable offer by the health care provider to provide services and it is the patient's or his surrogate's acceptance of the services. It is an offer, by the patient or the surrogate, to pay for the services, or at least acknowledge that they have a worth, and it is the health care provider's acceptance of the payment or acknowledgment.[13] Informed consent should also prevent unrealistic expectations from developing by informing the appropriate individuals of the possibility of the failure of the proposed therapeutic interventions.

Once the informed consent is provided and agreed to, the physician, and all those who are involved in the patient's care and treatment (e.g., nurse practitioners, nurses, respiratory therapists) have a responsibility to use sound judgment and provide quality medical care; the patient also has duty to reasonably cooperate with the care and treatment.[14] To create a valid contract, there is a legal requirement that an individual be legally competent and have the legal capacity or ability to enter into that contract.[15] Health care providers are sometimes faced with emotionally immature, incoherent, uncooperative, absent, or intoxicated parents. In such instances, assistance from the hospital attorneys and the courts may be required.

   b. Research. The Declaration of Helsinki, agreed to by the World Medical Association in 1964, distinguished between "clinical research combined with professional care" (that is, research that might directly benefit the patient) and "nontherapeutic clinical research."[16] Special and specific informed consent needs to be obtained for procedures conducted as part of research studies unless the procedures are considered to be a component of the "routine medical care" (see next section). The Department of Health and Human Services (DHHS) has promulgated a series of regulations to ensure that research subjects, especially children, are adequately protected when they are enrolled in clinical trials or other clinical experiments.[17,18] DHHS has the power to investigate and sanction investigators for violating its regulations.[19]

C. OBTAINING INFORMED CONSENT

The person obtaining consent should:

1. Be aware that there are two levels of informed consent
   a. General informed consent (often referred to as a "blanket consent"). The parent or guardian must understand that admission to a hospital entails active clinical intervention by a number of health care providers. While the parent or guardian can expect explanations of many of the procedures that will be used to help their child or ward, they cannot expect to be informed about every intervention. Routine medical care does not require a specific informed consent. Each medical facility needs to define (within the limits of what is reasonable for the type of care provided, as well as what is reasonable, given the social context of the community) the components of routine care. For instance, in an extensive care nursery, placing an arterial line in a critically ill infant for the purpose of obtaining blood gases is not a unique procedure requiring a specific informed consent, whereas placing a neonate on extracorporeal membrane oxygenation (ECMO) would generally require a specific informed consent form. However, it is the procedures in the "gray" area that require definition by the facility as standard or otherwise. Both a lumbar puncture and the percutaneous placement of a central venous catheter may be considered standard routine procedures in a critical care unit. However, on an infectious disease unit the percutaneous placement of a central venous line might require a specific informed consent form as it is not a usual and customary procedure.
   b. Specific informed consent. The parent or guardian must recognize that beyond the routine medical care provided in a nursery there are specialized medical and surgical procedures that require specific additional information be provided to them to assist them in determining whether they should permit their infant to undergo the recommended procedures. For each such procedure, a description of the procedure and the risks and benefits of performing the procedure versus not performing the procedure should be provided to the parent or guardian.

2. Understand the basic *principles* of informed consent as it pertains to neonates[13,17]
   a. The decision is free of coercion or undue influence. The health care provider has a duty to ensure that the parent or guardian voluntarily assents to permit the treatment or clinical research. As neonates are not in a position to maintain voluntary control over their environment and their body, their parent or guardian is assumed to protect them from harm by being kept informed. If there is a definite indication that the parent or guardian is not competent, then the health care provider should not accept consent. At that time, the hospital attorney and the local court may become intimately involved in the case.
   b. Mental capacity of the parent or guardian. The parent or guardian is presumed to be competent and have the capacity to understand the medical information, to remember that information, and to make logical inferences and conclusions from the information.
   c. The knowledge base of the parent or guardian. The more severe the consequences of the proposed diagnostic test or therapeutic intervention, the greater the need for information to be given in language that the parent or guardian can understand.
   d. The risk/benefit for a given therapeutic intervention. The parent or guardian must be provided with information regarding the frequency and severity of the adverse potential consequences as compared with the likelihood, duration, and degree of anticipated benefit from the treatment(s). Where relevant benefits are questionable, the option of no treatment should also be discussed.
   e. The emotional stability or maturity of the parent or guardian. Advice that includes information about very unlikely and undesirable consequences is not consistent with good medical care. Thus, the health care professional may withhold dis-

closure of information regarding untoward consequences of treatment when full disclosure may be detrimental to patient's total care and best interests. There are circumstances in which too much information may prevent the parent or guardian from making a decision. Because of underlying personal problems, they may become overwhelmed with the options or potential adverse consequences and therefore unable to make any decision.

f. The limits of medical confidentiality. Current legal, medical, policy, and social considerations would suggest that an informed consent contract with a parent or guardian needs to be defined in terms of relative rather than absolute confidentiality. Local, state, or federal regulations and laws may permit or require the reporting of medical and other information to third parties (e.g., state and federal law enforcement agencies, state and federal health agencies, insurance companies).

g. The duty to warn and protect obligation. A health care professional may have an ethical or legal duty to warn an identifiable individual that they have been or may be exposed to disease or violence. There are some states that forbid physician notification of the sexual partners of patients with AIDS that they may have been exposed to HIV. However, while the health care provider cannot force the infant's mother to inform the infant's biological father that she is infected with HIV, the health care provider can inform the infant's father that the infant is infected, regardless of whether the parents are married.

h. Duty to impute consent. There is a long-standing general medical principle that informed consent may be imputed to an unconscious accident victim who has a life-threatening condition that requires surgery. In an emergency, such rational behavior can also be imputed to the "absent parent" of an infant. However, imputed consent may not be viable when chronic care is required. Consultation with the hospital administration and/or hospital attorney is recommended in matters involving infants whose parents or guardians are not available, or are unable to make the necessary acute or long-term medical decisions concerning the infant. In such in-

stances, the hospital may be forced to petition the court to appoint a legal guardian. The court may accept its historic role of parens patriae (substitute parent) and make such an appointment.

i. Court petitions for guardianship. The court can be petitioned for the appointment of a temporary legal guardian, if the parents are unavailable or unwilling to consent to a routine medical treatment such as a life-saving blood transfusion (even if the refusal is based on sincere religious convictions such as those held by Jehovah's Witnesses[20]). If the parents are unavailable, and a reasonable attempt has been made to contact them, then continuing to withhold the emergency treatment because of the failure to obtain their consent may be the basis for malpractice liability.

3. Understand the basic *elements* of informed consent as it pertains to neonates[21,22]

a. A description of the patient's diagnosis, the procedure, and an explanation of why the procedure is necessary for the treatment of the neonate

b. A description of the reasonably foreseeable risks or discomforts to the neonate

c. A description of the benefits to the neonate. In the case of participation in a research protocol, the informed consent must contain a statement that there may be no benefit to the infant or the family.

d. A disclosure of appropriate alternative procedures or course(s) of treatment, if any, that might be advantageous to the neonate. This includes a description of what will happen to the neonate if the procedure is not performed.

e. A statement describing the extent, if any, to which the records will be protected and whether the research subjects, or their parent or guardian, can be identified from the medical records during or after the conclusion of the research. The statement should also indicate that research records may be inspected by the Food and Drug Administration, and other federal agencies.

f. A statement defining who can be contacted for additional information about the treatment procedure(s)

g. A signature of the health care provider who has discussed the contents of the informed consent with the parent or guardian, and a signature of the parent or guardian, dated, and usually witnessed by at least one person (which may be the health care provider who has also signed the form)

h. Traditionally, informed consent has been a written document, prepared and then signed by the consenting parent or guardian and the health care provider who has provided the information to the parent or guardian. Even with a signed informed consent form, the author recommends that the health care provider write a note in the chart indicating that the critical elements contained in the informed consent were explained to the parent or guardian. This note should also include the name(s) of those who signed and witnessed the consent. The most important aspect of an informed consent is the process of communication; the document is simply a record of what has occurred.

i. In instances in which written consent cannot be directly obtained, consent may be obtained by telephone. In such an instance, a copy of the consent form, co-signed by any witness(es) (at least one) who heard the explanation and the consent being given, should be legally sufficient to document that the consent was in fact given and that relevant and useful information was provided to the parent or guardian to assist in their decision-making process. A separate note, in the patient's chart, should also document the parties involved in the informed consent process and the general content of the material provided to the parent or guardian during the telephone conversation.

4. Be sure the individual who provides the necessary details of the planned procedure is qualified to do so.

a. The health care provider who is going to perform or direct the treatment or therapeutic intervention is in the best position to obtain the informed consent.

b. Consent can be obtained by anyone with the necessary training to understand and explain the details of the procedure and the relevant risks.

D. UNRESOLVED PROBLEMS

1. When emotional stability, maturity, or sobriety (the patient, parent, or guardian is intoxicated, regardless of the nature of psychoactive substance) is an issue in obtaining informed consent for treatment, the physician has a duty to inform a third party (the hospital legal department and the hospital department of social services) and to document his or her actions in the medical record.

2. Generally, the informed consent of the mother is considered more substantive than that of the father, if the parents are not legally married. However, when the parents are married, and they are in conflict as to the course of action to be taken, both parents' consent should be obtained before proceeding. Grandparents may advise the neonate's mother, but they cannot overrule her decision unless they have legal custody of the infant.

3. A non-pregnant teenager, living at home and attending school, is not considered emancipated. She may not have the right, under law, to make the ultimate decisions about her own medical care. A teenager becomes emancipated when she reaches the age of majority (in most states, age 18) or is a member of the Armed Forces, or is living away from home and economically supporting herself, or can otherwise demonstrate financial independence from her family. However, regardless of age and financial independence, once her child is born, she has the legal right to make medical decisions for her child. Thus a 13- or 14-year-old unwed mother usually has the ultimate legal responsibility for the care of her child, unless the court is petitioned for custody.

E. CONSULTATION WITH HOSPITAL ATTORNEYS

The author recommends that when the health care provider has any doubt as to an appropriate course of action that in any manner involves, or may involve, a legal issue, he or she should promptly consult with the hospital attorney or other designated legal expert.

References

1. Darling v. Charleston Community Memorial Hospital, 33 Ill.2d 326, 211 N.E.2d (1965); cert. denied, 383 U.S. 946 (1966)
2. 51 Fed. Reg. 22,010 (June 17, 1986)
3. Medicare Conditions of Participation for Hospitals, 42 CFR 403 et. seq. (1985)

4. Canterbury v. Spence, 464 F.2d 772 (D.C.Cir. 1972), cert. denied, 409 U.S. 1064 (1972)

5. Cooper v. Roberts, 286 A.2d 647, 650 (1971)

6. Davis v. Wyeth, 399 F.2d 121 (9th Cir. 1968)

7. Getchell v. Mansfield, 260 Or. 174, 489 P.2d 953 (1971)

8. LEVINE RJ: Informed consent: Some challenges to the universal validity of the western model. Law Medicine & Health Care, 19:207, 1991

9. LEVINE RJ: Ethics and Regulation of Clinical Research, 2nd ed. Baltimore, Urban & Schwarzenberg, 1986

10. Schloendorf v. Society of New York Hospital, 149 A.D. 415, 133 N.Y.S. 1143 (1912), affirmed Schloendorf v. Society of New York Hospital, 211 N.Y. 125, 105 N.E. 92 (1914)

11. INGELFINGER F: Informed (but uneducated) consent. N Engl J Med 287:465, 1972

12. Zebarth v. Swedish Hospital Medical Center, 81 Wash.2d 12, 499 P.2d 1 (1972)

13. GINZBURG HM: The evolution of psychiatric-legal diagnostic dilemmas, In: Simon RI ed., Annual Review of Clinical Psychiatry and the Law, Volume 1, pp. 239–294, Washington DC, American Psychiatric Press, 1989

14. KEETON WP, DOBBS DB, KEETON RE, OWEN DR (eds): Prosser & Keeton on Torts, Fifth Ed. St. Paul, MN, West Publishing Co, 1984, p. 114

15. Markowitz v. Arizona Parks Board, 146 Ariz. 352, 706 P.2d 365 (1985)

16. OPRR, 45 CFR (1988)

17. GINZBURG HM: Protection of research subjects in clinical research. In Vevaina JR, Bone RC, Kassoff E (eds): Legal Aspects of Medicine. New York, Springer-Verlag, 1989, pp 51–60

18. GINZBURG HM: Legal issues in the medical care of HIV infected children, In Pizzo PA, Wilfert C (eds): Baltimore, MD, Pediatric Aids: The Challenge of HIV Infection in Infants, Children and Adolescents. Williams & Wilkins, 1991, 133–46

19. Office of Protection of Research Risks, Division of Human Subject Protections, "Findings and required actions regarding investigation of noncompliance with HHS regulations for the protection of human subjects involving the National Institutes of Health Intramural Research Program," July 3, 1991

20. Application of President & Directors of Georgetown College, 331 F.2d 1000, reh'g denied, Application of President & Directors of Georgetown College, 331 F.2d 1010, and cert. denied, Jones v. President & Directors of Georgetown College, Inc., 377 U.S. 978 (1964)

21. 21 CFR 50 et seq. (1986)

22. REISER SJ, DYCK AJ, CURRAN WJ: Ethics in Medicine: Historical Perspectives and Contemporary Concerns. Cambridge, MA, MIT Press, 1977

2 Maintenance of Homeostasis

Mhairi G. MacDonald
Arthur J. Engler

A. THERMAL HOMEOSTASIS

All neonates undergoing a procedure must be ensured an environment that protects their thermal integrity.

1. Factors influencing heat loss
   a. Large surface area to body weight ratio
   b. Relatively large head with highly vascular fontanelle (Fig. 2-1)
   c. Metabolic demands of disease process
   d. Inability to signal discomfort
   e. Effects of pharmacologic agents, e.g., vasodilating drugs, maternal analgesics, and unwarmed infusates, including blood products
2. Adverse effects of cold stress
   a. Apnea and bradycardia
   b. Mobilization of catecholamines and free fatty acids
   c. Pulmonary hypertension
   d. Metabolic acidosis
   e. Depletion of caloric reserves
3. Equipment and techniques for temperature maintenance (Table 2-1)
4. General considerations for procedure outside the nursery
   a. Use heated, battery-operated transport incubator to move infant.
   b. Plug incubator into wall outlet during procedure, to allow battery to charge.
   c. Use heating pads or overhead radiant warmer during procedures. Preset temperature of heating pads should not exceed 40°C.
   d. Use continuous temperature monitor throughout procedure; or, check infant's axillary or rectal temperature at least every 15 minutes.

   Continuous monitoring is mandatory for small premature infants and/or during major procedures (see Chap. 6).

   e. Other considerations
      (1) Regulate room temperature to one optimal for infant (28–30°C).
      (2) Prewarm all heating units.
      (3) Give slow parenteral infusions at room temperature (28–30°C).
      (4) Warm rapid infusions (e.g., blood products for exchange transfusion) to body temperature (37°C).

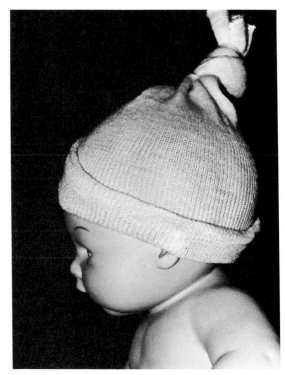

FIG. 2-1
Stockinette cap to reduce heat loss from the head.

TABLE 2–1
Practical Use of Mechanical Warming Devices During Procedures*

Considerations	Use of Incubator via Portholes	Radiant Warmer	Heat Lamp	Warming Mattress†
Maintenance of neutral thermal environment	Possible for short procedures	1. Inefficient for infants under 1200 g 2. Increased radiant heat loss	As for radiant warmer	May require ancillary heat source to minimize heat loss
Insensible water loss	Minimized	Increased 50% or more; the smaller the baby, the greater the loss	Increased	Not significantly affected
Accessibility	Poor	Excellent	Limited by other equipment used (e.g., with incubator)	Excellent
Maintenance of asepsis	Very difficult	Unimpeded	Limited by other equipment used	Unimpeded
Indications	1. Duration of procedure <10 min 2. No more than one assistant required 3. No special positioning required 4. Wide sterile field not required	1. Procedure requiring more than one assistant 2. Special positioning required 3. Wide sterile field required 4. As an alternative to open incubator with heat lamp	1. Infant unclothed in bassinette or on treatment table 2. Open incubator	Procedures that would be hindered by infant warmer or incubator (e.g., cardiac catheterization, CT scan, surgery)
Precautions	1. Take the infant's temperature‡ before and after the procedure. 2. Use infant servocontrol (ISC). Make sure that thermistor remains in place. 3. Have heat lamps or	1. Take the infant's temperature every 5–10 min or use continuous monitor. 2. Use ISC. Make sure that thermistor does not dislodge. 3. Do not place oily substances on	1. Take the infant's temperature every 5 min. For small premature or procedure >10 min, continuous temperature monitor should be used. 2. Do not place oily substances on skin—may cause burns. 3. Use a lamp a. No less than 20″ from the infant	Fluid-filled mattress: 1. Manual mode a. Set temperature of fluid reservoir to desired skin temperature (36.5°C). (Heat sensor in the reservoir will maintain temperature set.) b. Use continuous temperature monitor or

other heat source available for unstable infants or stressful procedures. Clinical deterioration may require lifting the protective shield.	skin—may cause burns.	b. Directed at the infant c. Placed to avoid heating incubator thermometer d. Placed to avoid obstructing or burning personnel e. With protective covering in case of exploding bulb 4. Remove the ISC thermistor and set the incubator thermostat on manual 33°–35° C when using an open incubator. 5. Cover the genital area for male infants. 6. Cover infant's eyes as for phototherapy.	take infant's temperature every 5–10 min. 2. Servocontrol mode: a. Set servocontrol to maintain temperature appropriate to site of thermistor placement (e.g., axillary, rectal, etc.). (See Chap. 6.) b. Take care that the thermistor does not dislodge. c. Be aware that some older heat mattresses have a tubular design. When a kink occurs, flow is stopped and the mattress will cool. Newer models are capillary in design. If an area kinks, the fluid flow continues through collateral pathways.	
Complications	1. Hyperthermia owing to displacement of thermistor 2. Hypothermia	1. Increased insensible water loss 2. Hyperthermia owing to displacement of thermistor 3. Equipment failure 4. Hypothermia owing to obstruction of radiant-heat shield by personnel 5. Increased oxygen consumption	1. Hypothermia or hyperthermia, because heat source is not controlled 2. Burns to staff or infant 3. Explosion of bulb owing to urination on heat source 4. Cooling or overheating of isolette owing to failure to detach thermistor from infant a. ISC will shut off if thermistor overheated by lamp b. Incubator will overheat if thermistor inadvertently displaced 5. Increased insensible water loss	1. Hypothermia or hyperthermia 2. Burns

*For technical operation of automated temperature-control and monitoring devices, see Chap. 6.

†Fluid-filled mattress with heat sensor (e.g., Gorman-Rupp American [Hamilton, Two Rivers, Wisconsin] or Blanketrol Cincinnati Sub-Zero [Cincinnati]); disposable chemical heat mattress (e.g., Porta-warm, Baxter-Health Care Corp., Valencia, CA 91355–8900 and Aquamatic K Module, Hamilton Industries, Cincinnati, OH 45238)

‡Use a digital thermometer. Glass thermometer must be kept in place for a minimum of 5 minutes for accuracy.

(5) Warm irrigation fluids and radiographic contrast materials to body temperature.

(6) Be aware that anesthesia may inhibit the infant's thermoregulatory capabilities.

(7) Warm all anesthetic gases to body temperature and humidify.

B. FLUID HOMEOSTASIS

1. When infant is dependent on parenteral infusion, ensure maintenance of reliable intravenous access during procedure.
   a. Check
      (1) For infiltration or extravasation
      (2) Flow rate
      (3) Volume remaining to be infused
   b. Keep intravenous site accessible during procedure.
   c. Check intravenous site frequently during procedure, especially if infant is active.
   d. Ensure continuous infusion of glucose if infant is at risk for hypoglycemia (e.g., premature infants, infants of diabetic mothers, infants that are small for gestational age, infants who have suffered cold stress).
   e. Ensure continuation of supportive drugs that have short half-lives (e.g., dopamine, dobutamine, tolazoline, prostaglandin E_1).
2. Use appropriate infusion rate to prevent dehydration or fluid overload.
   a. Use infusion pump to ensure constant planned delivery rate.
   b. If "catch-up" volume is needed, spread over several hours.
3. Consider impact of infusate temperature on infant.
4. Have adequate quantity of blood available prior to procedure that has risk of significant blood loss.

C. CARDIORESPIRATORY HOMEOSTASIS

See also Chap. 7.
1. Arrange for adequate number of assistants for observation of infant during procedure.
2. Do not obscure view of infant with drapes. Use transparent drapes whenever possible.
3. Have all necessary equipment for resuscitation (including resuscitation bag and mask of appropriate size) readily available.
4. Maintain airway.
   a. Ensure that restraint/positioning does not compromise airway.
   b. Stabilize artificial airway.
   c. Ensure access to airway at all times.
5. Use cardiorespiratory monitor, especially
   a. For unstable infants
   b. For preterm infants less than 36 weeks' gestation
   c. For prolonged or complex procedures
   d. When positioning for procedure might compromise cardiorespiratory function.
6. Use transcutaneous oxygen saturation or pO_2 monitor to detect inadvertent hypoxia or hyperoxia.
7. When using invasive blood pressure monitoring
   a. Be prepared to use indirect means in event of line failure.
   b. Be familiar with both venous and arterial pressure tracings so that abnormalities can be quickly recognized (see Chap. 8).
8. Be prepared to stop procedure if necessary
   a. To check endotracheal tube patency and/or position
   b. To initiate resuscitative efforts
   c. Because infant is unduly stressed by procedure

3 Methods of Restraint

Mhairi G. MacDonald
Arthur J. Engler

Improper position and inadequate restraint are the most common sources of failure or difficulty in the performance technical procedures.

A. INDICATIONS

1. During procedures to
   a. Expedite access
   b. Maintain safety of infants
   c. Ensure asepsis
   d. Minimize movement and discomfort
2. To prevent infants from displacing life-support devices and infusions

B. CONTRAINDICATIONS

1. When restraint not required
2. Where use may compromise clinical condition
3. When restraint by an assistant is more appropriate
4. When sedation is preferable
5. When close observation is more suitable

C. PRECAUTIONS

1. Do not use mechanical restraints as a substitute for observation.
2. Explain the purpose of the restraint to parents.
3. Mechanical restraints are not without risk and must be checked frequently to make sure they are accomplishing the purpose for which they were intended, that they are applied correctly, and that they do not impair circulation.
4. Use adequate additional manual restraint during procedure.
5. Restrain in position of function, being careful to maintain normal body alignment.
6. Always provide for quick release from restraint(s).
7. Make sure that restraint has no potential for tightening.
8. Pad pressure points adequately.
9. Remove restraint as soon as it is no longer needed; do not immobilize for longer than necessary.
10. Reposition infants as frequently as possible when prolonged restraint is required.
11. Never attach restraints to side rail of crib or warmer.
12. Immobilize heel for procedure on ankle or foot.
13. Weigh board and other equipment, and take into account when weighing infants.

    A list of the weights of common equipment can be made and updated as necessary.

14. When taping limb to a board, do not impede circulation; do not apply tape too tightly.
15. Always leave tips of fingers and toes visible; use transparent tape whenever possible.
16. Check distal circulation frequently, at least once per hour, when using limb restraints. Assess digits and extremity for
    a. Temperature
    b. Color
    c. Capillary refill
    d. Pulse
    e. Erythema/excoriation
    f. Edema
17. Release limb restraints every 4 hours to check for skin irritation and give range of motion exercises
    a. Put joint through as full range of motion as possible.
    b. Do not force joint.
    c. Position hands above and below the joint to reduce stress on long bones.
    d. Do not perform if to do so will compromise infant's condition.

13

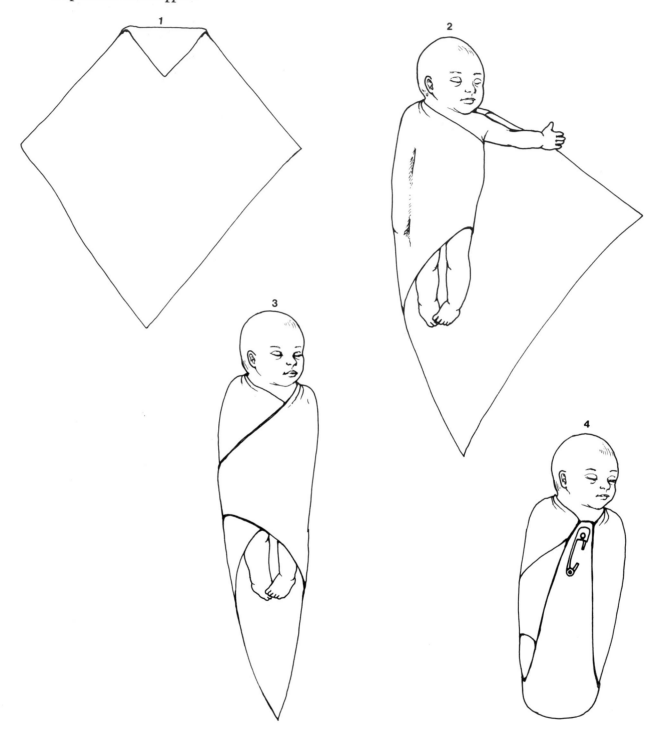

FIG. 3-1
Application of a mummy restraint.

General Methods of Restraint

D. EQUIPMENT

1. Mummy restraint
   a. Clean blanket or sheet
   b. Safety pin(s)
2. Limb restraint
   a. Gauze pads
   b. Safety pins
   c. Adhesive tape

   Tape selection should be based on knowledge of the characteristics of neonatal skin and on the adhesive qualities of the tape. Use of tape should be minimized and extreme care should be used when removing tape.

   d. 5 cm orthopedic stockinette

E. TECHNIQUE

1. Mummy restraint (Fig. 3-1)

   Useful for procedures on the head and neck. A single, upper limb may also be left free, e.g., for intravenous placement. In addition, the chest can be exposed by pulling the lateral wings of the blanket firmly over both arms and tucking under the infant's back. (A commercially available variation of this restraint is known as a "papoose board.")

2. Wrist/ankle restraint
   a. Method A (Fig. 3-2, A)
   b. Method B (Fig. 3-2, B)
   c. Method C
      The *clove hitch* restraint is fashioned from a length of gauze or muslin tape. When properly applied, the restraint should provide a snug fit with minimum danger of tightening with movement.
   d. Pin restraint to mattress or light sandbag.

F. COMPLICATIONS

1. Failure of restraint
2. Vascular compromise
3. Pressure necrosis (Fig. 3-3)
4. Interference with cardiorespiratory function
5. Positional deformity resulting from prolonged fixation in nonfunctional position
6. Limb fracture/dislocation caused by moving infants with restraint fastened to stationary object or moveable crib rail
7. Agitation

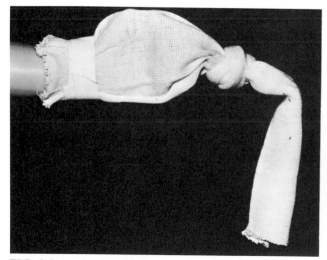 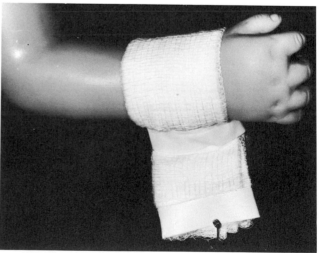

FIG. 3-2
A   B
(A) Wrist restraint using orthopedic stockinette. *(B)* Wrist restraint using gauze pads.

A *B*

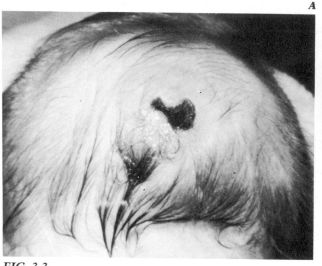 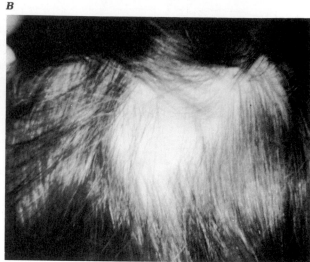

FIG. 3-3
(A) Occipital pressure necrosis caused by prolonged restraint in supine position. *(B)* Same patient showing failure of hair growth on follow-up.

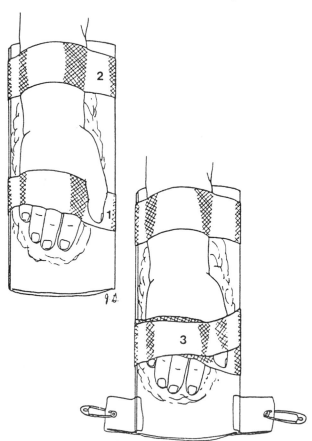

Restraint for Vascular Access

Regardless of the type of restraint used, the amount of tape and adhesive used should be minimized, particularly with preterm infants. The use of a protective pectin-based barrier (such as those used around stomas) between the skin and the tape and avoidance of adhesive skin preps and adhesive removers may reduce skin breakdown in very small infants.[1]

D. EQUIPMENT

1. Procedure light
2. Scissors
3. Roll of 1.25–2.5 cm porous adhesive tape, or semipermeable transparent dressing or tape.

FIG. 3-4
Forearm restraint with arm in prone position. Tapes are placed in order, 1 to 3, as shown. A longer restraint board, to allow immobilization above the elbow joint, may be necessary for large, active infants.

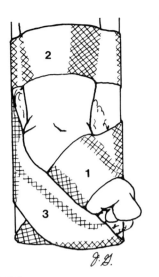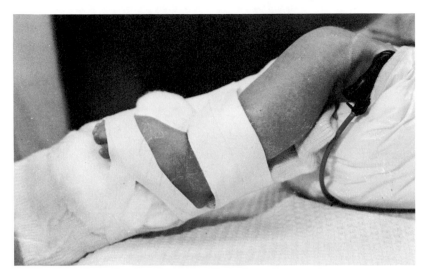

FIG. 3-5
(A) Foot and ankle restraint in equinovalgus position. Tapes are applied in order as numbered 1 to 3. *(B)* Foot and ankle restraint in equinovarus position, for procedures on the dorsum of the foot.

4. Light-weight, covered restraint board, 1–2 cm wider than breadth of hand or length of foot. Board should be of adequate length to extend from elbow or midcalf to approximately 2 cm beyond fingers or toes.
5. Padding, e.g., 2″ × 2″ gauze pads

E. TECHNIQUE

1. Forearm and hand restraint
   a. Cut 4 pieces of tape, each at least 10 cm long.
   b. Tape limb to board and insert padding as shown in Fig. 3-4.
   c. Check peripheral circulation (see General Restraints—Precautions).
   d. Attach tape wings to board, or place pins through coverings of board, if immobilization of limb is desired.

   Whenever possible, avoid immobilization since there is a risk of trauma if infants move or are inadvertently moved without first releasing the restraint

2. Ankle and foot restraint
   a. Cut 4 pieces of tape, 15–20 cm long.
   b. Place foot on board in slight equinovarus or equinovalgus position, with leg rotated according to proposed intravenous site.
   c. Tape lower leg and foot to board and insert padding as shown in Fig. 3-5A,B.

F. COMPLICATIONS

1. See General Restraints
2. Sloughing of tissue secondary to extravasation of parenteral fluid, if tight proximal tape causes pressure buildup in subcutaneous tissue
3. Peripheral nerve palsy[2,3] (see Chap. 27, Fig. 27-10)
4. Compromised peripheral circulation

References

1. NAACOG: OGN nursing practice resource. Neonatal Skin Care. Washington, DC, NAACOG Publication, 1992
2. FAHRNI WH: Neonatal sciatic palsy. J Bone Joint Surg 32B:42, 1950
3. FISCHER AQ, STRASBURGER J: Footdrop in the neonate secondary to the use of footboards. J Pediatr 101:1003, 1982

4 Aseptic Preparation

Mhairi G. MacDonald
Ayman A.E. El-Mohandes

A. DEFINITIONS

1. Antiseptic
   a. Bactericidal or bacteriostatic substances that can be safely applied to skin.
   b. Not reliable as a sporicidal.[1]
   c. Reduces, but does not eliminate, bacterial counts on the skin.
      (1) All have an immediate effect.
      (2) Some may have variable residual activity by binding to the stratum corneum of the skin.[2]
   d. Should be differentiated from disinfectants, which are chemical germicides used for objects and environmental surfaces.
2. Resident flora
   a. Organisms, usually of low virulence, that survive and multiply on skin and can be cultured repeatedly, e.g. *Staphylococcus epidermidis*.
   b. Cannot be completely eradicated without destroying the skin.
   c. Regenerate rapidly on skin when surgical gloves are worn.
3. Transient flora
   a. Organisms that are sometimes pathogenic but do not survive and multiply on skin, e.g., gram negative organisms such as *Escherechia coli*.
   b. Can be transmitted to patients on the hands of health care workers.
   c. Do not usually remain on the skin for more than 24 hours.
   d. Can be eradicated completely by hand washing with antiseptic solutions.

B. INDICATIONS

1. Preparation of patient's skin and hands of personnel prior to procedure
   a. To remove transient pathogenic organisms
   b. To remove and temporarily suppress most resident skin flora
2. Decontamination of hands after procedures
3. Prevention and treatment of local skin infection, for example
   a. Scalp laceration at birth
   b. Insertion site of indwelling line

C. CONTRAINDICATIONS

See also G, Complications.

1. Iodine solutions for preparation of skin in newborns
2. Halogenated bisphenols (e.g., hexachlorophene) for preparation of skin in premature infants (see D7)
3. Chlorhexidine for preparation of external auditory meatus

D. PRECAUTIONS

1. Universal[3,4]
   a. Definition: a method of infectious control in which all human blood and certain human body fluids are treated as if known to be infectious for HIV, HBV, and other blood born pathogens.
   b. Indications: reasonably anticipated skin, eye, mucous membrane, or parenteral contact with blood or other potentially infectious materials, including semen, vaginal secretions, cerebrospinal fluid, synovial fluid, pleural fluid, pericardial fluid, peritoneal fluid, amniotic fluid, saliva in dental procedures, and any body fluid that is visibly contaminated with blood.
   c. Major components
      (1) Use gloves when touching blood, body fluids, mucous membranes, or nonintact skin and when handling items or surfaces soiled with blood or body fluids.

(2) Use a mask and eye protection during procedures that might generate splashing or droplets in the air.

(3) Use a gown or use a plastic apron when splashing of blood or bloody fluid is likely.

(4) Wash hands carefully if they become contaminated with blood or body fluids.

(5) Take extraordinary care in handling needles and other sharp objects and dispose of them in puncture resistant containers.

(6) Exclude from patient care all personnel with exudative lesions or weeping dermatitis until these conditions have resolved.

2. Recognize that no antiseptic is totally effective or without risk (Table 4-1).

3. Always allow antiseptics to dry before starting procedure.

a. Drying time of at least 30 seconds[5] is required for optimal effect.

b. Contamination of instruments with antiseptic is undesirable and may invalidate specimens taken for culture.

4. Avoid removal of Iodophor preparations prior to procedure.

Removal negates the residual slow-release effect.

5. After the procedure, remove Iodophor from all but immediate area of procedure to prevent absorption through skin.[6–8]

6. Never allow antiseptic to pool under infant. Skin damage may result.[9]

7. Use hexachlorophene for skin preparation in newborns only as recommended by the American Academy of Pediatrics.[10]

a. Use only in term infants during outbreak of *Staphylococcus aureus* infection.

b. Do not apply more than twice to each infant, unless application is restricted to diaper area.[11]

c. Wash off solution completely.

8. Reapply alcohol prior to each attempt at procedure, or with any delay, as efficacy is short-lived and flora will regenerate quickly.

9. Keep all antiseptics away from eyes.

10. Store antiseptics in closed containers. Reusable dispensers should be thoroughly cleaned, dried, and refilled frequently. Disposable containers are available.

11. Remember that gloving cannot be used as an alternative to hand washing.

a. The warm, wet skin surface under gloves offers an ideal environment for bacterial multiplication.

b. Gloves are not completely impermeable to microorganisms.[12]

Latex and vinyl gloves offer comparable permeability but vinyl gloves leak more readily.

E. TECHNIQUE

A 3- to 5-minute scrub is necessary upon entering the nursery. Subsequently, a 15- to 30-second scrub is indicated prior to and after each patient contact.

1. Preparation for a minor procedure

a. Definition of a minor procedure

(1) Short duration (5–10 minutes); noncomplex

(2) Does not involve an area, such as the central nervous system (CNS), which is especially vulnerable to infection

(3) Does not require skin incision

(4) For example

(a) Blood drawing

(b) Placement of percutaneous peripheral venous line

(c) Bladder tap

(d) Punch-skin biopsy

b. Preparation of personnel

(1) Wear scrub cap/beard cover if hair is likely to contaminate the field.

(2) Remove all jewelry from hands and arms.

(3) Wash hands, wrist, forearms, and elbows using a small amount of antiseptic preparation (e.g., iodophor or chlorhexidine). Be sure to include between the fingers and the lateral surface of the fifth finger.

(4) Clean nails with stick.

(5) Wash/scrub hands and forearms to elbow with antiseptic for a further 2 to 3 minutes.

Iodophor preparations appear equally effective when applied with disposable sponges or brushes.[13] Vigorous scrubbing with a brush that leads to skin breakdown is contraindicated.

(6) Rinse hands and forearms with running water, keeping them elevated above elbows.

TABLE 4-1

A Comparison of Commonly Used Antiseptics

Considerations	Iodophor	Chlorhexidine (4%)	Alcohol (70%–90%)	Iodine (1%)	Hexachlorophene (3%)	Chloroxylenol (PCMX) (0.5%–3.5%)
1. Indications	Handwashing Skin preparation	Handwashing Skin preparation: 0.5% in 70% alcohol optimal	Skin preparation for minor procedures Preparation of external auditory canal	Surgical handwashing as tincture with alcohol	Handwashing Use limited to term infants during epidemics of *Staphylococcus aureus*	Handwashing Skin and wound disinfection
2. Effective concentration						
a. Nontoxic	Hypothyroidism	Yes*, but local ototoxicity Keratitis	Yes†	Hypothyroidism	CNS vacuolation	Yes*
b. Nonsensitizing	Yes	Yes	Yes	No	Yes	Low
c. Nonirritating	Yes	Yes	Burns in premature	No	Yes	Yes
3. Mode of Action	Oxidation	Cell wall disruption	Protein denaturation	Oxidation	Cell wall disruption	Cell wall disruption and enzyme inactivation
4. Bactericidal	Yes	Yes	Yes	Yes	No	Yes
5. May be used with detergent	Yes	Yes	No	No	Yes	Neutralized by nonionic surfactants
6. Persistent local action	Yes	Yes	No	Yes	Yes, but only with repeated use; reduced	Good

7. Effective against						by concomitant use of alcohol
a. Gram-positive bacteria	Yes	Yes	Yes	Yes	Yes (Bacteriostatic)	Good (better against Streptococcus than Staphylococcus)
b. Gram-negative bacteria	Yes	Yes	Yes	Yes	No	Fair, improved by EDTA
c. Spores	No	No	No	No	No	No
d. Tubercle bacillus	No	No	Yes	Yes	No	Fair
e. Viruses	Yes	Yes	Lipophilic viruses only	Yes	Yes	Fair
f. Fungi	Yes	Yes	Yes	Yes	Yes	Fair
8. Use associated with resistance	No	Contamination with *Pseudomonas* and *Proteus* species	No	No	Yes	Not effective against *Pseudomonas* species
9. Rapid action	No; Requires 4–5 min of scrubbing	Yes (better when combined with alcohol)	Yes (drying time)	Yes	No	Intermediate
10. Easily inactivated by extraneous organic matter	No; Low surface tension for good crevice and fat penetration	No	May be inactivated by nonbacterial protein	Yes	Yes	Minimal

*Skin absorption not studied in very low birth weight infants.

†Harpin V, Rutter N: Percutaneous alcohol absorption and skin necrosis in a premature infant. Arch Dis Child 57:477, 1982.

(7) Use towel to shut off water if knee- or foot-operated faucets are not available.

(8) Dry hands with clean towel prior to drying forearms.

(9) Wear gloves when obtaining specimens for culture.

c. Preparation of patient skin

(1) Shave area, if necessary, taking care not to nick skin.

(2) Apply antiseptic.

(a) Alcohol may be used. Preparation with Iodophor may be optimal, but color tends to obscure underlying vessels.

(b) Apply twice in circles progressing away from procedure site.

(c) Apply with some friction.

(d) Allow to dry.

(e) Reapply alcohol prior to every attempt at procedure.

2. Preparation for a major procedure

a. Definition of major procedure

(1) Invasive or involving skin incision

(a) central line placement

(b) cutdown

(c) chest tube

(d) lumbar puncture

(2) Duration longer than 5–10 minutes

b. Masks, drapes, and gowns

Clothing is an important barrier to microorganisms shed into the air from the skin and mucous membranes. The pore size of gowns and masks should prevent bacterial passage even when wet (use 140 thread count or higher unless plasticized[14]). Disposable gowns and drapes manufactured from nonwoven materials are effective in reducing infection.[15] When using woven reusable materials, they should be tightly woven and treated with a water repellant. It is recommended that woven materials should not be laundered more than 75 times.[16] There is no evidence that shoe covers reduce infection.[17]

(1) Put on cap and mask.

(2) Clean nails and scrub as for minor procedure, but continue for 4 to 5 minutes.

(3) Rinse forearms and hands, keeping them elevated above elbows.

(4) Dry hands, then forearms with two sterile towels. Keep wrists and hands elevated until drying is complete.

(5) Put on sterile gown with the aid of an assistant (Fig. 4-1).

(6) Put on sterile gloves, without contaminat-

FIG. 4-1
Correct technique for putting on a sterile gown. (*A*) Operator is assisted into gown. The assistant pulls the gown up and back over operator's shoulders by grasping the inside surface. (*B*) Operator hands tip of sterile tie to assistant, who will tie gown posteriorly.

A   B

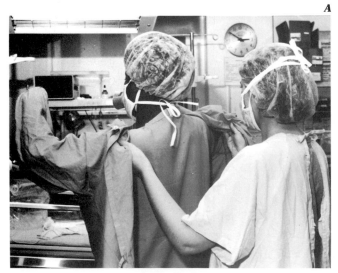
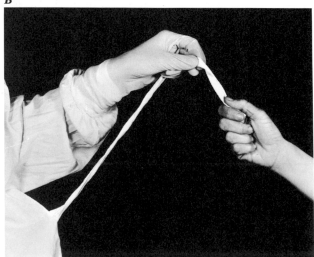

ing external surface with ungloved hand (Fig. 4-2).

  (a) Have assistant open packet without contaminating contents.

  (b) Pull gloves well over sleeve ends.

c. Preparation patient skin

  (1) Prior to procedure have assistant

   (a) Wash area, if soiled, with soap and water.

   (b) Shave area, if necessary, taking care not to nick skin.

  (2) Apply antiseptic with three separate sponges. Start at center of circle, and work centrifugally to at least 5 cm outside immediate area of procedure.

70% alcohol should not be used. An iodophor preparation is commonly used in nurseries in the United States.

  (3) Allow antiseptic to dry.

F. SPECIAL CIRCUMSTANCES

1. In clinical situations where traditional hand washing facilities are unavailable such as during patient transport, alcohol-based hand rinses, foams, or wipes may be used for hand cleaning. When alcohol solution is used, make three to five applications, of 3–5 ml each; rub hands well until completely dry.[2] Gloves should be used as otherwise indicated. This

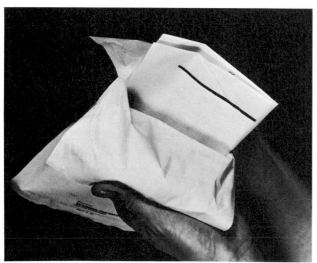
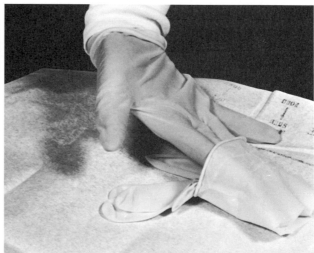
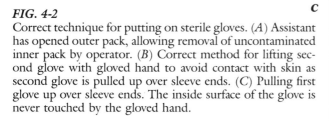
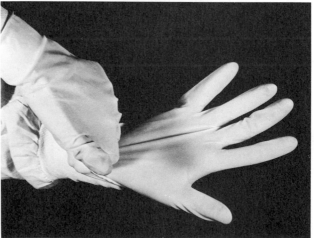

A B
C

FIG. 4-2
Correct technique for putting on sterile gloves. (*A*) Assistant has opened outer pack, allowing removal of uncontaminated inner pack by operator. (*B*) Correct method for lifting second glove with gloved hand to avoid contact with skin as second glove is pulled up over sleeve ends. (*C*) Pulling first glove up over sleeve ends. The inside surface of the glove is never touched by the gloved hand.

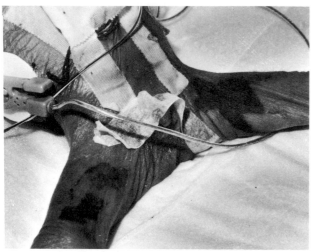

FIG. 4-3
Burns on thighs of premature infant caused by alcohol-impregnated pads placed under ECG recording electrodes.

technique is not adequate when hands are soiled with organic matter.

2. Personnel suffering from allergies to antimicrobial soaps may wash thoroughly for 3–5 minutes with plain soap or 70% isopropanol with glycerin prior to gloving.[18]

3. Personnel suffering from skin cracking due to frequent use of antiseptic soaps, may use skin lotions after hand washing. Products with a bacteriostatic ingredient, such as gels containing 60% ethanol, and emollients are safe and effective in reducing skin problems.[19] Containers with a flip-top rather than screw cap are recommended.[20]

> Doebbeling et al[21] have shown that a hand disinfection system using an antimicrobial agent (chlorhexidine) reduces the rate of nosocomial infection more effectively than one using alcohol and soap.

G. COMPLICATIONS

1. Dry skin with repeated use
2. Hexachlorophene
   a. Transcutaneous absorption with CNS vacuolation[22–29]
   b. *Possible* teratogenicity when used for handwashing by pregnant staff member[30–32]

3. Iodine
   a. Burns
   b. Skin absorption/hypothyroidism[6,7]
4. Iodophors
   a. Burns possible when allowed to pool under infant[9]
   b. Absorption through skin has been reported in burn patients and neonates.[8,33,34]
   c. Alteration of thyroid function[6,7]
5. Chlorhexidine

   Similarity in name and preparation has led to some confusion between chlorhexidine and hexachlorophene. These compounds are different in structure and properties (see Table 4-1).

   a. Ototoxicity when instilled into middle ear[35,36]
   b. Burns possible when allowed to pool under infant[9]
   c. Absorption through skin and from umbilical stump[37,38]

   No associated pathology was documented.

   d. Contamination with gram-negative organisms; in particular, *Pseudomonas* and *Proteus* species[39–41]

   There is no evidence that the detergent or alcohol preparations are susceptible to contamination.

6. Alcohol burns in premature infants[42] (see Fig. 4-3)
7. Mercurochrome: mercury poisoning[43]

References

1. KELSEY JC, MACKINNON IH, MAURER IM: Sporicidal activity in hospital disinfectants. J Clin Pathol 27:632, 1974
2. LARSON E: Guidelines for use of topical antimicrobial agents. Infect Control 16:253, 1988
3. Update: Universal precautions for prevention of transmission of human immunodeficiency virus, hepatitis B virus, and other blood borne pathogens in health-care settings. MMWR 37:377, 387, 1988
4. CDC guidelines for prevention of transmission of human immunodeficiency and hepatitis B virus to health-care and public safety workers. MMWR 38(5–6):1, 1989
5. Intravenous Nursing Standards of Practice. Intravenous Nurses Society, Revised 1990
6. CASTAING A, FOURIET JP, LEGER FA, et al: Thyroide du nouveau-ne et surcharge en iode après la naissance. Arch Fr Pediatr 36:356, 1979

7. CHABROLLE JP, MONOD N, PLOUIN P, et al: Surcharge iodee post-natal avec hypothyroidie et pauses respiratoires. Danger de l'application cutanee de produites iodes. Arch Fr Pediatr 35:432, 1978

8. PYATI SP, RAMAMURTHY RS, KRASS MT, PILDES RS: Absorption of iodine in the neonate following topical use of povidone iodine. J Pediatr 91:825, 1977

9. WILKINSON AR, BAUM JD, KEELING JW: Letter to the Editor: Superficial skin necrosis in babies prepared for umbilical arterial catheterization. Arch Dis Child 56:237, 1981

10. Committee on Fetus and Newborn: Standards and Recommendations for Hospital Care of Newborn Infants, 6th ed, pp 111, 112, 129. Evanston, Illinois, American Academy of Pediatrics, 1977

11. Report of the Committee on Infectious Diseases, 19th ed, p 243. Evanston, Illinois, American Academy of Pediatrics, 1982

12. More vinyl gloves leak, but test similar to latex in permeability. Hosp Infect Control Jan:12, 1989

13. BORNSIDE GH, CROWDER VH, COHN I: A bacterial evaluation of surgical scrubbing with disposable iodophore impregnated polyurethane scrub sponges. Surgery 64:743, 1968

14. Recommended practice: guideline for selection and processing of aseptic barrier material; January 1982 revision. Arlington, Virginia, Association for the Advancement of Medical Instrumentation.

15. MOYLAN JA, FITZPATRICK KT, DAVENPORT KE: Reducing wound infections. Arch Surg 122:152, 1987

16. LAUFMAN H, EUDY WW, VANDERNOOT AM, et al: Strike-through of moist contamination by woven and non-woven surgical materials. Ann Surg 181:857, 1975

17. HAMBREUS A, MALMBORG AS: The influence of different footwear on floor contamination. Scand J Infect Dis 11:243, 1979

18. ROTTER ML: Hygienic hand disinfection. Infect Control 5:211, 1984

19. NEWMAN JL, SEITZ JC: Intermittent use of an antimicrobial hand gel for reducing soap-induced irritation of health care personnel. Am J Infect Control 18:194, 1990

20. LARSON ELAINE: Letter to Editor. Ped Infect Dis J 8:732, 1989

21. DOEBBELING BN, STANLY GL, SHEETZE CT, et al: Comparative efficiency of alternative hand-washing agents in reducing nosocomial infections in intensive care units. N Engl J Med 327:88, 1992

22. ANDERSON JM, COCKBURN F, FORFAR JO, et al: Neonatal spongiform myelinopathy after restricted application of hexachlorophene disinfectant. J Clin Pathol 34:25, 1981

23. CURLEY A, HAWK RE, KIMBROUGH RD, et al: Dermal absorption of hexachlorophene in infants. Lancet ii:296, 1971

24. GREAVES SJ, FERRY DG, MCQUEEN EG, MALCOLM DS: Serial hexachlorophene blood levels in the premature infant. NZ Med J 81:334, 1975

25. INNES JRM: Stratum spongiosum and hexachlorophene toxicity in children, experimental monkeys, rats and other species. Bulletin of the Society of Pharmacological and Environmental Pathologists 2:8, 1973

26. KOPELMAN AE: Cutaneous absorption of hexachlorophene in low birth weight infants. J Pediatr 82:972, 1973

27. MARTIN-BAUYER G, LEBRETON R, TOGA M, et al: Outbreak of accidental hexachlorophene poisoning in France. Lancet i:91, 1982

28. ROSSITER EJR: Hexachlorophene—time to stop. Aust Paediatr J 16:236, 1980

29. TYRALA EE, HILLMAN LS, HILLMAN RE, DODSON WE: Clinical pharmacology of hexachlorophene in newborn infants. J Pediatr 91:481, 1977

30. CHECK W: New study shows hexachlorophene is teratogenic in humans. JAMA 240:513, 1978

31. HALLING H: Suspected link between exposure to hexachlorophene and malformed infants. Paper presented at the New York Academy of Science, July 1978

32. IARC monograph on the evaluation of the carcinogenic risk of chemicals to humans. International Agency for Research on Cancer 20:241, 1979

33. JAVELLE KJ, DOEDENS DJ, KLETT SA, JORNEY RB: Iodine absorption in burn patients treated topically with povidone iodine. Clin Pharmacol Ther 17:355, 1975

34. REITSCH J, MEAKINS JL: Complications of povidone-iodine absorption in topically treated burn patients. Lancet i:1976

35. BRICKWELL PG: Sensorineural deafness following myringoplasty operations. J Laryngol Otol 85:957, 1971

36. Hearing damage by chlorhexidine. Lakartidningen 73:3002, 1976

37. AGETT PJ, COOPER LV, ELLIS SH, MCAINSH J: Percutaneous absorption of chlorhexidine in neonatal cord care. Arch Dis Child 56:878, 1981

38. COWAN J, ELLIS SH, MCAINSH J: Absorption of chlorhexidine from the intact skin of newborn infants. Arch Dis Child 54:379, 1979

39. BASSETT DC, STOKES KJ, THOMAS WRG: Wound infection with *Pseudomonas multivorans*. Lancet 1:1188, 1970

40. BURDON DW, WHITBY JL: Contaminations of hospital disinfectants with *Pseudomonas* species. Br Med J [Pract Obs] 2:153, 1967

41. WISHART MM, RILEY TV: Infection with *Pseudomonas maltophilia*. Hospital outbreak due to contaminated disinfectant. Med J Aust 2:710, 1976

42. BONACCI H: Letter to the Editor: Hazard in the nursery. N Engl J Med 282:633, 1970

43. YEH TF, PILDES RS, FIROR HV, SZANTO PB: Letter to the Editor: Mercury poisoning from mercurochrome therapy of infected omphalocele. Lancet i:1978

5 Analgesia and Sedation in the Newborn

Lucienne S. Sanchez

A. INTRODUCTION

Adequate pain management is an essential component of compassionate, humane medical care. Traditionally barriers to adequate pain management in neonates have been related to the question of pain perception in the newborn. This question is no longer debated.[1–4] The American Academy of Pediatrics and the American Society of Anesthesiologists currently advocate the administration of adequate anesthesia to newborn infants undergoing surgery.[5] However, the question of analgesia for other painful procedures has not been addressed directly.[6] This chapter offers general guidelines for the management of analgesia and sedation in newborn infants. Pain control methods specific to circumcision and cryotherapy are discussed in Chapters 43 and 48 respectively.

B. DEFINITIONS

1. Anesthesia: a state characterized by loss of sensation as a result of either pharmacologic depression of nerve function or a primary neurologic disorder.[7]

   Further discussion of anesthesia is beyond the scope of this chapter.

2. Analgesia: a condition in which nociceptive stimuli are perceived but are not interpreted as pain; usually accompanied by sedation without loss of consciousness.[7]

3. Sedation: the act of calming, especially by the administration of a sedative drug; the state of being calm.[7]

4. Tolerance: the ability to resist the action of a drug, or the requirement for increasing doses of a drug, with time, to achieve a desired effect.[6,7]

5. Withdrawal: the development of a substance-specific syndrome that follows the cessation of, or reduction in, intake of a psychoactive substance previously used or administered regularly.[8]

6. Neonatal abstinence syndrome: onset of withdrawal symptoms in neonates on cessation of an agent associated with physical dependence.

C. GENERAL INDICATIONS

1. Any procedure known to be painful (see precautions)
2. Physiologic indications consistent with perception of pain[9]
   a. Tachycardia
   b. Tachypnea
   c. Elevated blood pressure (with secondary increase in intracranial pressure)
   d. Decreased arterial oxygen saturation
   e. Hyperglycemia secondary to hormonal and metabolic stress responses (see precautions)
3. Behavioral indications consistent with perception of pain[4,6,10]
   a. Simple motor responses (i.e., withdrawal of an extremity from a noxious stimulus)
   b. Facial expressions (i.e., grimace)
   c. Altered cry (primary method of communicating painful stimuli in infancy)
   d. Agitation

D. SPECIFIC INDICATIONS

In general, the potency of analgesic treatment selected should be directly related to the assessed level of pain.[11]

1. Mild pain
   a. Oral agents (e.g., acetaminophen)
   b. Local and/or topical anesthesia
   c. Non-pharmacologic approaches (see Section H)
2. Moderate and severe pain
   a. Intravenous opioid analgesics

b. Benzodiazepines (in combination with 2a.)
c. Local and/or topical anesthesia (in combination with 2a. or 2b.)
3. Sedation
   a. Chloral hydrate (see Precautions)
   b. Benzodiazepines
   c. Non-pharmacologic approaches (see Section H)

E. PRECAUTIONS

1. Be aware that
   a. The clinical assessment of pain in the newborn is imprecise.
   b. The physiologic and behavioral parameters cited in this chapter are *nonspecific* indicators of pain and may be related to many other factors.
   c. In sick neonates receiving muscle relaxants, physiologic indicators may be altered and the ability to assess behavioral indicators completely ablated.

   Consequently, a high index of suspicion is required to identify newborn infants in pain.[11]

2. Both the duration of the procedure and the pain assessed should be considered in selecting appropriate analgesia. For example, for a short procedure with mild to moderate associated discomfort (e.g., lumbar puncture) the risks of analgesia may outweigh the benefits.[12]
3. Minimize the number of painful episodes.

   Whenever feasible, schedule multiple procedures at the same time to avoid the need for repeated administration of analgesics.[11]

4. Be aware of the potential complications associated with the analgesic agent employed (Table 5-1).
5. Resuscitation equipment should be readily available. Be prepared to support ventilation; respiratory depression is a common side-effect of a number of analgesic agents.
6. Be aware that
   a. Newborn infants who have developed tolerance to a sedative or analgesic agent may exhibit symptoms of the neonatal abstinence syndrome upon abrupt cessation of the administered agent.[6,13]
   b. Chronic analgesic therapy with agents known to induce tolerance should be weaned gradually, with strict monitoring for evidence of the abstinence syndrome.[4,6,13]
   c. Naloxone (Narcan®, neonatal), an opioid antagonist, may be used to reverse the acute effects of morphine-like opioid agonists. Opioid antagonists should *not* be used in patients receiving chronic analgesic therapy because acute, severe withdrawal symptoms may be precipitated.
7. Chloral hydrate, previously regarded as a nontoxic sedative, should be used with caution in neonates (particularly premature neonates) for the following reasons
   a. Prolonged use of the drug has been associated with nonhemolytic direct hyperbilirubinemia in neonates.[14]
   b. The active metabolite, trichloroethanol, may compete with bilirubin for the glucuronide conjugating system, resulting in an elevation of the indirect fraction of total bilirubin. The half-life of trichloroethanol is prolonged in neonates, hence accumulation of this agent could increase the risk of toxicity.[15,16]
   c. Chloral hydrate should be used with caution in patients with hepatic or renal disease because it is metabolized in the liver and excreted in urine (see Table 5-1; for additional information on the common drugs and some less common drugs, see Appendix A).

F. ADVANTAGES AND DISADVANTAGES OF COMMONLY USED AGENTS IN THE NEWBORN

See Table 5-1.

G. COMPLICATIONS

See Table 5-1.

H. NON-PHARMACOLOGIC APPROACHES

1. Swaddling during heel-stick procedures has been shown to reduce behavioral pain responses.[17]
2. Non-nutritive sucking has been demonstrated to significantly reduce crying in response to painful stimuli.[18]

TABLE 5-1

Sedative and Analgesic Agents Commonly Used in the Newborn [6,9–11,13–16,20,21]

Agent	Category	Mechanism of Action	Advantages	Disadvantages	Recommended Dose	Metabolism
Acetamino-phen	Oral analgesic	Inhibition of peripheral afferent pain signals	No respiratory depression	Mild analgesia	10–20 mg/kg PO, PR	Hepatic
Fentanyl (Sub-limaze)	Synthetic narcotic analgesic	Opioid receptor agonist	Rapid onset of action (3–5 min) More potent than morphine Easily reversible with narcotic antagonist	Short duration (30–60 min) Respiratory depression Hypotension Risk of seizures Chest wall rigidity with rapid infusion Tolerance and withdrawal	1–5 μg/kg IV bolus 0.5–5 μg/kg/hr continuous infusion (analgesia) 10–50 μg/kg IV (anesthesia)	Hepatic
Morphine	Narcotic analgesic	Opioid receptor agonist	Longer duration than fentanyl (4 hours) Easily reversible with narcotic antagonist	Slower onset of action than fentanyl (10–15 min) Respiratory depression More adverse cardiovascular side effects than fentanyl Tolerance and withdrawal	0.05–0.2 mg/kg IV	Hepatic
Meperidine (Demerol)	Narcotic analgesic	Opioid receptor agonist	Longer duration than fentanyl (2–4 hours) Easily reversible with narcotic antagonist Less respiratory depression than morphine	Slower onset of action than fentanyl (10 min) Tolerance and withdrawal	0.5–1.5 mg/kg IV or IM	Hepatic

(continued)

TABLE 5-1 (*Continued*)

Agent	Category	Mechanism of Action	Advantages	Disadvantages	Recommended Dose	Metabolism
Diazepam* (Valium)	Benzodiaze-pine sedative/ hypnotic	Brain stem re-ticular for-mation depressant	Sedation Muscle relaxa-tion	No analgesic effect Respiratory depression Hypotension Withdrawal symptoms may occur	0.1–0.2 mg/kg IV	Hepatic
Lorazepam* (Ativan)	Benzodiaze-pine sedative/ hypnotic	Brain stem re-ticular for-mation depressant	Sedation Longer dura-tion than diazepam (8–12 h)	No analgesic effect Respiratory depression Hypotension Withdrawal symptoms may occur	0.05–0.1 mg/kg IV	Hepatic
Midazolam* (Versed)	Benzodiaze-pine sedative/ hypnotic	Brain stem re-ticular for-mation depressant	Sedation Rapid onset of action (2–5 min)	No analgesic effect Respiratory depression Hypotension Withdrawal symptoms may occur	0.05–0.2 mg/kg loading dose 0.4–6 u/kg/min continuous infusion	Hepatic
Phenobarbital	Barbiturate sedative	Nonspecific CNS de-pressant	Sedation Long half-life Serum levels easily monitored Reduces serum bili-rubin levels	No analgesic effect Slower onset of action than other barbiturates (> 5 min) No specific antagonist Respiratory depression	2–10 mg/kg IV, IM, PO	Hepatic
Chloral hy-drate	Sedative	Central de-pressant effect	Sedation Minimal car-diorespira-tory side-effects	No analgesic effect Gastrointesti-nal irritant May accumu-late in neonates May cause myocardial depression Associated with hyper-bilirubin-emia	25–50 mg/kg PO, PR	Hepatic

*Limited data available in newborns.

3. Sucrose
   a. Infants who drank 2 ml of a 12% sucrose solution prior to blood collection via heel stick cried 50% less than control infants during the same procedure.[19]
   b. Infants who received sucrose on a pacifier prior to and during circumcision cried significantly less than control infants.[19]

I. CONTRAINDICATIONS

There are no absolute contraindications to using analgesia and/or sedation when deemed clinically appropriate.

Be aware of the potential side-effects associated with the specific agent selected and take the proper precautions.

References

1. ANAND KJS, HICKEY PR: Pain and its effects in the human neonate and fetus. N Engl J Med 317:1321, 1987
2. FLETCHER AB: Pain in the neonate. N Engl J Med 317:1347, 1987
3. ANAND KJS, HICKEY PR: Halothane—morphine compared with high-dose susentanil for anesthesia and postoperative analgesia in neonatal cardiac surgery. N Engl J Med 326:1, 1992
4. ROGERS MC: Do the right thing: Pain relief in infants and children. N Engl J Med 326:55, 1992
5. American Academy of Pediatrics: Committee on Fetus and Newborn, Committee on Drugs, Section on Anesthesiology, Section on Surgery. Neonatal anesthesia. Pediatrics 80:446, 1987
6. TRUOG R, ANAND KJS: Management of pain in the postoperative neonate. Clin Perinatol 16:61, 1989
7. Stedman's Medical Dictionary, 25th Ed. Baltimore, Williams & Wilkins, 1990
8. Diagnostic and Statistical Manual of Mental Disorders, Third Ed. Revised (DSM-III-R). Washington, DC, American Psychiatric Association, 1987
9. SUKHANI R: Anesthetic management of the newborn. Clin Perinatol 16:43, 1989
10. MARSHALL RE: Neonatal pain associated with caregiving procedures. Pediatr Clin North Am 36:885, 1989
11. WEISMAN SJ, SCHECHTER NL: the management of pain in children. Pediatr Rev 12:237, 1991
12. PORTER FL, MILLER JP, SESSIONS CF, MARSHALL RE: A controlled clinical trial of local anesthesia for lumbar punctures in newborns. Pediatrics 88:663, 1991
13. CARON E, MAGUIRE DP: current management of pain, sedation, and narcotic physical dependency of the infant on ECMO. J Perinatal Neonatal Nursing July:63, 1990
14. LAMBERT GH, MURASKAS J, ANDERSON CL, MYERS TF: Direct hyperbilirubinemia associated with chloral hydrate administration in the newborn. Pediatrics 86:277, 1990
15. REIMCHE LD, SANKARAN K, HINDMARSH KW, et al: Chloral hydrate sedation in neonates and infants—Clinical and pharmacologic considerations. Dev Pharmacol Ther 12:57, 1989
16. MAYERS DJ, HINDMARSH KW, SANKARAN K, et al: Chloral hydrate disposition following single-dose administration to critically ill neonates and children. Dev Pharmacol Ther 16:71, 1991
17. CAMPOS R: Soothing pain-elicited distress with swaddling and pacifiers in early infancy. Presented at Sixth International Conference on Infant Studies. Washington, DC, April 1988
18. GUNNAR MR, FISCH RO, MALONE S: The effects of a pacifying stimulus on behavior and adrenocortical responses to circumcision in the newborn. J Am Acad Child Psychiatry 23:34, 1984
19. BLASS EM, HOFFMEYER LB: Sucrose as an analgesic for newborn infants. Pediatrics 87:215, 1991
20. BELL SG, ELLIS LJ: Use of fentanyl for sedation of mechanically ventilated neonates. Neonatal Network October:27, 1987
21. ARNOLD JH, ANAND KJS: Anaesthesia and pain control in the newborn. In Avery GB, Fletcher MA, MacDonald MG (eds): Neonatology: Pathophysiology and Management of the Newborn, 4th ed. Philadelphia, Lippincott (in press)

Part 2
Physiologic Monitoring

6 Temperature Monitoring

Andrea Lotze
Oswaldo Rivera

Intermittent Temperature Monitoring

A. BACKGROUND

1. Mercury-in-glass thermometer
   a. Benchmark standard
   b. Determination time greater than 3 minutes
2. Electronic thermometers most widely used
   a. Temperature sensor may be a thermistor or thermocouple.
   b. Temperature is sensed by the probe; the signal is then electronically processed and digitally displayed.
   c. Determination time under 45 seconds
   d. Small hand-held device
3. Infrared electronic thermometry
   a. Sensitive infrared sensor detects infrared energy radiation from the tympanic membrane.
   b. Sensor converts the infrared signal to an electrical signal.
   c. Electrical signal is then processed and digitally displayed as temperature.
   d. Determination time under 2 seconds

B. CONTRAINDICATIONS

Rectal route in tiny infants.

C. EQUIPMENT

1. Glass thermometers
   a. Sterile
   b. Disposable, single patient use
2. Electronic thermometers should provide
   a. Resolution of 0.1°C.
   b. Audible signal at the end of the determination time window
3. Probe-type electronic thermometers designed to be used with disposable probe covers
4. Infrared thermometers
   a. Primarily designed for tympanic membrane temperature
   b. Measures infrared energy emitted by the tympanic membrane

   Aural temperature measured either in the external auditory canal or on the tympanic membrane has been found to correlate well with rectal temperature in both term and preterm infants.[1–5] The tympanic membrane is situated close to the internal carotid artery; its temperature therefore reflects that of the blood flow into the hypothalamus.[6]

   c. Designed to be used with disposable sensor head covers

D. PRECAUTIONS

1. Glass thermometers
   a. Must be held in place during the entire determination time to prevent accidental breakage
   b. Do not force thermometer.
2. Probe-type electronic thermometers
   a. Always use disposable probe cover.
   b. Do not force probe.
3. Infrared thermometers
   a. Always use disposable sensor head covers.
   b. Do not force sensor head into the ear canal.
   c. Do not use in infants with middle ear disease.
   d. Do not use in the very low birth weight infant because of inappropriate speculum size.

   Sensor head may not be small enough for low birth weight infants <1000 gm.

e. Erroneous readings may result from
  (1) Not having the probe lined up with the tympanic membrane
  (2) The presence of heavy cerumen
  (3) The presence of serous otitis media[7]

E. TECHNIQUE

1. Glass thermometer
   a. Vigorously shake the thermometer to ensure that mercury column is down.
   b. For core temperature lubricate and insert into the rectum to a depth of 2 cm.
   c. For noninvasive approximation of core temperature, place bulb at the apex of the mid axilla.
   d. For both sites, the thermometer must be held in place for a period no shorter than 4 minutes.[8,9]
2. Probe-type electronic thermometers
   a. Apply disposable probe cover to the probe.
   b. For core temperature insert probe into the rectum (2–3 cm).
   c. For noninvasive approximation of core temperature place the probe in the axilla (Fig 6-1).[10]
   d. Hold probe in place and wait for an audible beep before removing the probe.
   e. Read temperature, and return the probe to its compartment to deactivate the unit.

3. Infrared thermometers
   a. Apply disposable cover to the sensor head.
   b. Gently insert tapered end into the ear canal.
   c. While holding the unit steady, depress trigger.
   d. Remove from the ear canal and read temperature.
   e. Remove used disposable cover

F. COMPLICATIONS

1. Inaccurate reading[11,12]
   a. Cracked glass thermometer[11,13]
   b. Insufficient application time[11,12]
2. Tissue trauma
   a. Rectal or colonic perforation[11,14,15]
   b. Pneumoperitoneum[16]
   c. Peritonitis
   d. Retention of glass fragments in the rectum from a broken glass thermometer
3. Risk of trauma to the tympanic membrane

Continuous Temperature Monitoring

A. BACKGROUND

1. Provides
   a. Reliable continuous monitoring of neonatal body temperature

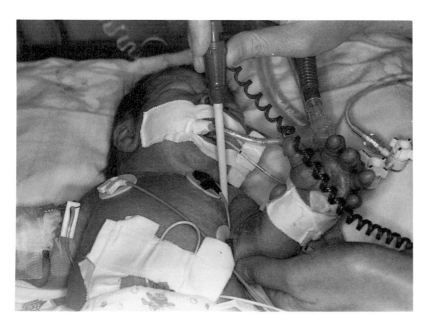

FIG. 6-1
Axillary temperature being taken with electronic probe thermometer. The probe is held perpendicular to the patient, and the arm is held securely against the side of the chest.

b. Trending of temperature over time

c. Automated environmental control (Fig. 6-2).

2. Thermistor probe (most widely used)

a. The thermistor is a resistive component, having a high negative temperature coefficient of resistance, so that its resistance decreases proportionately as the temperature increases.

b. As the resistance of the thermistor changes the electrical current flowing through the probe changes proportionally.

c. The level of current detected by the electronic monitor is converted to thermal units.

2. Thermocouple probes

a. Thermocouple probe is a very small bead made up of the junction of two dissimilar metals.

b. The bead generates a very small voltage proportional to temperature.

c. The voltage generated by the bead is measured by the monitor and converted to thermal units.

3. The thermocouple and the thermistor are not interchangeable.

The thermocouple is voltage generating, whereas the thermistor is a resistive device. Battery powered interface devices are available that allow the use of thermocouple probes with thermistor compatible monitors (Fig. 6-3).

4. Thermocouple probes are less expensive.

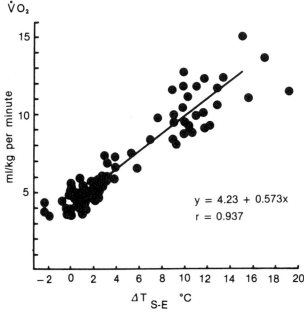

$$y = 4.23 + 0.573x$$
$$r = 0.937$$

FIG. 6-2
Oxygen consumption as a function of temperature gradient between skin and environment. (Adamsons K Jr, Gandy GM, James LS: The influence of thermal factors upon oxygen consumption of the newborn human infant. J Pediatr 66:495, 1965)

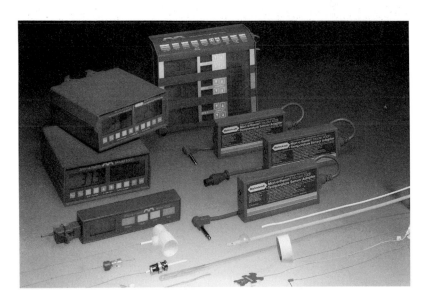

FIG. 6-3
Portable temperature monitors. Temperature sensor adapters allow thermocouple probes to be used with the bedside monitor. Disposable temperature probes (skin, airway, tympanic, esophageal, rectal) (courtesy of Mallinckrodt and Mon-a-therm).

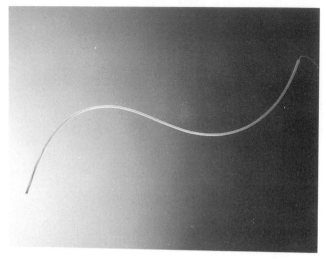

FIG. 6-4
Disposable esophageal/rectal probe (courtesy of Mon-a-therm).

B. CONTRAINDICATIONS

Rectal route in tiny infants.

C. EQUIPMENT SPECIFICATIONS (HARDWARE AND CONSUMMABLES)

Temperature monitoring may be a component of the bedside monitor, free standing or incorporated into a radiant warmer or incubator.

1. Capabilities of the neonatal temperature monitor should include
   a. A resolution to 0.1°C
   b. Temperature display in both fahrenheit and centigrade
2. Most free standing temperature monitors are battery powered.
3. The monitor will employ a thermistor or thermocouple.
4. Monitors using thermistors will be identified as YSI 400 or YSI 700 compatible.
   a. YSI 400 compatible probes are single element devices.
   b. YSI 700 compatible probes are dual element devices.

   The probes are physically identical and are available in the same configurations, but are elec-

trically different and will not work interchangeably.
5. Monitors using thermocouple probes will be identified as such, and the probe connection is different from the thermistor type.
6. Probes for both thermistors and thermocouples are available in different configurations for different sites. For example,
   a. Surface skin, rectal, esophageal, and bladder probes (Fig. 6-4)
   b. Tympanic membrane thermocouple probe

   Disposable probes are recommended for infection control reasons.

D. PRECAUTIONS

1. Do not apply skin probes to broken or bruised skin.
2. Do not apply skin probes over clear plastic dressings.
3. Do not use finger nails to remove skin surface probes.
4. Do not force core probes during insertion.
5. Do not reuse disposable probes.
6. Shield skin probes with reflective pad if used with radiant warmers or heat lamps.
7. When using servocontrol mechanisms for environmental control, take intermittent temperatures at other sites to monitor effect.[17]
8. Do not use core temperature to servoregulate the patient's environment.[18]

E. TECHNIQUE

1. Skin surface probe (Table 6-1)
   a. Prep the skin using an alcohol pad to ensure good adhesion to the skin.
   b. Cover probe with a reflective cover pad (foil covered foam adhesive pad, incorporated in the disposable probe) (Fig. 6-5).

   Probe must be covered with an aluminum foil disc to reflect back added heat from devices such as radiant warmers, phototherapy lights, infrared warming lights, and any other external radiant heat-generating source.[23]

   c. Apply probe over the liver in the supine infant.
   d. Apply probe to the flank in the prone infant.
   e. Ensure that skin probe is free of contact with bed (Fig. 6-6).

TABLE 6-1

Site for Temperature Monitoring[11,19–22]

Site	Rate (°C)	Application
Surface		
1. Abdomen over liver	36.0–36.5	Servocontrol
2. Axillary	36.5–37.0	Noninvasive approximation of core temperature
Core		
1. Sublingual	36.5–37.5	Quick reflection of body change
2. Esophageal	36.5–37.5	Reliable reflection of changes
3. Rectal	36.5–37.5	Slow reflection of changes

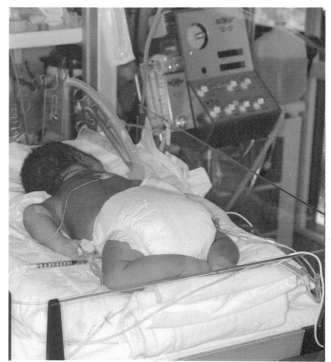

FIG. 6-5
Skin probe properly placed on infant under radiant warmer (note that probe has protective foil cover and lies flat on the skin surface).

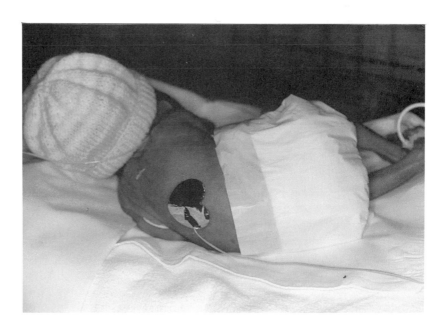

FIG. 6-6
Premature infant in an incubator with skin probe free of contact from bed surface.

TABLE 6-2
Potential Pitfalls of Servo-Controlled Heating Devices [12,21,24,25]

	Skin << Core	Skin ≅ Core	Skin > Core
Increased Heater Output	Cold stress Shock (vasoconstricted) Hypoxia Acidosis	Dislodged probe (early) Servo fails to shut off Vasodilators (e.g., tolazoline) Shock (vasodilated)	Dislodged probe (late) Servo fails (late)
Decreased Heater Output	Probe uninsulated (radiant heat) Servocontrol malfunction Onset of fever	Baby overheated Fever	Internal cold stress (e.g., unheated endotracheal oxygen, exchange transfusion)

Note: Changes in heater output may not be indicated; therefore, it is necessary to intermittently monitor the infant's *core* temperature (axillary optimal).

2. Application of core probe (Table 6-1)
   a. Choose probe size according to site, i.e., rectum or esophagus.
   b. Place in esophagus by inserting the probe through the nostril.
      (1) Esophageal probe does not need lubrication prior to placement.
      (2) Estimate the length of insertion using the sum of the distance from the mouth to the tragus of the ear, and the distance between the ear to the xiphisternal angle.
   c. Lubricate the probe before placing in rectum.

   Probe needs to be placed approximately 3 cm beyond anal sphincter; avoid further advancement due to risk of perforation.

   d. Do not force probe.
4. Connect the probe to the monitor.
5. Monitor energy output changes.
6. Reposition or replace the probe if temperature recorded does not correlate with that recorded using a standard temperature measuring device such as a glass or electronic thermometer.

   Skin surface temperature will be cooler than core temperature.

F. COMPLICATIONS

1. Tissue trauma caused by core temperature probe
   a. Rectal or colonic perforation
   b. Pneumoperitoneum
   c. Peritonitis
2. Unsafe environmental temperature control caused by unshielded skin probes or loosely adhered probe, when monitoring is used to servoregulate temperature (Table 6-2).

References

1. MAYFIELD SR, NAKAMURA KT, BHATIA J, et al: Tympanic membrane temperature of term and preterm neonates. Early Hum Dev 9:241, 1984
2. BENZIGER TH, TAYLOR GW: Cranial measurements of internal temperature in man. In Hardy JD (ed): Temperature: Its Measurement and Control in Science and Industry, Vol. 3. New York, Reinhold 1963, p 111
3. COOPER KE, CRANSTON WI, SNELL ES: Temperature in the external auditory meatus as an index of central temperature changes. J Appl Physiol 19:1032, 1964
4. STRATTON D: Aural temperature of the newborn infant. Arch Dis Child 52:865, 1977

5. BENZIGER M: Tympanic thermometry in surgery and anesthesia. JAMA 209:1207, 1969

6. JOHNSON KJ, BHATIA P, BELL EF: Infrared thermometry of newborn infants. Pediatrics 87:34, 1991

7. WEIR MR, WEIR TE: Are 'hot' ears really hot? Am J Dis Child 143:763, 1989

8. HADDOCK B, VINCENT P, MERROW D: Axillary and rectal temperatures of full-term neonates: Are they different? Neonatal Network 5:36, 1986

9. STEPHEN SB, SEXTON PR: Neonatal axillary temperatures: Increases in readings over time. Neonatal Network 5:25, 1987

10. MAYFIELD SR, BHATIA J, NAKAMURA KT, et al: Temperature measurements in term and preterm neonates. J Pediatr 104:271, 1984

11. GREENBAUM EI, CARSON M, KINCANNON WN, O'LOUGHLIN BJ: Hazards of temperature taking. Br Med J 3:4, 1970

12. GREENBAUM EI, CARSON M, KINCANNON WN, O'LOUGHLIN BJ: Mercury vs. electronic thermometers. Health Devices 2:3, 1972

13. FERGUSON GT, GOHRKE C, MANSFIELD L: The advantages of the electronic thermometer. Hospitals 45:62, 1971

14. MERENSTEIN GB: Rectal perforation by thermometer. Lancet i:1970

15. FRANK JD, BROWN S: Thermometers and rectal perforations in the neonate. Arch Dis Child 53:824, 1978

16. GREENBAUM EI, CARSON M, KINCANNON WN, O'LOUGHLIN BJ: Rectal thermometer-induced pneumoperitoneum in the newborn. Pediatrics 44:539, 1969

17. BELGAUMBAR TK, SCOTT K: Effects of low humidity on small premature infants in servocontrol incubators. Biol Neonate 26:348, 1975

18. SCOPES JW: Thermoregulation in the newborn. In Avery GB (ed): Neonatology, Philadelphia, JB Lippincott, 1981, p 176

19. BLAINEY CG: Site selection in taking body temperature. Am J Nurs 74:1859, 1974

20. NICHOLS GA, RUSKIN MM, GLOR BAK, KELLY WH: Oral, axillary and rectal temperature determinations and relationships. Nurs Res 15:307, 1966

21. SMITH RM: Temperature monitoring and regulation. Pediatr Clin North Am 16:643, 1969

22. STRATTON D: Aural temperature of newborn infant. Arch Dis Child 52:865, 1977

23. DODMAN N: Newborn temperature control. Neonatal Network 5:19, 1987

24. POMERANCE JJ, BRAND RJ, MERIDITH JL: Differentiating environmental from disease-related fevers in the term newborn. Pediatrics 67:485, 1981

25. SILVERMAN WA, ZAMELIS A, SINCLAIR JC, AGATE FJ JR: Warm nape of the newborn. Pediatrics 33:986, 1964

7 Cardiac/Respiratory Monitoring

Andrea Lotze
Oswaldo Rivera

Continuous neonatal monitoring has progressed to the stage of what is referred to as the multiparameter monitoring system. Microprocessor technology has made possible the integration of multiple parameters into a single system that comprises the bedside monitor. In this section, the individual parameters are outlined separately for clarity.

Cardiac Monitoring

A. PURPOSE

1. Reliable and accurate monitoring of neonatal cardiac activity
2. Monitoring beat to beat heart rate with a short rate display update period[1,2]
3. Trending of heart rate over time

B. BACKGROUND

1. Detection of the electrical signal emanating from the heart by the surface electrodes
2. Low level signal is amplified and filtered to eliminate high frequency interference and artifacts from the ECG bandpass.
3. Vectors (i.e., lead I, II, III) are selected by changing the lead input to the monitor.
4. Electrical signal is defined in millivolts (mv).
5. QRS, defined and detected from the signal, is used to determine heart rate.

C. CONTRAINDICATIONS

1. None

D. EQUIPMENT

Hardware—Specifications

1. The neonatal cardiac monitor should have the appropriate frequency response and sensitivity to accurately track the fast and narrow QRS complex of the newborn infant.

   Heart rate processed on a beat to beat basis with a short updating interval

2. Startup default heart rate alarm limits should be tailored to the neonatal population.

   Low rate (bradycardia) limit of 100 BPM; high rate (tachycardia) limit 175 to 200 BPM.

3. Waveform display of the ECG wave
   a. Cathode ray tube (CRT) oscilloscope has the highest resolution and the best definition.

   Display can either be monochromatic or color.

   b. Liquid crystal display (LCD): a flat, thin display
      (1) The resolution of this device leaves much to be desired when displaying the fast and narrow complex of the neonate.
      (2) Backlighting is necessary for viewing in low-light environments.
      (3) Viewing angle is critical, unlike the CRT.
4. Heart rate display can be any of following
   a. Alpha numeric part of waveform display
   b. Light emitting diode (LED) display
   c. Other separate numerical display window
5. Recorder (optional)
   a. Real time ECG
   b. Delayed ECG (Stored retrospective display mainly used for the short time interval prior to the occurrence of the alarm condition.)
   c. Printed record of trend information
   d. Free standing (directly connected to or part of a bedside monitor serving that monitor only)
   e. Central station recorder serving all the monitors connected to that station (remotely located from the bedside)
   f. On many monitoring systems, paper recording of the delayed ECG is activated automatically on alarm condition.

Consummables—Specifications

1. Disposable neonatal ECG electrodes
   a. Silver–silver chloride electrode
   b. Specifically designed for the neonatal population

   Supplied in muliple configurations: pregelled, conductive adhesive, pre-attached lead wires, foam body, paper body, fabric body, nonradiopaque and a variety of shapes and colors.

   c. In the selection of the electrode attention should be given to the following
      (1) The ability to remain adhered to the skin of an active infant
      (2) The quality of the signal attained
      (3) Minimally irritating to the skin
      (4) Ease of removal using water or skin adhesive remover without damage to or removal of skin
      (5) Performance in the warm, moist environment of an infant incubator
      (6) Adhesive–skin interaction under overhead infant warmers
2. Lead wires and patient cable
   a. All cables should be clean and the insulation free of nicks or cuts.
   b. Lead wires should lock or snap into the patient cable, preventing easy disconnections.
   c. Use infant/pediatric lead wires with small electrode clips.

   Standard adult-size clips will place too much torsion on the infant electrode, tugging on the skin and possibly peeling off the electrode.

E. PRECAUTIONS

1. Do not use alcohol wipes as conductors under electrodes (see Fig. 4-3).
2. Do not apply electrodes to broken or bruised skin.
3. Do not apply electrodes to clear film plastic dressings.

   Plastic dressing will act as an insulator between the skin and the electrode.

4. Do not deactivate heart rate alarm.
5. Do not use finger nails to remove electrodes from the skin surface, to avoid skin damage.
6. Secure the patient cable to patient's environment to prevent tugging.

7. Do not use monitors that have not been checked for safety and performance (dated sticker on the monitor will verify the monitor's condition).
8. Do not use monitors with any sign of defects such as exposed wires, broken or dented enclosure, broken knobs or controls, cracked display.

F. TECHNIQUE

1. Familiarize yourself with the monitor before proceeding.
2. Placement of electrode
   a. Skin preparation: prepare the skin using an alcohol pad.
   b. Allow the skin to dry before adhering the electrodes.
   c. Remove all substances from the skin surface to provide the best electrode-to-skin interface (monitor performance is only as good as the interface obtained).
   d. The basic 3 lead configuration for ECG/respiration (Figs. 7-1 and 7-2).
      (1) Right arm (white)—nipple line lateral chest right
      (2) Left arm (black)—nipple line lateral chest left
      (3) Left leg (red)—left lower rib cage

   Note monitor manufacturer's placement instructions. Usually, the same set of electrodes will be used for both cardiac and respiratory monitoring.

   e. The use of tape for electrode adherence should be avoided.

   Electrodes must adhere to skin without tape to perform correctly and provide proper electrical interface.

3. Attach lead wires
   a. White—right arm—to right chest electrode
   b. Black—left arm—to left chest electrode
   c. Red—left leg—to left lower rib cage electrode
4. Turn monitor on (modern monitors will go through an automatic power-on self test).
5. Connect the patient cable to the monitor.
6. Select the lead that provides the best signal and QRS size (most monitors use lead II for default).
7. Ensure that the QRS indicator flashes with each

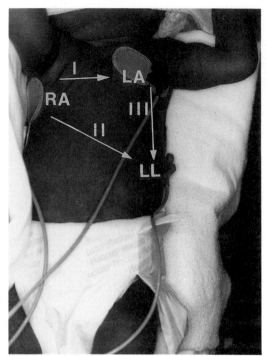

FIG. 7-1
Basic lead clip placements and lead vectors for optimal ECG signal detection. RA/LA positions also provide maximal signal for impedance pneumography.

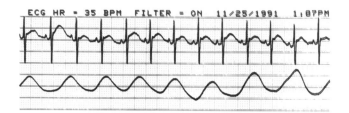

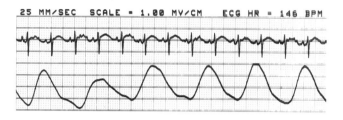

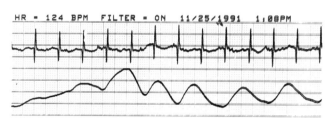

FIG. 7-2
Typical ECG tracings: (top) lead I; (middle) lead II; (bottom) lead III.

TABLE 7-1

Heart Rates in Premature and Fullterm Neonates

	1 to 7 Days			1 to 4 Weeks		
	Min	**Mean**	**Max**	**Min**	**Mean**	**Max**
Premature (<1500 g)	125	145	168	110	161	192
Premature (1500–2500 g)	100	147	195	123	157	190
Term	100	133	175	115	163	190

(From Goldsmith JP, Karotkin EH: Assisted ventilation of the neonate. Philadelphia, WB Saunders, 1988, p 455, with permission.)

QRS seen on the display (make sure that the QRS detector is not counting high T or P waves).

8. Set the low and high rate alarms accordingly (Table 7-1).

G. COMPLICATIONS

1. Skin lesions (rare)
   a. Skin irritation from electrolyte gel when it is incorrectly formulated
   b. Skin irritation from alcohol, especially with immature skin[3] (see Fig. 4-3)

   This complication may occur even with a short-term application of alcohol preparation to immature skin. It is probably the combined result of immature squamous-cell layer, and excessive vigor used to rub skin during electrode site preparation. During emergency application of ECG limb plate electrodes on the extremities for monitoring in resuscitation or performance of procedures that interfere with routine chest lead placement, use of electrolyte gel, rather than alcohol pads, is imperative.

   c. Cellulitis (after prolonged application) (Fig. 7-3).
   d. Abscess
   e. Hypo- or hyperpigmentation marks (Fig. 7-4).

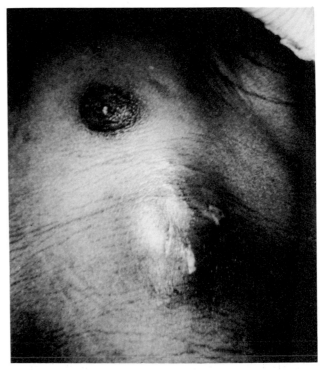

FIG. 7-3
Cellulitis with abscess formation after electrode fixation with tape.

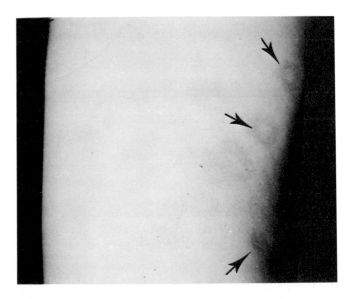

FIG. 7-4
Residual markings more than 1 year after applications of ECG leads for cardiorespiratory monitoring. Hyperpigmented marks on extremities.

2. Erroneous readings caused by artifact[4]
  a. 60 cycle electrical interference (Table 7-2).
    (1) Poor contact of electrode
    (2) Dried electrode gel
  b. Decreased signal amplitude with motion artifact
  c. Electrical interference from other equipment used in the patient's immediate environment
  d. Electrical spikes generated by piezoelectric effect when certain types of polyvinyl chloride tubing are mechanically deformed by infusion pump devices (rare)[5]

  These spikes may appear as ectopic beats on the monitor.

  e. Incorrect vectors because of inaccurate lead placement
  f. Inappropriate sensitivity settings will cause erroneous heart rate readings.

  This only applies to non-automated monitors (Fig. 7-5, Table 7-2).

TABLE 7-2
Steps to Minimize Artifact Interference

Problem	Treatment
Poor electrode contact	Gently clean skin with alcohol wipe and allow to dry prior to electrode reapplication.
Dried electrode	Replace
Equipment interference	a. Systematically turn off one piece of adjacent equipment at a time while observing monitor for improvement in signal quality. b. Once source for interference identified, increase distance between that equipment and patient while rerouting power cords and any cables connected to the patient. c. If above maneuver does not help, replace equipment.
60 Hertz interference	a. Follow procedure for poor electrode contact. b. Replace patient cable. c. Try another monitor if a and b don't work.

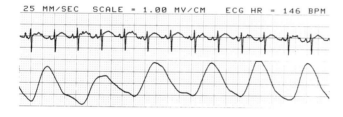

25 MM/SEC   SCALE = 1.00 MV/CM   ECG HR = 146 BPM

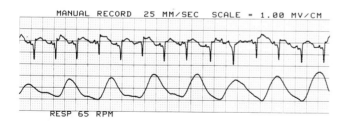

MANUAL RECORD   25 MM/SEC   SCALE = 1.00 MV/CM

RESP 65 RPM

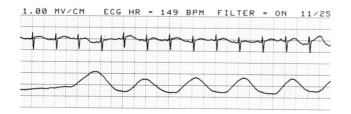

1.00 MV/CM   ECG HR = 149 BPM   FILTER = ON   11/25

FIG. 7-5
Normal P, QRS, and T wave detection. (Top) lead II tracing with electrodes properly located. Note normal P, QRS, and T wave detection. (Middle) lead II tracing with electrodes close together on anterior chest wall. Note altered QRS and decreased T wave amplitude. (Bottom) lead II tracing with electrodes placed laterally on the abdomen. Note decreased wave amplitude and flattened P wave.

Respiration Monitoring

A. PURPOSE

1. Reliable and accurate monitoring of neonatal respiratory activity[6]
2. Monitoring of breath to breath activity with a short rate display update period
3. Trending of respiration activity over time
4. Detection of apnea

B. BACKGROUND

1. Transthoracic impedance measurement is the most commonly and widely used.
2. Technique involves the passage of a low level high frequency signal through the patient's chest (Fig. 7-6).
3. Signal is passed by the same electrodes used for cardiac monitoring. In most cases the RA (right arm—white) and the LA (left arm—black) are used as the path for the high frequency signal.
4. As the density of the chest cavity changes due to lung inflation, the impedance of the chest cavity also changes (impedance = the electrical resistance to the high frequency signal).
5. The high frequency signal is transmitted through the chest and undergoes an amplitude change proportional to the impedance change of the thorax.
6. This impedance change, as seen by the modulation of the high frequency signal, is detected and quantified by the monitor and counted as respiratory activity per minute or breaths per minute.
7. The monitor will set an impedance threshold limit for valid respiratory activity because cardiac pumping (pulmonary blood flow) action will also cause thoracic impedance changes (usually much smaller than changes with respiration).
8. The monitor will separate the ECG signal from the high frequency carrier signal used for detection of respiration.

C. CONTRAINDICATIONS

None

D. EQUIPMENT

Hardware—Specifications

1. Same as for the cardiac monitor. The most basic neonatal monitor is a combination heart rate/respiration monitor.

   Low level threshold for breath validation should not be below 0.2 ohms (minimizes cardiogenic artifact).

2. Should have coincidence alarm and rejection (when the respiration rate being picked up is equal to the heart rate activity being detected by the cardiac portion of the system).
3. Should have variability in apnea time delay setting (= apnea length in seconds before alarming).

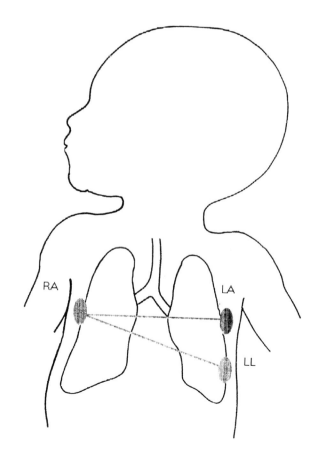

FIG. 7-6
Transthoracic impedance pneumography. Path of the high-frequency signal through the patient's chest. (Note: Most monitors use RA → LA; others may use RA → LL).

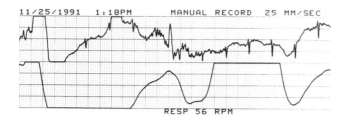

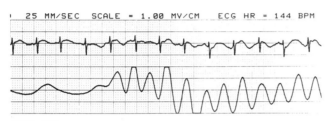

FIG. 7-7
Tracings of artifacts affecting ECG/respiration. (Top) loose electrode affected by motion; (bottom) motion artifact caused by patient's moving arm coming in contact with chest electrodes (note change in respiratory frequency signal).

4. Start-up default limits should be tailored to the neonatal population.

> Start-up default apnea time delay usually 15 to 20 seconds.

Consummables—Specifications
Same as for cardiac monitor.

E. PRECAUTIONS

1. Same as for cardiac monitor.
2. Electrodes can pick up muscular activity and may count this as respiration; as a result, alarm may not occur during an apneic episode (see G1) (Fig. 7-7).

F. TECHNIQUE

1. Same as for cardiac monitor.
2. Ensure that the breath detector flashes with each breath seen on the display, coincident with the initiation of inspiration.
3. Move the right and left arm electrodes up towards the axillary area if respiration pickup is marginal due to shallow breathing.
4. Set desired low—high respiratory rate and apnea delay alarm limits.

G. COMPLICATIONS

1. False positive "respiratory" signal in the absence of effective ventilation[7]
   a. Chest-wall movement with airway obstruction
   b. Nonrespiratory muscular action giving motion artifact
      (1) Stretching
      (2) Seizure
2. False alarm
   a. Improperly set sensitivity not detecting respiratory activity
   b. Electrodes not correctly placed
   c. Loose electrodes
3. Skin lesions (see Cardiac Monitoring)

Cardiorespirograph Monitoring

A. INDICATIONS

Monitoring of infants for identification and quantification of apnea, periodic breathing, bradycardia, and O_2 desaturation episodes.

1. Combination heart rate with compressed or trended respiration activity
2. Chronological order of relationship of bradycardia and apnea. Some systems may provide continuous SaO_2 information to show time relationship of bradycardia, apnea, and desaturation.
3. Detection, real time identification and quantification of heart rate activity, respiration activity and, in some cases, arterial O_2 saturation on the same time frame

B. BACKGROUND

1. Heart rate value is plotted on a graph ("Y" axis, heart rate in beats per minute), with time graphed on the "X" axis (usually minutes and seconds).
2. Respiration wave is compressed to allow approximately 2 minutes of activity to be displayed.

FIG. 7-8
Typical stand-alone beside monitor with integrated recorder. (Courtesy Medical Data Electronics)

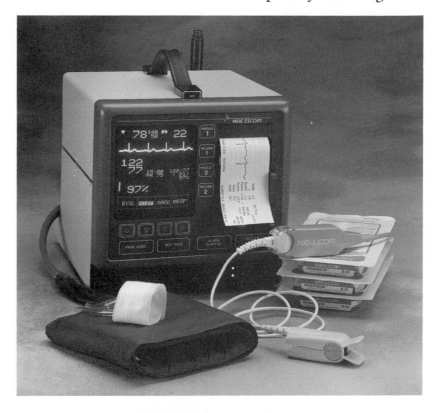

3. Both heart rate and respiration activity are updated at the same point in time, allowing appreciation for time relationship between the two parameters (Fig. 7-8).
4. The SaO_2 value is plotted in the same fashion as the heart rate (2nd "Y" axis).
5. This technique allows for visualization of entire apneic episodes and the identification of precipitating factors (e.g., a drop in respiratory rate may precede bradycardia).
6. Short-term trending is constantly updating and displacing the oldest piece of information. Short-tern trending is usually based on a 2-minute window o time (Fig. 7-9).

C. CONTRAINDICATIONS

None

D. EQUIPMENT

Standard feature for most current neonatal monitors

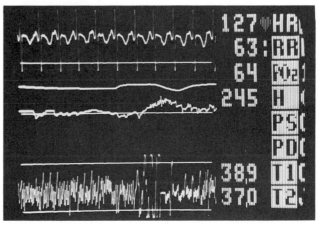

FIG. 7-9
Typical cardiorespirogram display. Traces from top to bottom: 5 sec ECG activity (25 mm/sec); $TcPO_2$ (2 min); heart rate (2 min); respiration waveform (2 min). HR—heart rate; RR—resp rate; PO_2—$TcPO_2$; M—heat output $TcPO_2$; PS—systolic blood pressure; PD—diastolic blood pressure; T—temperature. (Courtesy of Siemens Medical Systems, Inc.)

References

1. CABAL LA, SIASSI B, ZANINI B, et al: Factors affecting heart rate variability in preterm infants. Pediatrics 65:50, 1980
2. VALIMAKI IA, RAUTAHARJU PM, ROY SB, SCOTT KE: Heart rate patterns in healthy term and premature infants and in respiratory distress syndrome. Eur J Cardiol 1:411, 1974
3. SCHICK JB, MILSTEIN JM: Burn hazard of isopropyl alcohol in the neonate. Pediatrics 68:588, 1981
4. JACOBS MK: Sources of measurement error in noninvasive electronic instrumentation. Nurs Clin North Am 13:573, 1978
5. SAHN DJ, VAUCHER YE: Electrical current leakage transmitted to an infant via an IV controller: An unusual ECG artifact. J Pediatr 89:301, 1976
6. NEUMAN NR: The biophysical and bioengineering bases of perinatal monitoring. Part V: Neonatal cardiac and respiratory monitoring. Perinatology/Neonatology 3:17, 1979
7. SOUTHALL DP, RICHARDS JM, LAU KC, SHINEBOURNE EA: An explanation for failure of impedance apnea alarm systems. Arch Dis Child 55:63, 1980

8 Blood Pressure Monitoring

Andrea Lotze
Oswaldo Rivera

Noninvasive (Indirect) Methods

Auscultatory Measurement

A. BACKGROUND

1. This technique employs a blood pressure cuff, insufflator, manometer, and stethoscope.
2. Sphygmomanometer uses a pneumatic cuff to encircle the upper arm or leg, and a pressure gauge (manometer) to register the pressure in the cuff.
3. There are two types of manometers
   a. Aneroid (mechanical air gauge)
   b. Mercury (mercury column)
4. Encircling pneumatic cuff is inflated to a pressure higher than the systolic pressure in the underlying artery. The cuff pressure compresses the artery and stops blood flow.
5. A stethoscope placed distal to the cuff, over the occluded artery, will pick up the Korotkoff sounds when the pressure of the cuff is decreased to the point at which blood flow resumes.

   > Korotkoff sounds are the noise generated by blood spurting from the compressed artery, producing turbulence and vibration within the vessel.

6. The pressure observed while the cuff pressure is falling that coincides with the artery Korotkoff sounds is the systolic pressure. The point at which the Korotkoff sound disappears completely is defined as the diastolic pressure.

   > In patients in whom the sound does not disappear, the point at which the sound changes abruptly to a muffled tone can be accepted as an approximation of the diastolic pressure, but is slightly higher than true diastolic pressure.

7. An 8 to 9 MHz doppler device can be used in place of a stethoscope.

   > This device will only detect systolic blood pressure levels.

B. CONTRAINDICATIONS

None

C. EQUIPMENT

1. Neonatal Cuff (Table 8-1)[1] Largest cuff that will fit comfortably around upper arm or leg; inflatable bladder should completely encircle extremity without overlapping.
2. Mercury manometer or aneroid-type gauge
3. Stethoscope with diaphragm, or doppler system

TABLE 8-1
Neonatal Cuff

Cuff No. (Size)	Limb Circumference
#1	3–6 cm
#2	4–8 cm
#3	6–11 cm
#4	7–13 cm
#5	8–15 cm

From: American Academy of Pediatrics Task Force Pressure Control: Report. Pediatrics 59: 797, 1977.

TABLE 8-2

Sources of Error in Indirect Blood-Pressure Measurements[8]

Problem	Effect on Blood Pressure	Precaution

Defective manometer
  1. Air leaks
  2. Improper valve function
  3. Dry rotted tubing
  4. Loss of mercury
	Falsely low values	1. Check level of mercury at zero cuff pressure.
		2. Check for clear definition of meniscus.
		3. Verify that pressure holds when tightened.

Inappropriate cuff size
  1. Too narrow
  2. Too wide
	1. Falsely high values
	2. Falsely low values
		Verify appropriate size cuff.

Cuff applied loosely	Falsely high values owing to ballooning of bag and narrowing of effective surface	Apply cuff snugly.
Cuff applied too tightly	Inaccurate reading owing to impedance of flow through artery	Apply cuff snugly without undue pressure.
Rapid deflation of cuff	1. Falsely low values owing to inaccurate detection of beginning of sounds, or 2. Falsely high values owing to inadequate equilibration between cuff pressure and manometer pressure	Deflate cuff at rate of 2 mm Hg/sec–3 mm Hg/sec.
Active or agitated patient	Variable	Recheck when patient is quiet.

D. PRECAUTIONS (TABLE 8-2)

1. Carefully select the appropriate cuff size because incorrect size can significantly alter the blood pressure recorded.[2]

   Cuff too small, BP higher; cuff too large, BP lower

2. Check functional integrity of manometer.
3. Speed of cuff deflation

   If deflation is too rapid, accuracy may be compromised.

4. Patient must be quiet and still during measurements.
5. For optimal infection control, use disposable cuff issued to the patient.

E. TECHNIQUE

1. Place infant supine, with the limb fully extended level with the heart.
2. Measure the circumference and select the appropriate size cuff for limb.

   a. Neonatal cuffs are marked with the size range (Fig. 8-1).
   b. When the cuff is wrapped around the limb, the end of the cuff should line up with the range mark.
   c. If the end of the cuff falls short of the range mark, the cuff size is too small.
   d. If the end of the cuff falls beyond the range mark, the cuff size is too large.
3. Apply the cuff snugly to the bare limb, above elbow or knee joint.
4. Place stethoscope or doppler over the brachial artery.
5. Inflate the cuff rapidly, to a pressure 15 mm Hg above the point at which the brachial pulse disappears.
6. Deflate cuff slowly.

F. COMPLICATIONS

1. Inaccurate measurements (see Table 8-2).
   a. Defective manometer
   b. Air leaks at the tubing connections or from dry rotted tubing

c. Inappropriate cuff size

d. Cuff applied loosely

e. Rapid deflation of cuff

f. Active or agitated patient

2. Nosocomial infection from multiple patient use of a cuff.

3. Pressure may not be detectable in low perfusion state or shock.

4. Prolonged repeated cycling has been associated with ischemia, purpura, and/or neuropathy.

5. Pressure not detectable or inaccurate in neonates experiencing convulsions or tremors.

Oscillometric Measurement of Arterial Blood Pressure (Automatic Noninvasive)

A. BACKGROUND

Oscillometric technique now offers a means for measuring all arterial blood pressure parameters (systolic, diastolic, mean, heart rate).[3-8] This technique is referred to as NIBP (noninvasive blood pressure).

1. This technique employs a blood pressure cuff interfaced to computerized blood pressure monitor.

2. The pneumatic cuff is used in the same fashion as with the auscultatory technique.

3. The monitor employs a miniature computer-controlled air pump and bleed valve to control inflation and deflation of the cuff.

4. A pressure transducer interfaced to the cuff tubing senses the pressure pulsations transmitted to the cuff by the underlying artery and also the inflation pressure of the cuff.

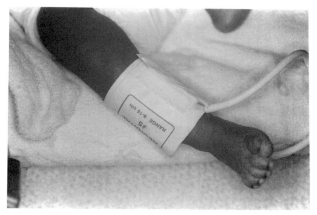

FIG. 8-1
Infant blood pressure cuff to demonstrate use of range mark.

5. The system will inflate the cuff to level above the point at which no pulsations are detected.

6. As the cuff is being deflated to the level of the systolic pressure, arterial pulses are transmitted to the cuff.

   The systolic pressure is assigned the value of the cuff pressure at the time pulsations were initially detected.

7. With most systems the mean pressure value is determined by the highest pulsation level detected at the lowest cuff pressure.

8. The diastolic value is determined by the lowest cuff pressure before baseline arterial pulsations are detected (Fig. 8-2).

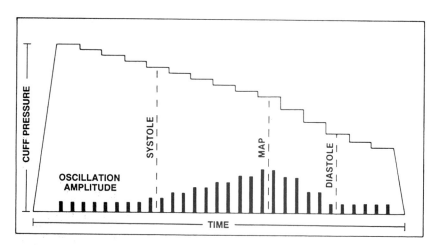

FIG. 8-2
Determination sequence for oscillometric measurement.

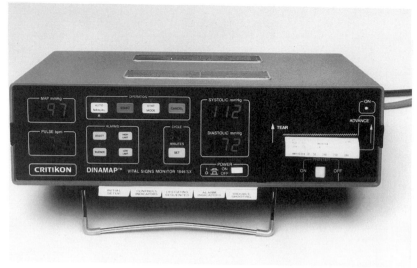

FIG. 8-3
Oscillometric blood pressure monitor (Courtesy of Johnson & Johnson).

9. Heart rate values are calculated by computing the mean value of the time interval between pulsations.
10. Higher detection sensitivity allows this technique to be used on parts of the extremities where auscultatory methods are not possible (i.e., distal arm and lower leg).

B. EQUIPMENT

1. Neonatal noninvasive blood pressure monitor. Display should include systolic, diastolic, mean, and heart rate values (Fig. 8-3).
2. Neonatal cuff (designed for use with the specific monitor). Cuff may be the single-tube or double-tube type, provided the appropriate adapter is used. Cuff size range #1 to #5 (see Table 8-1).

C. PRECAUTION

1. Carefully select appropriate cuff size, because incorrect size can significantly alter the blood pressure value obtained.

    Oversized cuff will yield lower blood pressure values. Undersized cuff will produce higher pressure values.

2. Patient must be still during measurements.

3. For optimal infection control, cuffs should be single-patient use.
4. Caution should be exercised when used with the preterm, very low birth weight infant in a hypotensive state.[9]

D. TECHNIQUE

1. Become familiar with the monitor and the consummables to be used.
2. Measure the circumference of the extremity where the cuff is to be applied. Select the appropriate size cuff for the limb (Fig. 8-4).
3. Apply the cuff snugly to the limb. Cuff can be applied over thin layer of clothing if necessary; however, bare limb is recommended.
4. Attach the monitor air hoses to the cuff.
5. Turn the monitor on and ensure that it passes the power-on self test before proceeding.
6. Press the appropriate button to start a blood pressure determination cycle.
7. If the values obtained from the initial cycle are questionable, repeat step 6.

    Multiple readings with similar values yield the optimal assurance of accuracy.

FIG. 8-4
Cuff of correct size applied to upper arm.

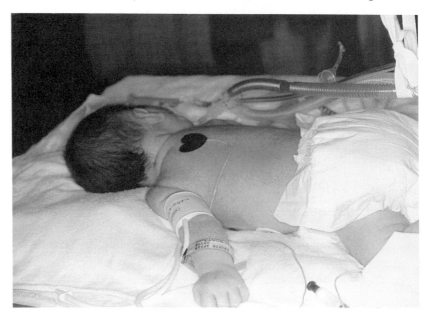

8. If after repeating the cycle, readings are still questionable, reposition the cuff and repeat the measurement.
9. Periodic inspection of the cuff and extremity is critical to avoid problems such as cuff detachment or shift in extremity position.
10. Most NIBP systems can be programmed by the user to automatically measure blood pressure at user-determined intervals.

> The interval between measurements should be as long as possible to ensure adequate circulation and minimize trauma to the limb and skin distal to the cuff.

E. COMPLICATIONS

1. Inaccurate measurements due to motion artifact or inappropriate cuff size
2. Nosocomial infection from multiple-patient use of a cuff
3. Pressure not detectable in neonates experiencing convulsions or tremors.
4. Aborted determination cycle due to air leaks in the cuff, air hoses, or the connection points
5. System malfunction alarms
6. Repeated continuous cycling can cause ischemia, purpura, and/or neuropathy.

Blood Pressure—Invasive

A. PURPOSE

Blood pressure measurement from the vascular system via a catheter that has been introduced into a vein or artery

B. INDICATIONS

To monitor intravascular pressure

1. In very small or unstable infants, particularly those with severe hypotension (shock)
2. During major procedures that could cause or exacerbate intravascular instability
3. To monitor infants on aggressive ventilator support or ECMO

C. BACKGROUND

1. The catheter is coupled to a pressure transducer outside the body by a fluid-filled conduit.
2. Because fluid is noncompressible, it is the medium used to transmit the pressure from the vessel to the transducer.
3. The tubing used to couple the catheter to the transducer is special high-pressure tubing. This tubing

has low compliance and is capable of withstanding high pressures without bursting and with very little stretch.

4. A blood pressure transducer is a device that converts mechanical forces (pressure) to electrical signals. There are two major types of transducer

   a. Strain gauge pressure transducer: composed of metal strands or foil that is either stretched or released by the applied pressure on the diaphragm.

   Applied pressure causes a proportional and linear change in electrical resistance. Problems associated with strain gauges include drift due to temperature changes (departure from the real signal value), fragility, and cost.

   b. Solid state pressure transducers (semiconductor): composed of a silicone chip that undergoes

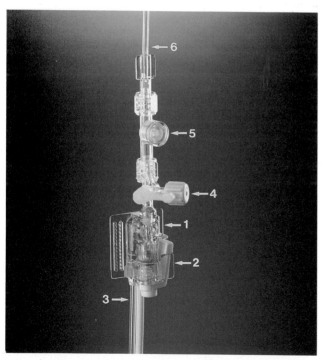

FIG. 8-5
Representative disposable blood pressure transducer setup. 1) pressure transducer; 2) integral continuous flush device; 3) infusion port (connects to infusion pump); 4) stopcock; 5) optional anti-resonnating device; 6) high-pressure tubing. Reusable transducer systems use similar components but the transducer is detachable.

electrical resistance changes as a result of the applied pressure.

   (1) Because of its low cost it has made possible inexpensive, accurate disposable transducers.

   (2) Because of the miniature integration on the silicone chip, the circuitry necessary to minimize temperature drift is incorporated in the device. This technology offers a superior alternative to the strain gauge.

   c. Pressure transmitted to the transducer causes a micro mechanical displacement of the diaphragm (receptor of mechanical energy linked to the transducer element) or directly to the transducer.

   d. This mechanical displacement causes a proportional change in the electrical resistance of the transducer.

   e. Excitation voltage applied to the transducer is responsible for the signal produced in relation to the pressure applied.

   f. The standard medical blood pressure transducer output rating is 5uv/v/cm Hg.

5. Miniature transducer-tipped catheters are available that do not depend on fluid-filled lines for the transmission of pressure.

   Microtransducer catheters in general have better fidelity characteristics, but at a much higher cost than conventional fluid-filled systems.

6. The pressure monitor processes the electrical signal generated by the transducer and converts it to blood pressure units in either mm Hg or kPa. Part of this processing involves the detection of systolic, diastolic, and mean values.

D. CONTRAINDICATIONS

None absolute except for those specific to catheter placement.

E. EQUIPMENT

1. Neonatal physiologic monitor (multiparameter monitoring system).

   a. Minimum configuration should have the capability of displaying systolic, diastolic, and mean pressures.

   b. Should have provision for high and low alarm settings.

2. Mechanical infusion device (infusion pump).

Pressurized IV bag should never be used.

3. Fluid to be infused via the pressure line

4. Appropriate sized catheter and supplies

5. Pressure monitoring kit with integrated disposable transducer and continuous flush device (Fig. 8-5).

    a. Pressure monitoring tubing should not exceed 48 inches from the transducer to the patient connection.

    b. Distal end of the kit should have a stopcock or an arterial extension no longer than 12 inches, that can be used for drawing blood samples.

    c. New advances in pressure monitoring kits (disposable) offer closed-loop systems for sampling.

        (1) The system employs a mechanism for aspirating and holding a fixed amount of blood in the pressure tubing, rather than in a syringe.

        (2) The distal end is equipped with a small chamber with a rubber septum that allows a self-guiding short blunt syringe adapter to penetrate and aspirate blood for the sample.

The initial volume pulled back is sufficient to ensure that the blood drawn into the sample chamber is greater than the catheter/distal tubing volume and is not diluted by the fluid being infused. The absence of stopcocks at the distal end eliminates a possible site for contamination. In addition, the blood pulled back is conserved and the amount of fluid used to flush the sample line is reduced.

F. TECHNIQUE

For catheter placement, see Part V, Vascular Access.

1. Familiarize yourself with the bedside monitor and the pressure zero/calibration procedure.

2. If using discrete components, assemble the pressure monitoring circuit maintaining the sterile integrity.

    a. A basic circuit configuration will consist of a transducer dome, flush device, stopcock, pressure tubing, and an optional arterial extension set (short length of pressure tubing, less than 12 inches in length, inserted between the catheter and the pressure tubing).

    b. If using pressure monitoring kit, ensure that all the luer lock connections are tight and free of any defects.

    c. If possible, avoid the use of IV tubing components in the pressure monitoring circuit.

3. Set up the infusion pump that will be used for the continuous infusion through the flush device. Contininous flush devices limit flow rates to 3 or 30 ml/hr, depending on the model.[10] For neonatal arterial lines the infusion pump supplying the flush device should be set to 1 to 3 ml/h and never exceed the flow rating of the flush device. When pump flow exceeds flush device rating it will cause an occlusion alarm in most IV pumps. A pump flow rate of 1 mm/h is recommended for most arterial lines.

4. For circuit priming, use the solution that will be used for the continuous infusion. Prime the circuit slowly, in order to avoid trapping air bubbles in the flush device inlet. Ensure that the entire circuit and all the ports are filled and bubble free (Fig. 8-6).

5. If using disposable transducers, connect the reusable interface cable to the transducer and to the monitor. Turn the monitor on.

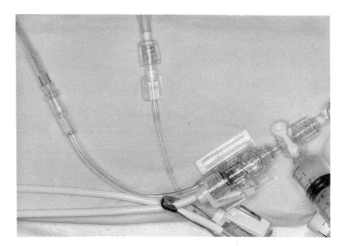

FIG. 8-6
Infusion lines hooked up to continuous infusion port of a disposable transducer. Note fluid-filled syringe is used for system flushing.

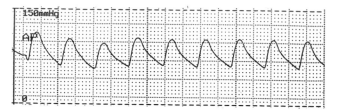

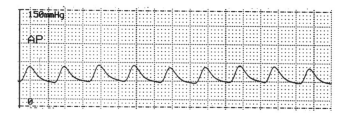

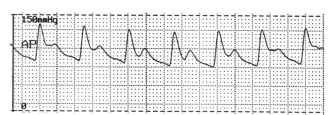

FIG. 8-7
Arterial pressure waveforms: (Top) normal arterial waveform; (middle) dampened arterial waveform; (bottom) arterial waveform with spike caused by catheter whip or inappropriate tubing. (Note that figure demonstrates waveform appearance only, and not actual pressure values.)

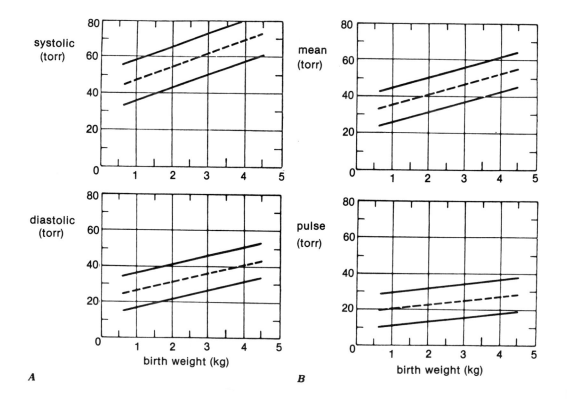

6. Secure the transducer at the patient's reference level, defined as the mid axillary line (heart level). If using transducer holders, level the reference mark on the holder at the patient's reference level.
7. Connect the distal end of the circuit to the patient's catheter, ensuring that the catheter hub is filled with fluid and is bubble free.
8. Start the infusion pump. Pump rate cannot exceed the flow rate of the flush device.
9. Open the stockcock connected to the transducer to air (shut off to the patient, open to atmosphere).
10. Zero/calibrate the monitor, as per manufacturer instructions.
11. Close the stopcock connected to the transducer (open to the patient).
12. Set the monitor pressure waveform scale to one that accommodates the entire pressure wave.
13. Observe the waveform obtained. If the wave appears to be dampened (flattened, poorly defined with slow rise time), check the circuit for air bubbles starting at the distal end. If no air bubbles detected, then gently flush the catheter (Fig. 8-7). (For central venous waveforms see Chap. 26.)
14. Once stable pressure reading is obtained, set the alarm limits. Mean pressure value is optimally used to set alarm limits (Fig. 8-8).
15. Zero the transducer every shift, or every 8 hours.
16. When blood samples are drawn from the line, flushing should be done gently with a syringe using a minimal amount of heparinized saline solution.

G. COMPLICATIONS (TABLE 8-3)

1. Defective transducer
2. Cracked luer lock connections causing leaks, low pressure readings, or blood to back up in the line
3. Air in the line
4. Malfunctioning infusion pump not providing continuous flush; causing the line to clot off
5. Defective reusable transducer interface cable (disposable transducer system)
6. Erroneous readings caused by the transducer not being properly set at the patient's reference level

   Lower readings when the transducer is high; higher readings when the transducer is low.

7. Problems associated with catheters
8. Tip of the catheter lodging against the wall of the vessel (will cause the pressure wave to flatten and the pressure to slowly rise, as a result of the continuous infusion)
9. Transducer not zeroed to atmosphere (static pressure trapped by stopcock valve and a syringe stuck in the port that should be opened to air)

   Will cause lower or negative pressure readings

10. Loss of blood if stopcock is left opened to the patient and air.
11. Fluid overload if a pressurized IV bag is used instead of an infusion pump and the *fast* flush mode is used to clear the line.[10]

FIG. 8-8
Pressures obtained by direct measurement through umbilical artery catheter in healthy newborn infants during first 12 hours of life. Broken lines represent linear regressions; solid lines represent 95% confidence limits. *(A)* Systolic pressure *(top)* and diastolic pressure *(bottom)*. *(B)* Mean aortic pressure *(top)* and pulse pressure (systolic–diastolic pressure amplitude) *(bottom)*. (Versmold HT, Kitterman JA, Phibbs RH et al: Aortic blood pressure during the first 12 hours of life in infants with birth weight 610 to 4220 grams. Pediatrics 67, No. 5:611, May 1981. Copyright © American Academy of Pediatrics, 1981)

TABLE 8-3
Complications and Precautions for Intravascular-Pressure Monitoring

Problem	Cause	Prevention	Treatment
Damped pressure tracing	Catheter tip against vessel wall	Usually unavoidable	Reposition catheter while observing wave form.
	Partial occlusion of tip by clot	Use continuous infusion of 5% dextrose in water or add heparin (1 unit/ml IV fluid)	Aspirate clot with syringe and flush with heparinized saline.
	Clotting in stopcock or transducer, or blood in system	Flush catheter carefully after blood withdrawal and re-establish IV drip; back-flush stopcocks to remove blood. Use continuous flush device.	Flush stopcock and transducer; if no improvement, change components.
Abnormally high or low readings	Change in transducer level	Maintain patient in same position for serial pressure measurements.	Recheck patient and transducer positions.
	Leaks in transducer system	Assemble transducer carefully, ensuring that dome is attached snugly; use Luer-Lok fittings and disposable stopcocks.	Check all fittings, transducer dome, and stopcock connections.
	External vascular compression	Secure catheter firmly without putting tape circumferentially on extremity.	Loosen tape, securing catheter in place.
	Strained transducer	Attention to stopcocks when aspirating or flushing	Replace transducer.
	Loose dome on transducer, producing low blood pressure without leak or change in waveform[9]	Attach transducer dome securely to module.	Vent system and retighten dome.
	High intrathoracic pressure secondary to ventilation; particularly influences central venous pressure	Be aware of problem.	Take pressure readings off ventilation or in expiratory phase.
Damped pressure without improvement after flushing	Air bubbles in transducer or connector tubing	Flush transducer and tubing carefully when setting up system and attaching to catheter; handle system carefully.	Check system; rapid flush; attach syringe to transducer and aspirate bubble.
No pressure available	Transducer not open to catheter, or settings on monitor amplifiers incorrect—still on zero, cal, or off	Follow routine, systematic steps for setting up system and pressure measurements.	Check system—stopcocks, monitor, and amplifier set-up.

References

1. American Academy of Pediatrics Task Force Pressure Control: Report. Pediatrics 59:797, 1977
2. Moss AJ: Indirect methods of blood pressure measurement. Pediatr Clin North Am 25:3, 1978
3. KIRKENDALL WM, FEINLEIB M, FREIS ED, et al: Recommendation for human blood pressure determination by sphygmomanometers: Subcommittee on the American Heart Association postgraduate education committee. Circulation 62:1145A, 1980
4. SADOVE MS, SCHMIDT G, WU H-H, KATZ D: Indirect blood pressure measurement in infants: A comparison of four methods in four limbs. Anesth Analg 52:682, 1973
5. RAMSEY M III: Automatic oscillometric noninvasive blood pressure: Theory and practice. In Meyer-Sabellak W (ed): Blood Pressure Measurements. Steinkopff Verlag Darmstadt, 1990 p 15
6. KIMBLE KJ, DARNALL RA JR, YELDERMAN M, et al: An automated oscillometric technique for estimating mean arterial pressure in critically ill newborns. Anesthesiology 54:423, 1981
7. FRIESEN RH, LICHTOR JL: Indirect measurement of blood pressure in neonates and infants utilizing an automatic noninvasive oscillometric monitor. Anesth Analg 60:742, 1981
8. PARK MK, MENARD SM: Accuracy of blood pressure measurement by the Dinamap monitor in infants and children. Pediatrics 79:907, 1987
9. WEINDLING AM: Blood pressure monitoring in the newborn. Arch Dis Child 64:444, 1989
10. MORRAY J, TODD S: A hazard of continuous flush systems for vascular pressure monitoring in infants. Anesthesiology 38:187, 1983

9 *Continuous Blood-gas Monitoring*

Andrea Lotze
Oswaldo Rivera

Pulse Oximetry

A. PURPOSE

1. Noninvasive arterial oxygen saturation monitoring
2. Pulse rate monitoring
3. Trending of SaO_2 and pulse rate over time

B. BACKGROUND

1. Principles of oxygen transport
   a. Approximately 98% of the oxygen in the blood is bound to hemoglobin.

   The amount of oxygen carried in the blood is directly related to the amount of hemoglobin in the blood as well as to the partial pressure of unbound, dissolved oxygen in the blood ($= PO_2$).[1] The relationship of arterial PO_2, in near-term infants, to percent saturation measured by pulse oximeter is shown in Fig. 9-1.

   b. The relationship between blood PO_2 and the amount of oxygen bound to Hb is graphically presented as an oxygen–hemoglobin affinity curve. Percent oxygen saturation is calculated below (see Fig. 9-2):

   $$\frac{Oxyhemoglobin}{Oxyhemoglobin + Deoxyhemoglobin} \times 100$$

2. Principles of pulse oximetry
   a. Based on the principles of spectrophotometric oximetry and plethysmography[2]
   b. Determines arterial saturation and pulse rate by measuring the absorption of selected wavelengths of light.

   Oxygenated hemoglobin (oxyhemoglobin) and reduced hemoglobin (deoxyhemoglobin) absorb light as known functions of wavelengths. By mea-

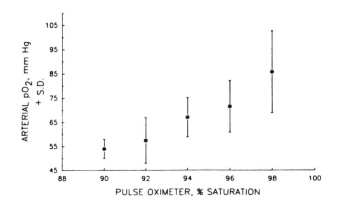

FIG. 9-1
Arterial PO_2 versus pulse oximeter percent (%) saturation in near-term newborn infants in whom pulse saturation was fixed by adjusting F_IO_2 first and then measuring PaO_2. Values are mean ± SD. (From Brockway J, Hay WW Jr: Ability of pulse O_2 saturations to accurately determine blood oxygenation. Clin Res 36:227A, 1988, with permission.)

suring the absorption levels at different wave-lengths of light, the relative percentage of these two constituents and SaO_2 is calculated.

c. Sensor is composed of two light emitting diodes (LEDs) as light sources and one photodetector as a light receiver. The photodetector is an electronic device that produces a current proportional to the incident light intensity.[3]

(1) One LED emits red light with an approximate wavelength of 660 nm.

Red light is absorbed selectively by deoxyhemoglobin.

(2) The other LED emits infrared light with an approximate wavelength of 925 nm.

Infrared light is absorbed selectively by oxyhemoglobin.

d. Absorption of the light wavelengths takes place when transmitted through tissue and blood (Fig. 9-3).

(1) The photodetector measures the level of light that passes through without being absorbed.

(2) During the absence of pulse (diastole) the detector establishes baseline levels for the absorption of tissue and nonpulsatile blood.

(3) With each heart beat, a pulse of oxygenated blood flows to the sensor site.

(4) Absorption during systole of both the red and infrared light is measured to determine the percentage of oxyhemoglobin.

(5) Because the absorption change measurements are made during a pulse (systole), these pulses are counted and displayed as heart rate.

C. INDICATIONS

1. To monitor oxygenation in infants suffering from conditions associated with

a. Hypoxia

b. Apnea/hypoventilation

c. Cardiorespiratory disease

d. Bronchopulmonary dysplasia

Pulse oximetry is the optimal mode of monitoring for larger infants with bronchopulmonary dysplasia. Whereas $P_{tc}O_2$ monitors may under-

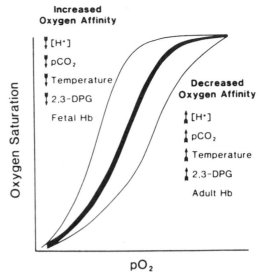

FIG. 9-2
Factors affecting hemoglobin–oxygen affinity. 2,3-DPG = 2,3-diphosphoglycerate. (From Hay WW Jr: Physiology of oxygenation and its relation to pulse oximetry in neonates. J Perinatol 7:309, 1987, with permission.)

FIG. 9-3
Tissue composite showing dynamic as well as static components affecting light absorption. (From Wukitch MW, Petterson MT, Tobler DR et al: Pulse Oximetry: Analysis of theory, technology and practice. J Clin Monit 4:290, 1988, with permission.)

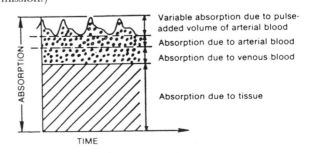

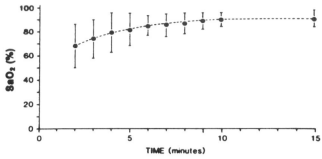

FIG. 9-4

Mean arterial oxygen saturation (SaO_2) values measured by pulse oximetry from the time of cord-clamping. Values are mean ± SD. (From House JT, Schultetus RR, Gravenstein N: Continuous neonatal evaluation in the delivery room by pulse oximetry. J Clin Monit 3:96, 1987, with permission.)

estimate PaO_2 in this population, oximetry has been found to be reasonably accurate for these infants.[4]

The pulse oximeter requires no patient preparation or calibration time, has a rapid response time, and is readily adaptable to different patient populations.[5]

2. To monitor response to therapy
   a. Resuscitation[6]

Pulse oximetry is a significant adjunct to monitoring in the delivery room as well. With the use of pulse oximetry, SaO_2 values can be obtained within 1 minute after birth[7-9] (Fig. 9-4).

   b. Monitoring effectiveness of mask ventilation[10] or during placement of an endotracheal tube
3. Monitoring side-effects of other therapy
   a. Suctioning
   b. Position for laryngoscopy[6]
4. For low birth weight infants <1000 grams[11,12]

It is optimal to use pulse oximetry for oxygen monitoring in the very low birth weight infant because of its noninvasiveness. Pulse oximetry can be used reliably in very low birth weight infants with acute as well as chronic lung disease.[11]

5. Pulse oximetry also offers an advantage for precise F_1O_2 control during neonatal anesthesia due to the short response time to changes in SaO_2.[13]

D. LIMITATIONS

1. Decreased accuracy when arterial saturation is less than 65%.

Pulse oximetry will overestimate SaO_2 when at this level; therefore, blood gas confirmation is imperative.[14-16]

2. Not a sensitive indicator for hyperoxemia[1]

Pulse oximeter accuracy does not allow for precise estimation of PO_2 at saturations above 90%. Small changes in O_2 saturation (1–2%) may be associated with large PO_2 changes (6–12 mm Hg).[1]

3. Because pulse oximeters rely on pulsatile fluctuations in transmitted light intensity to estimate SaO_2, they are all adversely affected by movement.[3,17-19]

In some cases the pulse oximeter may calculate an SaO_2 value for signals caused by movement or it may reject the signal and not update the display.

Usually, the HR output from the oximeter will reflect the detection of nonarterial pulsations, either indicating "0" saturation or "low quality signal."[3]

4. Significant levels of carboxyhemoglobin or methemoglobin can yield erroneous readings (carboxyhemoglobin absorbs light in the 660 nm wavelength).[18] However, carboxyhemoglobin levels of less than 3% will not affect the accuracy of the instrument.

5. SaO_2 may be overestimated in darkly pigmented infants.

Some oximeters will give a message such as "insufficient light detected" if a valid signal is not obtained.[18,19]

6. Erroneous reading in the presence of high fetal hemoglobin (HbF)[18]

A smaller impact on accuracy is noted when HbF levels are less than 50%.[20-22]

With a predominance of fetal Hb, SaO_2s of >92% may be associated with hyperoxemia.[22] However, while saturations may appear adequate, PO_2 may be low enough to produce increased pulmonary vascular resistance (SaO_2/PO_2 curve shift to the left).

Because infants with chronic lung disease and prolonged oxygen dependence are older and have less HbF, SaO_2 readings obtained from these patients may be more accurate than those obtained from neonates with acute respiratory disorders.[23]

The same situation exists in infants who have undergone exchange transfusion due to decreased levels of fetal Hgb.[24]

7. Light sources that can affect performance include surgical lights, xenon lights, bilirubin lamps, fluorescent lights, infrared heating lamps, and direct sunlight.

Although jaundice does not account for variability in pulse oximeter accuracy,[25] phototherapy can interfere with accurate monitoring. Therefore, appropriate precautions should be taken, such as covering the probe with a relatively opaque material.[1]

8. Do not correlate SaO_2 values with laboratory hemoximeters.[18]

Most laboratory oximeters measure fractional oxygen saturation (all hemoglobin including dysfunctional hemoglobin) as opposed to functional oxygen saturation (oxyhemoglobin and deoxyhemoglobin excluding all dysfunctional hemoglobin).

Use of normal adult values for hemoglobin, 2-3-DPG, and, in some cases, PCO_2 can lead to errors in the algorithm to calculate SaO_2 with some blood gas analysis instruments.[18]

9. Although pulse oximeters can detect hyperoxemia, it is important that type-specific alarm limits are set.[26]

In order to avoid hyperoxemia, a minimal sensitivity of at least 95% is required.

10. In summary, it is optimal to make some correlation between SaO_2 and PO_2 throughout a reasonable range of SaO_2 (lower = 85–88%, higher = 95–97%) before relying completely on SaO_2 for oxygen and/or respirator management.[24]

E. EQUIPMENT

1. The manufacturer-specific sensor and monitor (see Fig. 9-5 for example) with
   a. Display of SaO_2 and pulse rate and a pulse indicator.
   b. Adjustable alarm limits for SaO_2 as well as pulse rate.
   c. Battery powered operation.
2. Neonatal sensor, either disposable or reusable
   a. Disposable sensors have become the standard from the standpoint of infection as well as quality control.
   b. Disposable neonatal sensors are available in different sizes, depending on the site to be used.

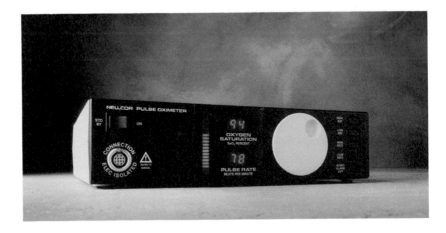

FIG. 9-5
Pulse oximeter. Vertical column indicates pulse. (Courtesy of Nellcor.)

F. PRECAUTIONS

1. Use only with detectable pulse.

   Cardiopulmonary bypass with nonpulsating flow, inflated blood pressure cuff proximal to the sensor, tense peripheral edema, hypothermia, low perfusion state secondary to shock or severe hypovolemia, and significant peripheral vasoconstriction may interfere with obtaining accurate readings.[5]

2. Assess the sensor site every 8 hours to be certain that the adherent bandage is not constricting the site, and that the skin is intact.[28]

3. Whenever possible, SaO_2 sensor should not be on the same extremity as the blood pressure cuff.

   When the cuff is inflated, the SaO_2 sensor will not detect a pulse, will not update SaO_2 values, and will alarm. Use of ace bandages on the extremities to increase central venous return may also interfere with the function of the sensor.

G. TECHNIQUE

1. Familiarize yourself with the system before proceeding.

2. Select an appropriate sensor and apply it to the patient.
   a. Ear lobe, finger, toe, the lateral side of the foot or across the palm of the hand in a position matching that of peripheral arterial line, if present, (avoids discrepancies caused by intracardiac or ductal shunts when trying to correlate SaO_2 with arterial PO_2).
   b. For neonates 500 g to 3 kg use the palm or anterior part of a foot (Fig. 9-6).[1]
   c. For infants >3 kg use palm, thumb, great toe, or index finger.[1]
   d. Align the LEDs (light source) and the detector so they are directly opposite each other.
   e. Reusable sensors should be applied with nonadhesive elastic wrap.
   f. Tighten sensor snugly to the skin but not so as to impede circulation.

   The probe should then be left in place for several seconds until extremity movement stops and the signal is stable.

   g. Secure the sensor to the site to prevent tugging or movement of the sensor independent of the body part.
   h. Cover the sensor to reduce the effect of intense light levels, direct sunlight, or phototherapy.

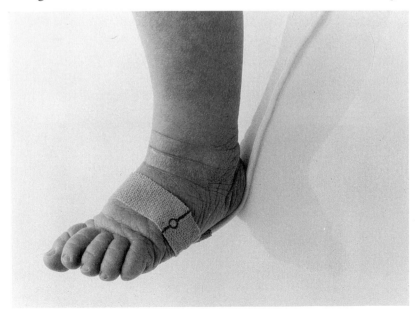

FIG. 9-6
Disposable sensor applied to foot.

3. Attach the sensor to the system interconnecting cable and turn the monitor on.
4. Calibration of the system is not required (internal autocalibration).
5. After a short interval, if all connections are correct the monitor will display the pulse detected by the sensor. If the pulse level is adequate, it will display SaO_2 and pulse rate. If the pulse indicator is not synchronous with the patient's pulse rate, reposition the probe. If after repositioning the sensor, the pulse detector is still not indicating properly, change the sensor site.
6. Once reliable operation is achieved set the high and low alarm limits.
   a. Although pulse oximeters can detect hyperoxemia, it is important that type-specific alarm limits are set and a low specificity is accepted.[26] Type-specific alarm limits should be guided by normative values for SaO_2 depending upon postnatal age (Fig. 9-7).
   b. The optimal alarm limit, defined as having a sensitivity of 95% or more, associated with maximal specificity, will differ depending on which particular monitor is used.

   In general, low limit SaO_2s are defined as 87 to 89%; higher limit SaO_2s are defined as 94 to 95%.

   c. Default (starting point) alarm limits for a newborn[27]:
   High limit = 94 to 95%
   Low limit = 87 to 90%
   Note that SaO_2 is a more sensitive indicator of hypoxemia and decreased tissue oxygenation than is PaO_2. Lower alarm limits should be individualized to alert the user when the oxygenation requirements of the given patient are not satisfied.

H. COMPLICATIONS

1. Management based on erroneous readings caused by a misapplied sensor or conditions affecting instrument performance.
2. Burn due to electrical short[28a]

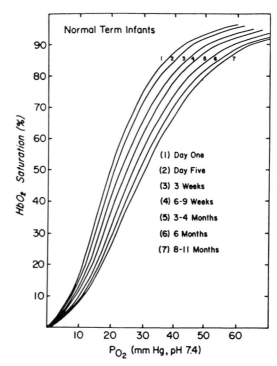

FIG. 9-7
The oxygen dissociation curve at various postnatal ages. (From Oski FA, Delivoria-Papadopoulos M, The red cell 2, 3-diphophoglycerate, and tissue oxygen release. J Pediatr 77:941, 1970.)

Transcutaneous Blood-gas Monitoring

A. PURPOSE

1. Noninvasive blood gas monitoring of $P_{tc}O_2$ and $P_{tc}CO_2$
2. Trending of PO_2 and PCO_2 over time

B. BACKGROUND

1. Accomplished by two electrodes contained in a heated block that maintains the electrodes and the skin directly beneath it at a constant temperature[29] (Fig. 9-8).
   a. Arterialized capillary oxygen levels are more accurately measured by heating the skin to establish hyperemia directly beneath the sensor.

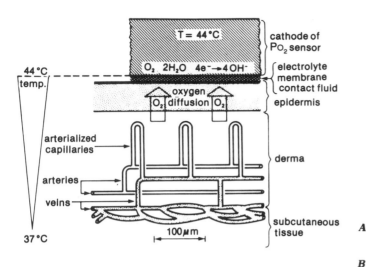

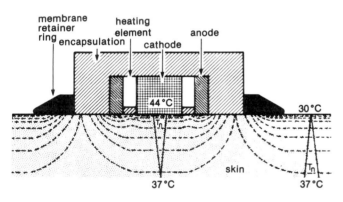

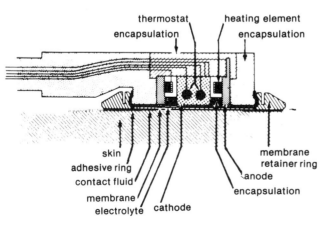

A

B

C

b. The electrodes are covered with an electrolyte solution and sealed with a semipermeable plastic membrane.
2. A modified Clark electrode is used to measure oxygen.
   a. Produces an electrical current proportional to PO_2
   b. Measured current is converted to PO_2 then corrected for temperature.
3. A Severinghaus electrode is used to measure CO_2.
   a. A pH-sensitive glass electrode
   b. CO_2 diffuses from the skin surface through the membrane. The CO_2 changes the pH of the electrolyte solution bathing the electrode.
   c. The measured pH is converted to PCO_2 then corrected for temperature

   Conversion of electric current and pH to PO_2 and PCO_2 respectively is based on conversion equations adjusted by a two-point calibration. This is part of the setup and calibration process.

C. INDICATIONS

1. To approximate arterial PaO_2 and $PaCO_2$ for respiratory management
   a. To monitor impact of therapeutic ventilatory maneuvers,[30-34] particularly in infants with a combined oxygenation/ventilation problem
   b. For stabilization and monitoring during transport[35,36]
2. To reduce the frequency of arterial blood-gas analysis[37]
3. To determine by a noninvasive and continuous method the regional arterial oxygen tension[38-40]
4. To infer regional arterial blood flow[40-43]

D. CONTRAINDICATIONS

1. Skin disorders (e.g., epidermolysis bullosum, staphlococcal scalded skin syndrome)

FIG. 9-8
(*A*) Principle of cutaneous PO_2 measurement by heated oxygen sensor. (*B*) Temperature profile cutaneous tissue. (*C*) Cross section of cutaneous oxygen sensor. (Courtesy of Kontron Medical Instruments.)

FIG. 9-9
Transcutaneous PO_2/PCO_2 monitor. (Courtesy of Kontron.)

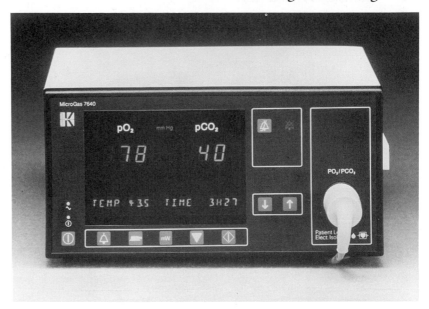

2. Relative contraindications
   a. The very low birth weight infant[44]
   b. Severe acidosis
   c. Significant anemia
   d. Decreased peripheral perfusion
   e. $P_{tc}O_2$ may underestimate PaO_2[45]

E. EQUIPMENT—SPECIFICATIONS

1. Transcutaneous monitor components
   a. Dual electrode
   b. Electrode cleaning kit
   c. Electrolyte and membrane kit
   d. Contact solution
   e. Double-sided adhesive rings
   f. Calibration gas cylinders with delivery apparatus
2. Digital display shows values for PO_2, PCO_2, and site or sensor temperature (Fig. 9-9).
3. Monitor with controls for both high and low alarm limits as well as for electrode temperature. The monitor may also have a site placement timer that will alarm as an indication to change the site of the electrode.

F. PRECAUTIONS

1. Be aware that
   a. Equilibration requires approximately 20 minutes once the electrode is placed, with the response time for $P_{tc}O_2$ being much faster than that for $P_{tc}CO_2$. Therefore, management changes based on transcutaneous values should be guided by values that have been consistent for at least 5 minutes.
   b. Periodic correlation with PO_2 from appropriate arterial sites is recommended.[46]
   c. $P_{tc}O_2$ may underestimate PaO_2 in the infant with hyperoxemia ($PaO_2 > 100$ mmHg) with reliability of $P_{tc}O_2$ measurement decreasing as PaO_2 increases.[47–51]
   d. $P_{tc}O_2$ may underestimate PaO_2 in older infants with bronchopulmonary dysplasia.[52,53]
   e. Transcutaneous blood gas measurements are affected by the state of the infant.

   Values during feeding or active sleep can be lower.[54]

   f. Pressure on the sensor (e.g., infant lying on sensor) may restrict blood supply, resulting in falsely low $P_{tc}O_2$ values.
   g. Manufacturers' parts are not interchangeable. Only supplies of the same brand and designated for the monitor should be used.
2. Change electrode location every 4 hours (maximum) to avoid burns.
3. Do not allow electrode temperature to exceed 44°C.

4. $P_{tc}O_2$ may underestimate PaO_2 in the presence of
   a. Severe acidosis
   b. Significant anemia
   c. Decreased peripheral perfusion

G. TECHNIQUE

1. Familiarize yourself with the system before proceeding.
2. Perform routine electrode maintenance, if there is any question as to the status of the electrode.
   a. Remove the membrane, rinse the electrode with deionized water, and dry with a soft lint-free tissue or gauze.
   b. Clean the electrode using the solution provided in the cleaning kit; abrasive compounds or materials should never be used (will permanently damage the electrode).
   c. Rinse the electrode with deionized water and dry with lint-free tissue.
   d. Apply the electrolyte solution.
   e. Place a new membrane on the electrode. Avoid finger contact and always handle the membrane inside its protective package or with plastic tweezers.

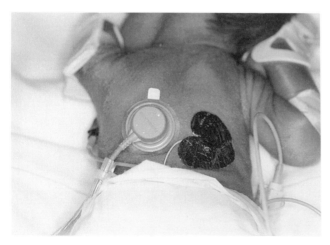

FIG. 9-10
Cutaneous PO_2/PCO_2 sensor applied to the back.

3. Perform two-point gas calibration using the device specific apparatus, as per manufacturer's instruction.
4. Use an alcohol pad to clean and degrease the skin site where the sensor is to be placed.
5. Apply double-sided adhesive ring to the sensor.
6. Apply one drop of contact solution to the skin site.
7. Peel protective backing from adhesive ring, place sensor on the skin over the contact solution, and press the sensor to the skin.
   a. For best results, place the sensor on a location with good blood flow.
      (1) Appropriate sites include the lateral abdomen, anterior or lateral chest, volar forearm, inner upper arm, inner thigh, or posterior chest (Fig. 9-10).[55]
      (2) Although large differences between pre- and postductal PaO_2s are uncommon in premature infants with hyaline membrane disease, preductal location of the electrode is optimal for prevention of hyperoxemia.[56]
   b. Choose site devoid of hair.
   c. Avoid bony prominences.
   d. Avoid areas with large surface blood vessels (Fig. 9-10).
8. Secure the sensor cable to prevent tugging of the electrode when the cable is manipulated.
9. Turn the site/sensor temperature control to 44°C.
10. Allow 15 to 20 minutes for site equilibration before taking readings.
11. Note the time at which the sensor was placed on the skin, so that the site can be changed after a 4-hour period (maximum site time). When changing the sensor site
    a. use an alcohol pad to help loosen the adhesive and peel gently from the skin.
    b. Inspect the skin site for signs of sensitivity to heat or to the adhesive. In the event of skin irritation, either lower the sensor temperature or change the site more frequently; mild erythema after sensor removal is typical.
    c. Peel adhesive ring off the sensor.
    d. Flush the membrane surface with deionized water.
    e. Gently blot excess water and dry the sensor.

f. Recalibrate if instructed to do so by the manufacturer's guidelines.

Most of the systems recommend recalibration every 4 to 8 hours.

12. Remember that response time for gas measurements is slow and values will not always immediately reflect physiologic changes.

   a. Average 90% response time for O_2 is 15 to 20 seconds.

   b. Average 90% response time for CO_2 is 60 to 90 seconds.

H. COMPLICATIONS

1. Skin blisters or burns[44,57,58]

2. Management based on erroneous readings if the unit was not calibrated properly or site precautions not adhered to (Table 9-1).

TABLE 9-1
Poor Correlation of $P_{tc}O_2$ and PaO_2

	Technical		Clinical
Problem	*Solution*		*Clinical*
$P_{tc}O_2 < PaO_2$			
1. Improper calibration	1. Recalibrate		1. Presence of shock
2. Insufficient warm-up period after electrode application	2. Allow longer warm-up period		2. Use with high dose tolazoline,* Isuprel, dopamine
3. Insufficient heating temperature	3. Increase heating temperature		3. Obstructive heart disease with hypoperfusion
			4. Edema
			5. Severe hypothermia
$P_{tc}O_2 > PaO_2$			
1. Improper calibration	1. Recalibrate		1. Right to left ductal shunt with preductal electrode and postductal arterial sample
2. $P_{tc}O_2$ reading taken immediately after electrode application	2. Allow longer warm-up period		2. General anesthesia†
3. Air bubble beneath membrane or leak to atmosphere	3. Reapply electrode		
4. Excessive heating temperature	4. Attempt calibration at lower temperature		

*In the presence of tolazoline, $P_{tc}O_2$ measurements appear to be accurate at lower doses (1–2 mg/kg/hr), becoming increasingly inaccurate as dosage increases.[43]

†Effect depends on concentration and type of membrane.

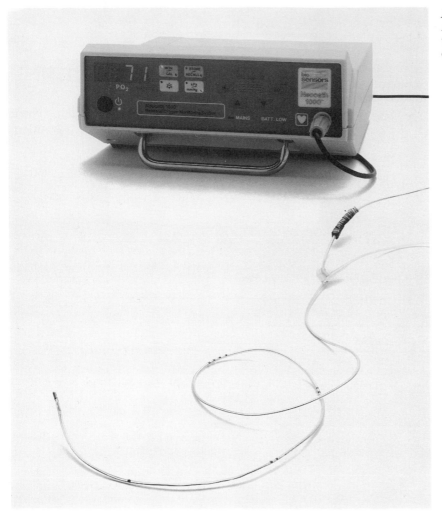

Continuous Umbilical Artery PO_2 Monitoring[59,60]

A. PURPOSE

1. Continuous arterial PO_2 monitoring from the umbilical artery (Fig. 9-11)

   Continuous PaO_2 monitoring through the umbilical artery offers a means for determining precise PaO_2 data on a continuous basis.

2. Trending of PaO_2 over time

B. BACKGROUND

1. Dual purpose biluminal catheter
   a. A miniature polarographic bipolar oxygen electrode is incorporated into the tip of a bilumen umbilical catheter (Fig. 9-12).
   b. The small lumen contains the wires for the electrode.
   c. The larger lumen can be used for blood sampling, infusion, blood pressure monitoring, and sampling for instrument calibration.

2. The electrode is covered by a gas-permeable membrane, under which is a layer of dried electrolyte. The probe is packed dry, and activated before use. Water vapor from the activating (hydrating) solution diffuses through the membrane to form a thin layer of liquid electrolyte on the surface of the electrode.
3. While in the artery, the electrode will produce an electrical current proportional to the PO_2 in the blood.
4. The device is calibrated to the PO_2 value obtained from a blood sample drawn from the catheter.

C. CONTRAINDICATIONS

1. Previous history of or evidence of compromise to the vascular supply of the lower extremity or the buttock area.
2. History of previous complications related to an umbilical arterial line.
3. Peritonitis
4. Necrotizing enterocolitis
5. Omphalitis
6. Omphalocele

D. EQUIPMENT

1. A manufacturer-specific, single-use sterile catheter
   a. Labelled with a serial and lot number
   b. Available in 4 and 5 Fr
2. Monitor
   a. Battery powered
   b. AC powered with backup battery
   c. Digital or analog display
   d. High and low alarm limits

E. PRECAUTIONS

See also umbilical artery catheterization, chap. 24.

1. Because this specialized catheter is stiffer and has a wider outer diameter than other UACs, there is the theoretical possibility of a higher rate of failure to insert and a higher risk of vascular spasm with interference to peripheral blood flow.
2. Failure to insert this catheter does not imply that

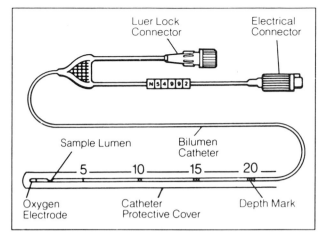

FIG. 9-12
Umbilical artery catheter for continuous measurement of arterial PO_2. (Courtesy of Shiley Incorporated.)

insertion of other arterial catheters will be unsuccessful.
3. The electrode may fail to activate or lose activation.
4. The catheter should be removed slowly to ensure that physiologic vasospasm occurs with removal.

F. TECHNIQUE

1. Use sterile procedure.
2. Hydrate the catheter according to the manufacturer's instructions.
3. The 4 Fr catheter is recommended for infants weighing less than 1500 g.
4. The technique for placement/insertion is the same as that used for the placement of conventional umbilical artery catheters. Either a high or low umbilical artery placement can be used. (See Chap. 24.)
5. Verify catheter position by x-ray.
6. Draw blood sample for calibration.
7. Calibrate the monitor according to manufacturer's instructions.

G. COMPLICATIONS

Same as for umbilical artery catheterization; see Chap. 24.

References

1. HAY WW: Physiology of oxygenation and its relation to pulse oximetry in neonates. J Perinatol 7:309, 1987
2. DZIEDZIC K, VIDYASAGAR D: Pulse oximetry in neonatal intensive care. Clin Perinatol 16:177, 1989
3. BARRINGTON KJ, FINER NN, RYAN CA: Evaluation of pulse oximetry as a continuous monitoring technique in the neonatal intensive care unit. Crit Care Med 16:1147, 1988
4. SOLIMANO AJ, SMYTH JA, MANN TK, et al: Pulse oximetry advantages in infants with bronchopulmonary dysplasia. Pediatrics 78:844, 1986
5. BOWES WA, CORKE BC, HULKA J: Pulse oximetry: A review of the theory, accuracy and clinical applications. Obstet Gynecol 74:541, 1989
6. SENDAK MJ, HARRIS AP, DONHAM RT: Use of pulse oximetry to assess arterial oxygen saturation during newborn resuscitation. Crit Care Med 14:739, 1986
7. HOUSE JT, SCHULTETUS RR, GRAVERSTEIN N: Continuous neonatal evaluation in the delivery room by pulse oximetry. J Clin Monit 96, 1987
8. PORTER KB: Evaluation of arterial oxygen saturation of the newborn in the labor and delivery suite. J Perinatol 7:337, 1987
9. DECKARDT R, SCHNEIDER K-T, GRAEFF H: Monitoring arterial oxygen saturation in the neonate. J Perinat Med 15:357, 1987
10. MAXWELL LG, HARRIS AP, SENDAK MJ, DONHAM RT: Monitoring the resuscitation of preterm infants in the delivery room using pulse oximetry. Clin Peds 26:18, 1987
11. RAMANATHAN R, DURAND M, LARRAZABAL C: Pulse oximetry in very low birth weight infants with acute and chronic lung disease. Pediatrics 79:612, 1987
12. DECKARDT R, STEWART DJ: Noninvasive arterial hemoglobin oxygen saturation versus transcutaneous oxygen tension monitoring in the preterm infant. Crit Care Med 12:935, 1984
13. MIYASAKA K, KATAYAMA M, KUSAKAWA I, et al: Use of pulse oximetry in neonatal anesthesia. J Perinatol 7:343, 1987
14. FANCONI S: Reliability of pulse oximetry in hypoxic infants. J Pediatr 112:424, 1988
15. LEWALLEN PK, MAMME MC, COLEMAN JM, BOROS SJ: Neonatal transcutaneous oxygen saturation monitoring. J Perinatol 7:8, 1987
16. PRAUD JP, CAROFILIS A, BRIDEY F, et al: Accuracy of two wavelength pulse oximetry in neonates and infants. Pediatric Pulmonol 6:180, 1989
17. SOUTHALL DP, BIGNALL S, STEBBENS VA, et al: Pulse oximeter and transcutaneous arterial oxygen measurements in neonatal and pediatric intensive care. Arch Dis Child 62:882, 1987
18. HAY WW: The uses, benefits and limitations of pulse oximetry in neonatal medicine: Consensus on key issues. J Perinatol 7:347, 1987
19. EMERY JR: Skin pigmentation as an influence on the accuracy of pulse oximetry. J Perinatol 7:329, 1987
20. DURAND M, RAMANATHAN R: Pulse oximetry for continuous oxygen monitoring in sick newborn infants. J Pediatr 109:1052, 1986
21. JENNIS MS, PEABODY JL: Pulse oximetry: An alternative method for the assessment of oxygenation in newborn infants. Pediatrics 79:524, 1987
22. WASUNNA A, WHITELAW GL: Pulse oximetry in preterm infants. Arch Dis Child 62:957, 1987
23. WALSH MC, NOBLE LM, CARLO WA, MARTIN RJ: Relationship of pulse oximetry to arterial oxygen tension in infants. Crit Care Med 15:1102, 1987
24. REYNOLDS GJ: Guidelines for the use of pulse oximetry in the noninvasive estimation of oxygen saturation in oxygen-dependent newborn infants. Aust Paediatr J 24:346, 1988
25. ANDERSON JV: The accuracy of pulse oximetry in neonates: Effects of fetal hemoglobin and bilirubin. J Perinatol 7:323, 1987
26. BUCHER H-U, FANCONI S, BAECKERT P, DUC G: Hyperoxemia in newborn infants: Detection by pulse oximetry. Pediatrics 84:226, 1989
27. HAY WW, BROCKWAY J, EYZAGUIRRE M: Neonatal pulse oximetry: Accuracy and reliability. Pediatrics 83:717, 1989
28. KOPOTIC RJ, MANNINO FL, COLLEY CD, HORNING N: Display variability, false alarms, probe cautions, and recorder use in neonatal pulse oximetry. J Perinatol 7:340, 1987
28a. SOBEL DB: Burning of a neonate due to a pulse oximeter: Arterial saturation monitoring. Pediatrics 89:154, 1992
29. GHAT R, DIAZ-BLANCO J, CHAUDHRY U, VIDYASAGAR D: Recent Instrumentation. Ped Clin North Am 33:503, 1986
30. HUCH R, HUCH A, ALBANI M, GABRIEL M: Transcutaneous PO_2 monitoring in routine management of infants and children with cardiorespiratory problems. Pediatrics 57:681, 1976
31. OKKEN A, RUBIN IL, MARTIN RJ: Intermittent bag ventilation of preterm infants on continuous positive airway pressure: The effect on transcutaneous PCO_2. J Pediatr 93:279, 1978
32. HANSEN TH, TOOLEY WH: Skin surface carbon dioxide tension in sick infants. Pediatrics 64:942, 1979
33. LAPTOOK A, OH W: Transcutaneous carbon dioxide monitoring in the newborn period. Crit Care Med 9:759, 1981
34. MONACO F, MCQUITTY J: Transcutaneous measurement of carbon dioxide partial pressure in sick neonates. Crit Care Med 9:756, 1981
35. CLARKE TA, ZMORA E, CHEN J-H, et al: Transcutaneous

oxygen monitoring during neonatal transport. Pediatrics 65:884, 1980

36. MILLER C, CLYMAN RI, ROTH RS, et al: Control of oxygenation during transport of sick neonates. Pediatrics 66:117, 1980

37. BEACHY P, WHITFIELD J: The effect of transcutaneous PO₂ monitoring on the frequency of arterial blood gas analysis in the newborn with respiratory distress. Crit Care Med 9:584, 1981

38. SLAVIN RE, COHEN A, EPSTEIN MF, ROOP E: Two-site non-invasive oxygen monitoring in a case of persistent fetal circulation. Respiratory Care 25:358, 1980

39. TATEISHI K, YAMANOUCHI I: Noninvasive transcutaneous oxygen pressure diagnosis of reversed ductal shunts in cyanotic heart disease. Pediatrics 66:22, 1980

40. VERSMOLD HT, LINDERKAMP O, HOLZMAN M, et al: Limits of TcpO₂ monitoring in sick neonates: Relation to blood pressure, blood volume, peripheral blood flow, and acid base status. Acta Anaesthesiol Scand 68:88, 1978

41. BERAN A, TOLLE C, HUXTABLE R: Cutaneous blood flow and its relationship to transcutaneous O₂/CO₂ measurements. Crit Care Med 9:736, 1981

42. ROWE MI, WEINBERG G: Transcutaneous oxygen monitoring in shock and resuscitation. J Pediatr Surg 14:773, 1979

43. PEABODY JL: Transcutaneous oxygen measurement to evaluate drug effects. Clin Perinatol 6:109, 1979

44. AVERY GB, BANCALARI EH, ENGLER A, et al: Task force on transcutaneous oxygen monitors: Report of consensus meeting December 5 to 6, 1986. Pediatrics 83:122, 1989

45. PEABODY JL: Historical perspective of noninvasive monitoring. J Perinatol 7:306, 1987

46. FANCONI S, SIGRIST H: Transcutaneous carbon dioxide and oxygen tension in newborn infants: Reliability of a combined monitor of oxygen tension and carbon dioxide tension. J Clin Monitoring 4:103, 1988

47. YIP WCL, HO TF, TAY JSH, WONG HB: The application of transcutaneous oxygen monitoring in paediatric intensive care: A critical appraisal of reliability and safety. J Singapore Paediatr Soc 25:33, 1983

48. FANCONI S, DOHERTY P, EDMONDS JF, et al: Pulse oximetry in pediatric intensive care: Comparison with measured saturations and transcutaneous oxygen tension. J Pediatr 107:362, 1985

49. BEACHY P, WHITFIELD JM: The effect of transcutaneous PO₂ monitoring on the frequency of arterial blood gas analysis in the newborn with respiratory distress. Crit Care Med 9:584, 1981

50. KRAUS AN, WALDMAN S, FRAYER W, AULD PA: Noninvasive estimation of arterial oxygenation in newborn infants. J Pediatr 93:275, 1978

51. ROOTH G, HUCH A, HUCH R: Transcutaneous oxygen monitors are reliable indicators of arterial oxygen tension (if used correctly). Pediatrics 79:283, 1987

52. ROME ES, STORK EK, CARLO WA, MARTIN RJ: Limitations of transcutaneous PO₂ and PO₂ measurements in infants with BPD. Pediatrics 74:217, 1984

53. SOLIMANO AJ, SMYTH JA, MANN TK, et al: Pulse oximetry advantages in infants with bronchopulmonary dysplasia. Pediatrics 78:844, 1986

54. MOK JYQ, McLAUGHLIN FJ, PINTAR M, et al: Transcutaneous monitoring of oxygenation: What is normal? J Pediatr 108:365, 1986

55. PALMISANO BW, SEVERINGHAUS JW: Transcutaneous PCO₂ and PO₂: A multicenter study of accuracy. J Clin Monitoring 6:189, 1990

56. PEARLMAN SA, MAISELS MJ: Preductal and postductal transcutaneous oxygen tension measurements in premature newborns with hyaline membrane disease. Pediatrics 83:98, 1989

57. GOLDEN SM: Skin craters—A complication of transcutaneous oxygen monitoring. Pediatrics 67:514, 1981

58. WIMBERLEY PD, FREDERIKSEN PS, WITT-HANSEN PS, et al: Evaluation of a transcutaneous oxygen and carbon dioxide monitor in a neonatal intensive care department. Acta Paediatr Scand 74:352, 1985

59. FINK SE: Continuous PaO₂ monitoring through the umbilical artery. Neonatal Intensive Care 3:16, 1990

60. PHILLIPS BL, QUITTY J, DURAND DJ: Blood gases: Technical aspects and interpretation. In Goldsmith JP, Karotkin EH, Barber S (eds): Assisted Ventilation of the Neonate (2nd Ed.). Philadelphia, WB Saunders, 1988, p 213

10 Pulmonary Function Monitoring

Andrea Lotze
Robert P. Howard

A. PURPOSE

1. Quantitative determination of pulmonary mechanics including lung compliance and tidal volumes
2. Qualitative evaluation of volume–pressure and flow–volume loops

B. INDICATIONS

1. To assist in ventilatory management[1]
2. To follow sequential changes in pulmonary mechanics[2]
3. To predict successful weaning from the ventilator or ECMO[3]
4. To monitor the effects of therapeutic interventions: exogenous surfactant, bronchodilators, steroids, diuretics[4–8]
5. To determine optimal continuous positive airway pressure (CPAP)[9]

C. BACKGROUND

1. Lung compliance (C_L) is the change in lung volume divided by the corresponding change in transpulmonary pressure.
   a. Change in lung volume
      (1) Equals all or part of tidal volume depending on the measurement technique
      (2) Is measured with a pneumotachograph (pneumotach) system or tidal volume monitor
   b. Change in transpulmonary pressure
      (1) Equals alveolar pressure minus pleural pressure
      (2) When airflow is zero, the pressure at the mouth, or upper airway pressure (P_{AW}) is equal to alveolar pressure.
      (3) Pleural pressure is measured with an esophageal balloon positioned just above the diaphragm.

   c. The unit of measure is ml/cm H_2O, or normalized to weight, ml/cm H_2O/kg.
   d. The normal range in the term neonate is 1.0 to 3.0 ml/cm H_2O/Kg.[1]
2. Respiratory system compliance (C_{RS}), or total compliance, has the following relationship to C_L and chest wall compliance (C_{CW}):

$$\frac{1}{C_{RS}} = \frac{1}{C_L} + \frac{1}{C_{CW}}$$

   C_{CW} is the change in thoracic volume divided by the change in pleural pressure, and C_{RS} equals the change in lung volume divided by the change in alveolar pressure.[10]
3. Compliance is measured either dynamically or statically.
   a. Dynamic compliance is described by a volume–pressure curve (Fig. 10-1).
      (1) The measurement is made by connecting the zero flow points (end inspiration and end expiration) with a straight line.
      (2) The slope of this line is the dynamic compliance.[10]
      (3) An esophageal balloon is required for measurement of pleural pressure during dynamic compliance measurements in a spontaneously breathing patient.
      (4) When the infant is being mechanically ventilated, the C_{RS} provides a good approximation of dynamic C_L, eliminating the need for an esophageal balloon when analyzing mechanical breaths only.[11]

   In neonates, the chest wall compliance contributes very little (less than 20%) to the compliance of the respiratory system.[8]

   b. For static compliance measurements, alveolar pressure is measured at the mouth for zero flow

FIG. 10-1

Normal dynamic volume–pressure curve is on the left and flow–volume loop is on the right. The diagonal line inside the volume–pressure loop connects the points of zero flow. The slope of this diagonal line is the dynamic compliance. (Note: These are actual recordings from a patient.)

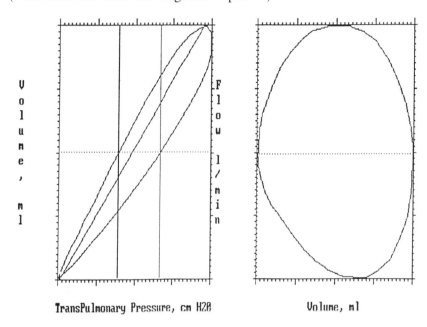

TransPulmonary Pressure, cm H2O   Volume, ml

conditions at several levels of lung inflation. The slope of the line described by this volume–pressure relationship is the static compliance.

4. Multiple occlusion technique during exhalation measures static compliance in both mechanically ventilated and spontaneously breathing patients.[12–15]

 a. Several periods of brief airway occlusion are produced at different lung volumes throughout the tidal range, always during expiration[10] (Fig. 10-2).

 b. The compliance is the slope of the volume–pressure relationship described by these occlusions.[15]

5. Lung overdistension can be readily identified by qualitative evaluation of the volume–pressure curve.

 a. Compliance during terminal 20% of insp (C_{20}) divided by C_L

 b. Normal C_{20}/C_L ratio: >1

 c. Overdistension: Volume changes outside the lin-

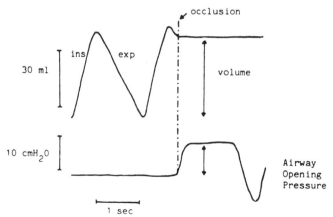

FIG. 10-2

Typical volume and proximal airway pressure wave forms resulting from a single airway occlusion. (From Stocks J, Nöthen U, Sutherland P, Hatch D, Helms P: Improved accuracy of the occlusion technique for assessing total respiratory compliance in infants. Pediatr Pulmonol 3:71, 1987, with permission.)

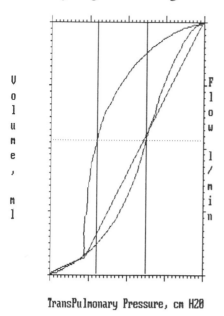

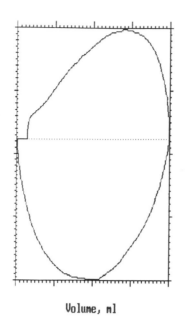

TransPulmonary Pressure, cm H2O   Volume, ml

FIG. 10-3
Lung over-distention produces this representative volume–pressure curve. The dynamic curve crosses the diagonal compliance line during the inspiratory phase. (Note: These are actual records from a patient.)

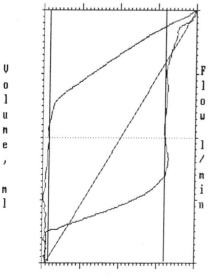

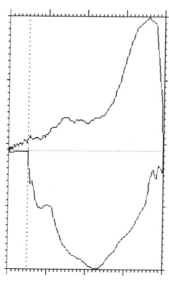

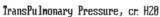

TransPulmonary Pressure, cr. H2O   Volume, ml

FIG. 10-4
Increased airway resistance will cause a "bulging" of the volume–pressure curve as increased pressures are needed to overcome the resistance to airflow. Note the concave nature of the flow–volume loop. Initial expiratory flows are high but fall rapidly.

ear portion of the curve $C_{20}/C_L \leq 1$ (Fig. 10-3)[16]

6. Increased airway resistance (Fig. 10-4)

D. CONTRAINDICATIONS

1. None

E. EQUIPMENT

1. Minimum requirements are a volume measurement device for tidal volume and a differential pressure transducer for transpulmonary pressure (Fig. 10-5).
2. Volume measurement devices
   a. Pneumotach
      (1) The pneumotach contains a flow-resistive element (such as a screen) that causes a pressure drop as air flows through it.
      (2) Throughout its linear range, the pressure drop, measured with a differential pressure transducer, is directly proportional to the airflow. It is linear to 10 ml/sec at a pressure drop of 1 cm H_2O.

For most neonatal measurements the 00 size pneumotach is sufficient.[17]

    (3) The pneumotach is connected between the endotracheal tube and the ventilator circuit to measure airflow in both directions.

    (4) Typical rebreathing deadspace of a pneumotach is 1 to 2 ml.

    (5) Most pneumotachs are heated to prevent condensation on the flow-resistive screen.

  b. "Heated wire" transducer[18,19]

    (1) As air flows across a heated filament, the heat loss from the filament varies directly with the velocity of air flowing past it.

    (2) The higher the velocity, the higher the electrical current required to maintain the heat of the filament.

    (3) The result is an output signal proportional to mass flow, which is then integrated for volume measurements.

  c. Flow transducers are reusable, and must be cleaned and disinfected between patients.

3. Transpulmonary pressure measurement
   a. Differential pressure transducer

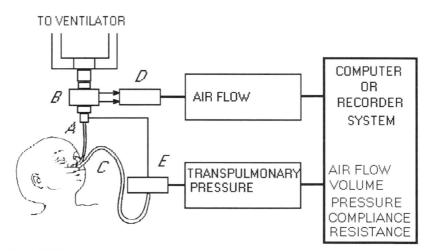

FIG. 10-5
Typical pulmonary mechanics system. The pneumotach (*B*) is connected between the endotracheal tube (*A*) and the ventilator circuit. The pressure changes from the pneumotach are measured by differential pressure transducer (*D*) with a range of ±2 cm H_2O. Transpulmonary pressure is determined with a differential pressure transducer (*E*) with a range of ±50 cm H_2O. Transpulmonary pressure is the difference between proximal airway pressure and esophageal pressure (*C*).

(1) One pressure port connected to the ventilator circuit proximal to the endotracheal tube

(2) Second port connected to the esophageal balloon.

(3) Typical range of this transducer is ±50 cm H_2O.

b. Esophageal balloons

(1) A small volume balloon (0.6 to 1.0 ml) is required for neonatal applications.

(2) Improper size, inflation, or placement of balloon, or catheter dimensions affects test results.

8-French catheters are most appropriate for the neonatal population.[20]

c. An intact balloon may be reused on the same patient. Otherwise, balloons are disposable.

4. Computerized pulmonary function systems are available which simplify the collection and analysis of the pressure, flow, and volume data. These systems consist of a flow measurement device and a differential pressure transducer that are interfaced to a microprocessor.

On-line displays of volume–pressure curves and flow–volume loops can be very useful in determining the validity of the test results.

5. Compliance measurement

a. Dynamic

(1) Mechanical breaths or spontaneous breaths (esophageal balloon required)

b. Static compliance: automatic shutter system

(1) Describes a static volume–pressure line from multiple occlusions, the slope of which equals respiratory system compliance.

(2) Does not require balloon.

c. Respiratory system compliance can be estimated with the use of an in-line tidal volume monitor, used in conjunction with ventilator pressure measurements.

$$C_{RS} = \frac{V_T}{PIP - PEEP}$$

Where V_T is tidal volume; PIP equals peak inspiratory pressure and PEEP is positive end expiratory pressure as supplied by the ventilator (Figs. 10-6 and 10-7).

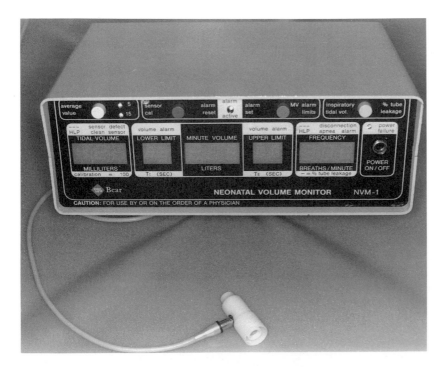

FIG. 10-6
Neonatal tidal volume monitor with a heated wire transducer.

F. PRECAUTIONS

1. Determine that the patient can tolerate the increase in deadspace associated with the measurement system hardware.
2. Be familiar with equipment usage and limitations.
3. Recognize limitations of equipment in that inaccurate data may be obtained if careful technique is not used.
4. Recognize causes of variable results.[21]
   a. Change in patient status[22]
      (1) Instability of lung volume
      (2) Uneven distribution of pleural pressure due to
         (a) Chest wall distortion
         (b) Sleep state
         (c) Changes in patient positioning
         (d) Lung water variations and atelectasis
   b. Inaccurate attachments or loose fittings
   c. Dirty pneumotach
   d. Malpositioned tubes (endotracheal or esophageal)
   e. Overinflation of balloon
4. Because of variability, perform multiple serial measurements for each patient for optimum information.
5. Show caution in using test results as sole criterion for extubation.[23]
   a. The ability to maintain adequate independent ventilation depends on the interaction of multiple complex factors including compliance, airway resistance, central respiratory drive, chest wall stability, and diaphragmatic endurance.
   b. Sequential compliance measurements may not accurately predict whether the patient will sustain adequate spontaneous ventilation.
6. In the presence of significant chest wall distortion the esophageal pressure may not accurately reflect changes in pleural pressure, resulting in inaccurate compliance measurements.[23–27]

   In this situation use of the occlusion technique may be indicated.

7. The dynamic measurement of compliance may underestimate the actual compliance of infants with high respiratory rates.

   This may occur at respiratory frequencies above 60 breaths per minute.[10]

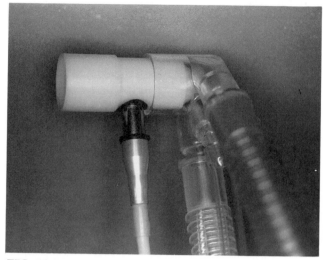

FIG. 10-7
Heated wire volume transducer connected to ventilator circuit.

8. For accurate measurements of dynamic compliance, the patient must have a tidal volume that is larger than the rebreathing deadspace of the flow transducer.
9. Compliance data calculated from spontaneous breath measurements tend to be greater than data calculated from mechanical breath measurements.[4] Therefore, spontaneous breath data should not be compared with mechanical breath data.

   For optimal consistency, either spontaneous or mechanical breaths should be chosen for sequential studies.

10. For the multiple occlusion technique, a tidal volume of at least 3 to 4 ml is needed to yield an accurate measurement.

G. TECHNIQUE

1. Familiarize yourself with the instrumentation of system to be used.
2. Following the manufacturer's instructions
   a. Set up test parameters.
   b. Input patient data (patient's current weight is a critical datum since reported values are indexed to body weight).
   c. Zero all the transducers.

3. Insert the esophageal balloon.
   a. Estimate the length of insertion to the lower third of the esophagus using the sum of the distance from the mouth to the tragus of the ear, and the distance between the ear to the xiphisternal angle.[28,29]

   The accuracy of the measurement is affected by the balloon and catheter dimensions.

   b. Connect the esophageal balloon to the pressure transducer and inflate with a small amount of air (typically 0.1 to 0.5 ml).
      (1) Do not overdistend the balloon.
      (2) Determine the correct amount of air by constructing a pressure–volume curve for the given balloon.[29]
   c. Observe for positive pressure fluctuations during spontaneous inspiration, suggesting the esophageal balloon is below the diaphragm.

   These pressure fluctuations will become negative when the balloon is pulled back to the optimal esophageal position.[1]

   d. Do not use with multiple occlusion technique (shutter).
4. Attach the pneumotach between the patient's endotracheal tube and the ventilator circuit.
5. Secure the pneumotach so that it does not exert undue torsion on the endotracheal tube.

   Due to its weight, an unsupported pneumotach can kink an endotracheal tube or cause accidental extubation or malposition.

6. For multiple occlusion technique, attach the shutter between the pneumotach and the ventilator circuit.
7. Initiate test sequence and review data on completion of the test interval.
8. Remove the pneumotach (and shutter assembly if used). Reattach to previous ventilator support if intubated.
9. Remove esophageal balloon and clean for reuse with the same patient.
10. Generate report if results appear valid.

   A valid test is characterized by well-defined (and repeatable) volume–pressure and flow–volume loops with minimal variance in compliance measurements.

11. Clean and disinfect pneumotach after each use (soak in antiseptic solution, rinse with water, and dry with forced air).

H. COMPLICATIONS

1. Tissue trauma caused by insertion of the esophageal balloon
2. Increased carbon dioxide retention due to increased rebreathing deadspace of the test apparatus

References

1. CUNNINGHAM MD: Bedside pulmonary function testing of infants. Respiratory Treatment Devices; In Levin DL, Morriss FC, Anas NG, Capron CC (eds): Essentials of Pediatric Intensive Care. St. Louis, Missouri, Quality Medical Publishing Inc., 1990, p 881
2. GREENSPAN JS, ABBASI S, BHUTANI VK: Sequential changes in pulmonary mechanics in the very low birth-weight ($\leq$1000 grams) infant. J Pediatr 113:732, 1988
3. LOTZE A, SHORT BL, TAYLOR GA: Lung compliance as a measure of lung function in newborns with respiratory failure requiring extracorporeal membrane oxygenation. Crit Care Med 15:226, 1987
4. DAVIS JM, VENESS-MEEHAN KA, NOTTER RH, et al: Changes in pulmonary mechanics after the administration of surfactant to infants with respiratory distress syndrome. N Engl J Med 319:476, 1988
5. ROOKLIN AR, MOOMJIAN AS, SHUTACK JG, et al: Theophylline therapy in bronchopulmonary dysplasia. J Pediatr 95:882, 1979
6. MAMMEL MC, GREEN TP, JOHNSON DE, THOMPSON TR: Controlled trial of dexamethasone therapy in infants with bronchopulmonary dysplasia. Lancet i:1356, 1983
7. SHICK JB, GOETZMAN BW: Corticosteroid response in chronic lung disease of prematurity. Am J Perinatol 1:23, 1983
8. RUSH MG, ENGLEHARDT B, PARKER RA, HAZINSKI TA: Double-blind, placebo-controlled trial of alternate-day furosemide therapy in infants with chronic bronchopulmonary dysplasia. J Pediatr 117:112, 1990
9. SCHULZE A, MÄDLER H-J, GEBHARDT B, et al: Titration of continuous positive airway pressure by the pattern of breathing: Analysis of flow–volume-time relationships by a noninvasive computerized system. Pediatr Pulmonol 8:96, 1990
10. BEARDSMORE CS, STOCKS J, HELMS P: Elastic properties of the respiratory system in infants. Eur Respir J 2, Suppl. 4, 135s, 1989

11. POLGAR G, WENG TR: The functional development of the respiratory system. Am Rev Respir Dis 120:625, 1979

12. STOCKS J, NÖTHEN U, SUTHERLAND P, et al: Improved accuracy of the occlusion technique for assessing total respiratory compliance in infants. Pediatr Pulmonol 3:71, 1987

13. ENGLAND SJ: Current techniques for assessing pulmonary function in the newborn and infant: Advantages and limitations. Pediatr Pulmonol 4:48, 1988

14. GERHARDT T, REIFERBERG L, SHAHNAZ D, BANCALARI E: Comparison of dynamic and static measurements of respiratory mechanics in infants. J Pediatr 114:120, 1989

15. MORTOLA JP, FISHER JT, SMITH B, et al: Dynamics of breathing in infants. J Appl Physiol 52:1209, 1982

16. FISHER JB, MAMMEL MC, COLEMAN JM, et al: Identifying lung overdistension during mechanical ventilation by using volume–pressure loops. Pediatr Pulmonol 5:10, 1988

17. CUNNINGHAM MD, DESAI NS: Methods of assessment and findings regarding pulmonary function in infants less than 1000 grams. Clin Perinatol 13:299, 1986

18. MACDONALD KD, WIRTSCHAFTER DD: Neonatal pulmonary monitoring goes on-line. Arkos 1:4, 1989

19. BABOOLAL R, KIRPALANI H: Measuring on-line compliance in ventilated infants using hot wire anemomentry. Crit Care Med 18:1070, 1990

20. MCCANN EM, GOLDMAN SL, BRADY JP: Pulmonary function in the sick newborn infant. Pediatr Res 21:313, 1987

21. ANDAY EK, GODART-WLODAVAR A, DELIVORIA-PAPADOPOULOS M: Sequential pulmonary function measurements in very low birthweight infants during the first week of life. Pediatr Pulmonol 3:392, 1987

22. STOCKS J, BEARDSMORE C, HELMS P: Infant lung function: Measurement conditions and equipment. Eur Respir J 2:Suppl. 4, 123s, 1989

23. VENESS-MEEHAN KA, RICHTER S, DAVIS JM: Pulmonary function testing prior to extubation in infants with respiratory distress syndrome. Pediatr Pulmonol 9:2, 1990

24. D'ANGELO E, SANT'AMBROGIO G, AGOSTONI E: Effect of diaphragm activity or paralysis on distribution of pleural pressure. J Appl Physiol 37:311, 1974

25. LE SOUEF PN, LOPES JM, ENGLAND SJ, et al: Effect of chest wall distortion on occlusion pressure and the preterm diaphragm. J Appl Physiol 55:359, 1983

26. GERHARDT T, BANCALARI C: Chest wall compliance in full term and preterm infants. Acta Paediatr Scand 69:359, 1980

27. LE SOUEF PN, LOPES JM, ENGLAND SJ, et al: Influence of chest wall distortion on esophageal pressure. J Appl Physiol 55:353, 1983

28. BHUTANI VK, SIVIERI EM, ABBASI S, SHAFFER TH: Evaluation of neonatal pulmonary mechanics and energenics: A two factor least mean square analysis. Pediatr Pulmonol 4:150, 1988

29. BEARDSMORE CS, HELMS P, STOCKS J, et al: Improved esophageal balloon technique for use in infants. J Appl Physiol 49:735, 1980

Part 3
Blood Sampling

11 Vessel Transillumination[1-5]

Billie Lou Short

A. INDICATION

To locate artery of vein for

1. Puncture for sampling
2. Vessel cannulation

See also Chapter 35, for use in diagnosing thoracic air leaks.

B. CONTRAINDICATIONS

None

C. PRECAUTIONS

1. Use fiberoptic light source with appropriate filters to cool light and prevent burns.[6]
2. Place sterile surgical glove over tip of probe to preserve sterile field.

D. EQUIPMENT

1. High intensity fiberoptic light
2. Black, soft tube around tip of probe if needed to make light seal
3. Alcohol
4. Sterile glove

E. TECHNIQUE

1. Wash end of light probe. Cover with sterile glove.
2. Dim light in room. Some residual light is necessary to visualize operating field.
3. Set light source at low intensity and increase as needed for visualization.
4. Position probe to transilluminate vessel.
   a. Directly opposite to puncture site, through extremity
   b. Adjacent to vessel but out of way of procedure

5. Identify vessel as dark, linear structure (see Color Fig. 11-1 at beginning of book)
   a. Edges may be indistinct.
   b. Arteries will be pulsatile.
6. Compensate for distortion if light is not directly opposite puncture site.

F. COMPLICATIONS

1. Burns from light probe (Fig. 11-1)
2. Cross contamination from breach of sterile technique

FIG. 11-1
Burn from transilluminator.

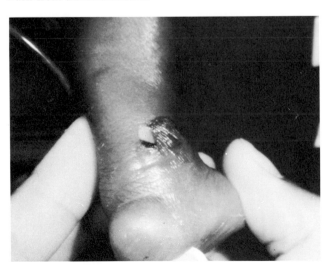

85

References

1. Cole FS, Todres ID, Shannon DC: Technique for percutaneous cannulation of the radial artery in the newborn infant. J Pediatr 92:105, 1978
2. Curran JS: A restraint and transillumination device for neonatal arterial/venipuncture: Efficacy and thermal safety. Pediatrics 66:128, 1980
3. Kuhns LR, Martin AJ, Gildersleeve S: Intense transillumination for infant venipuncture. Radiology 116:734, 1975
4. Stein RT, Kuhns LR: Letter to the Editor. J Pediatr 93:162, 1978
5. Wall PM, Kuhns LR: Percutaneous arterial sampling using transillumination. Pediatrics 59:1032, 1977
6. Uy J, Kuhns LR, Wall PM: Light filtration during transillumination. A method to reduce heat build-up in the skin. Pediatrics 60:308, 1977

12 Venipuncture

Billie Lou Short

A. INDICATIONS

1. Blood sampling
   a. Routine
   b. Blood culture
   c. If large quantities needed
   d. Central hematocrit
   e. Preferred (over capillary sample) for certain studies, for example[1-3]
      (1) Ammonia (arterial optimal)
      (2) Drug levels
      (3) Cross matching blood
      (4) Hemoglobin
      (5) Total neutrophil counts
2. Administration of drugs

B. CONTRAINDICATIONS

1. Use of deep vein in presence of coagulation defect
2. Local infection at puncture site
3. Femoral or internal jugular vein (see Complications)
4. External jugular vein in infants with respiratory distress, intracranial hemorrhage, or raised intracranial pressure

C. PRECAUTIONS

1. Observe universal precautions. Wear gloves.
2. When sampling from neck veins, place infant in head-down position to avoid cranial air embolus. Do not use neck veins in infants with intracranial bleeding or increased intracranial pressure, except as last resort.
3. Remove tourniquet before removing needle to minimize hematoma formation.
4. Apply local pressure with dry gauze to produce hemostasis (usually 2 to 3 minutes)
5. Avoid using alcohol swab to apply local pressure (painful, impairs hemostasis).

D. SPECIAL CONSIDERATIONS FOR NEONATES

1. Conserve sites to preserve limited venous access by using distal sites first.
2. Use small needle or scalp-vein butterfly. Hemolysis may occur with a 25 or smaller gauge.
3. Choice of veins (Fig. 12-1) in order of preference
   a. Dorsum of hands
   b. Dorsum of feet
   c. Medial wrist
   d. Antecubital fossa
   e. Scalp
   f. Medial ankle
   g. Proximal greater saphenous vein
   h. Neck

E. EQUIPMENT

1. Gloves
2. 23- to 25-gauge scalp-vein or venipuncture needle
3. Syringe with volume just larger than sample to be drawn
4. Prepared alcohol swabs
5. Gauze pads
6. Appropriate containers for specimens
7. Blood culture
   a. Iodophor preparation
   b. Sterile gloves
   c. Blood culture bottles (aerobic and anaerobic)
8. Tourniquet or sphygmomanometer cuff

F. TECHNIQUE

General Venipuncture[1,4]

1. Restrain infant appropriately.
2. Prepare area with antiseptic (see Chap. 4).
3. Occlude vein proximally using
   a. Tourniquet or cuff inflated to level between systolic and diastolic pressure (Fig. 12-2)

FIG. 12-1
The superficial venous system in the neonate.

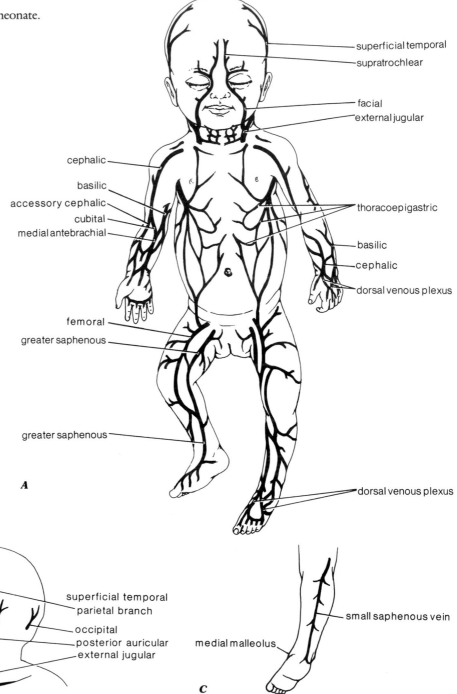

superficial temporal
supratrochlear

facial
external jugular

cephalic

basilic

accessory cephalic
cubital
medial antebrachial

thoracoepigastric

basilic
cephalic
dorsal venous plexus

femoral
greater saphenous

greater saphenous

dorsal venous plexus

A

superficial temporal
frontal branch

supratrochlear

superficial temporal
parietal branch

occipital
posterior auricular
external jugular

facial

B

small saphenous vein

medial malleolus

C

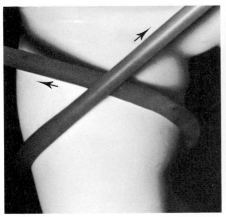
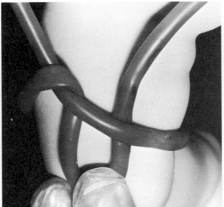
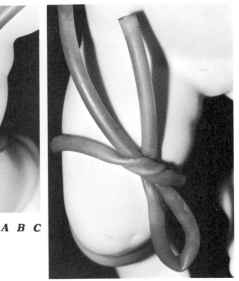

FIG. 12-2
Correct application of a tourniquet for quick release.

A B C

  b. Direct pressure over vessel
  c. Rubber band
4. Check syringe function and attach to needle.
5. Penetrate skin first and position for entry of vein (Fig. 12-3)
  a. Angle of entry 25 to 45 degrees
  b. Bevel up preferred for optimal blood flow (less chance of needle occlusion by vein wall)
  c. Direction of entry may be with or against direction of blood flow
6. Collect sample by gentle suction
  a. To prevent occlusion by vein wall
  b. To avoid hemolysis
7. Release tourniquet
8. Remove needle and apply local pressure with dry gauze for 3 minutes, or until complete hemostatis.

Scalp Vein
1. Shave adequate area of frontal or parietal scalp.
2. Use scalp-vein needle set.
3. Occlude vein proximally with finger.
4. Feel pulse to avoid tapping an artery.
5. Use shallow angle (15 to 20 degrees).
6. See technique for general venipuncture.

Proximal Greater Saphenous Vein[5]
1. Have assistant hold infant's thighs abducted with knees and hips slightly flexed.
2. Locate femoral triangle (Fig. 12-4, A).
  a. Proximal boundary inguinal ligament
  b. Lateral boundary: medial border of sartorius muscle
  c. Medial boundary: lateral border of adductor longus muscle

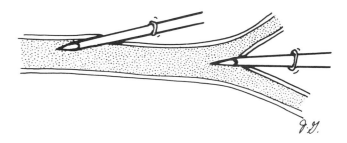

FIG. 12-3
Anterior wall of vein removed. Needle penetrating skin a short distance from site of venipuncture.

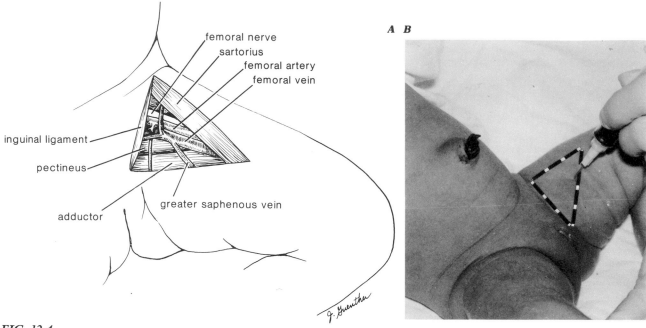

A B

FIG. 12-4

(A) Anatomy of the femoral triangle as defined in the text. (Adapted from Plaxico DT, Bucciarella RL: Greater saphenous vein venipuncture in the neonate. J Pediatr 93:1025, 1978) (B) Position of the femoral triangle on the abducted thigh.

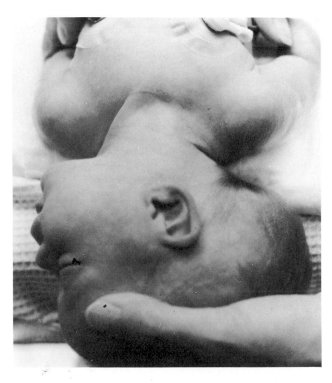

FIG. 12-5

Infant positioned for puncture of external jugular vein.

3. Enter skin and then vein at point approximately 2/3 along line from inguinal ligament to apex of triangle (Fig. 12-4, B).
   a. Use relatively steep angle (60 to 90 degrees).
   b. After entering skin, advance while applying gentle suction 1 to 4 mm until blood return is achieved.
4. See technique for general venipuncture.

External Jugular Vein
1. Position infant in head-down position with head extended and rotated away from selected vessel (Fig. 12-5).
2. Prepare skin over sternocleidomastoid muscle with antiseptic.
3. Make infant cry to distend vein.
4. Visualize external jugular vein running from angle of jaw to posterior border of sternocleidomastoid in its lower third.
5. Puncture vessel where it runs across anterior border of sternocleidomastoid muscle.
6. See technique for general venipuncture.

G. COMPLICATIONS[6–8,9,10]

1. Hemorrhage with
   a. Coagulation defect
   b. Puncture of deep vein
2. Venous thrombosis or embolus, with puncture of large, deep vein[10]
3. Laceration of adjacent artery
4. During femoral vein puncture
   a. Reflex arteriospasm of femoral artery with gangrene of extremity[7,10]
   b. Penetration of peritoneal cavity
   c. Septic arthritis of hip[6]

5. During internal jugular puncture
   a. Laceration of carotid artery
   b. Pneumothorax/subcutaneous emphysema
   c. Interference with ventilation owing to positioning for jugular vein puncture
   d. Raised intracranial pressure owing to head-down position aggravating intraventricular hemorrhage

References

1. BARAL J: Use of a simple technique for the collection of blood from premature and full-term babies. Med J Aust 1:97, 1968
2. SHOHAT M: Preterm blood counts vary with sampling site (letter). Arch Dis Child 62(11):1193, 1987
3. THUELBECK SM, McINTOSH N: Preterm blood counts vary with sampling site. Arch Dis Child 62:72, 1987
4. KUHNS LR, MARTIN AJ, GILDERSLEEVE S: Intensive transillumination for infant venipuncture. Radiology 116:734, 1975
5. PLAXICO DT, BUCCIARELLI RL: Greater saphenous vein venipuncture in the neonate. J Pediatr 93:1025, 1978
6. ASNES RS, ARENDAR GM: Septic arthritis of the hip. A complication of venipuncture. Pediatrics 38:837, 1966
7. GARROW E, KUSHNICK T: Management of femoral artery obstruction: Complication of femoral venipuncture. Am J Dis Child 110:570, 1965
8. KANTR RK, GORTON JM, PALMIERI K, et al: Anatomy of femoral vessels in infants and guidelines for venous catheterizations. Pediatrics 33:1020, 1989
9. McKAY RJ JR: Diagnosis and treatment: Risk of obtaining samples of venous blood in infants. Pediatrics 38:906, 1966
10. NABSETH DC, JONES JE: Gangrene of the lower extremities of infants after femoral venipuncture. N Engl J Med 268:1003, 1963

13 Arterial Puncture

Billie Lou Short

A. INDICATIONS[1-3]

1. Sampling for arterial blood-gas determination
2. Sampling for routine laboratory test when venous and capillary sampling not suitable[4]

B. CONTRAINDICATIONS

1. Coagulation defects
2. Circulatory compromise in the extremity
3. Inappropriate artery
   a. Femoral artery
   b. Use of radial artery if inadequate collaterals (see Allen's test)
4. Infection in sampling area
5. When cannulation of that vessel is anticipated

C. PRECAUTIONS

1. Select arterial sampling only when venous or capillary inappropriate.
   a. Ammonia levels
   b. Fungal blood cultures
2. Use smallest possible needle to minimize trauma to vessel (27 to 25 gauge)
3. Avoid lacerating the artery caused by puncturing both sides of arterial wall in exactly opposite locations.
4. Guarantee hemostasis at end of procedure.
5. Check distal circulation after puncture.
   a. Arterial pulse
   b. Capillary refill time
   c. Color, temperature
6. Take action to reverse arteriospasm, if necessary (see Chap. 15, Management of Vascular Spasm, Thrombosis, and Infiltrates).

D. SELECTION OF ARTERIAL SITE

1. Peripheral preferred over central
2. Radial artery preferred if ulnar collateral intact

3. Temporal, dorsalis pedis, posterior tibial arteries satisfactory
4. Brachial artery only as last resort; urgent indication

E. EQUIPMENT

Sterile

1. Gloves
2. Needle
   a. 23- to 25-gauge venipuncture
   b. 23- to 27-gauge scalp-vein set
3. Appropriate syringes (1-ml syringe for blood-gas sampling)
4. Materials for minor skin preparation; iodophor preparation preferred for blood culture.
5. Cotton balls or gauze pads

Unsterile

1. Plastic bag to cover transilluminator (A clean bag must be used for each infant.)
2. High-intensity fiberoptic light for transillumination (see Chap. 11, Vessel Transillumination)

F. TECHNIQUE

General Principles[1,2]

1. Transillumination may assist location of vessel (see Color Fig. 11-1 at the beginning of this book).[5]
2. Position needle for arterial puncture against direction of blood flow.
   a. Keep angle of entry more shallow for superficial vessels.
      (1) 15 to 25 degrees for superficial artery, bevel down
      (2) 45 degrees for deep artery, bevel up
   b. Penetrate skin first, then puncture artery to minimize trauma to vessel.
   c. Use fresh needle and repeat skin preparation if withdrawal from skin is necessary.
3. Apply firm, local pressure for 5 minutes to achieve complete hemostasis.

Radial-Artery Puncture[3]

1. Extend wrist, supine, not hyperextended (Fig. 13-1).
2. Locate radial and ulnar arteries at proximal wrist crease (Fig. 13-2).
   a. Radial artery is lateral to flexor carpi radialis tendon.
   b. Ulnar artery is medial to flexor carpi ulnarius tendon.
   c. Transillumination may be helpful.
3. Perform modified Allen's test for collateral supply.
   a. Elevate infant's hand.
   b. Occlude both radial and ulnar arteries at wrist.
   c. Massage palm toward wrist to cause bleeding.
   d. Release occlusion of ulnar artery only.
   e. Look for color to return to hand in less than 10 seconds, indicating adequate collateral supply.
   f. Do not puncture radial artery if color return takes more than 15 seconds.
4. Prepare area with antiseptic, as for minor procedure.

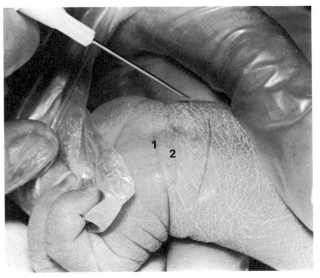

FIG. 13-1
Position of wrist for puncture of radial artery. (*1*, distal wrist crease; *2*, proximal wrist crease)

FIG. 13-2
Anatomy of the major arteries of the wrist and hand.

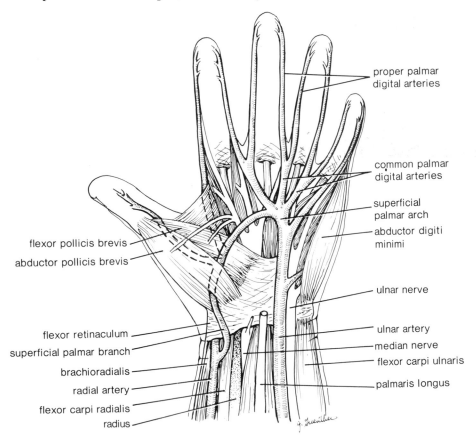

proper palmar digital arteries

common palmar digital arteries

superficial palmar arch

abductor digiti minimi

ulnar nerve

ulnar artery

median nerve

flexor carpi ulnaris

palmaris longus

flexor pollicis brevis

abductor pollicis brevis

flexor retinaculum

superficial palmar branch

brachioradialis

radial artery

flexor carpi radialis

radius

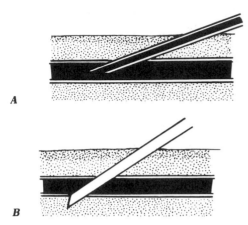

A

B

FIG. 13-3
(*A*) Penetration of artery at angle of 15 to 25 degrees with bevel down. Preferred method for small premature infants. (*B*) Penetration of artery at angle of 45 degrees with bevel up.

5. Check function of syringe.
6. Puncture skin and penetrate artery at 45 degrees with bevel up. For very small infants, use angle of 15 to 25 degrees with bevel down (Fig. 13-3).
   a. While maintaining gentle suction, advance until there is blood return or resistance from bone.
   b. If no blood prior to encountering resistance, withdraw needle cautiously until blood returns.
7. Collect sample and remove needle.
8. Compress site for 5 minutes or until hemostasis is complete.
9. Verify satisfactory peripheral blood flow.

Dorsalis-Pedis Puncture

1. Locate artery by palpation and transillumination on dorsum of foot between extensor hallucis longus and extensor digitorum longus tendons (Fig. 13-4).
2. Choose an angle of 15 to 25 degrees.
3. See radial-artery puncture.

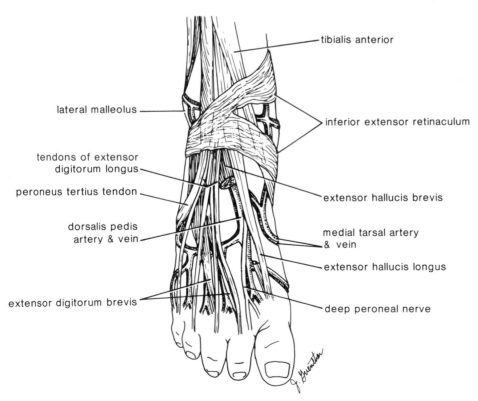

— tibialis anterior

lateral malleolus —

— inferior extensor retinaculum

tendons of extensor digitorum longus —

peroneus tertius tendon —

— extensor hallucis brevis

dorsalis pedis artery & vein —

— medial tarsal artery & vein

— extensor hallucis longus

extensor digitorum brevis —

— deep peroneal nerve

FIG. 13-4
Anatomical relations of the dorsalis pedis artery.

FIG. 13-5
Anatomical relations of the posterior tibial artery.

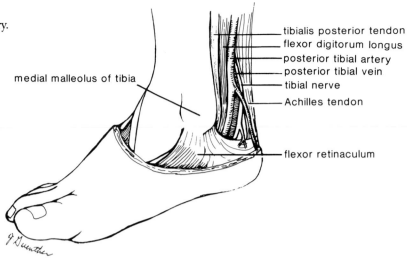

medial malleolus of tibia

tibialis posterior tendon
flexor digitorum longus
posterior tibial artery
posterior tibial vein
tibial nerve
Achilles tendon

flexor retinaculum

Posterior Tibial Puncture

1. Locate artery by palpation and transillumination between Achilles tendon and medial malleolus (Fig. 13-5).
2. Choose an angle of 45 degrees.
3. See radial-artery puncture.

Temporal-Artery Puncture[6,7]

1. Identify temporal artery anterior to tragus of ear (Fig. 13-6).
2. Select frontal or parietal branch.
3. Choose an angle of entry of 15 to 25 degrees.
4. See radial-artery puncture.

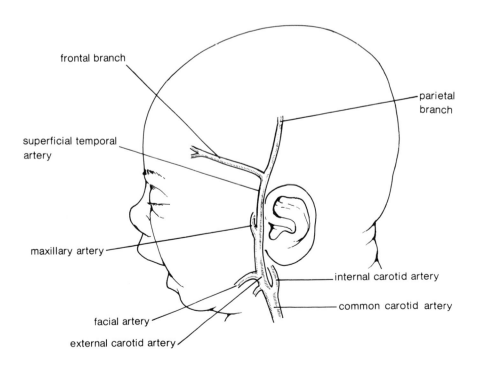

frontal branch

parietal branch

superficial temporal artery

maxillary artery

facial artery

external carotid artery

internal carotid artery

common carotid artery

FIG. 13-6
Temporal artery frontal and parietal branches.

G. COMPLICATIONS

See Chapter 30 for complications of arterial cannulation.

1. Distal ischemia from arteriospasm, hematoma, thrombosis, or embolism
2. Infection
   a. Osteomyelitis[8]
   b. Infected hip joint after femoral puncture[8]
3. Hemorrhage or hematoma
4. Nerve damage[9]
   a. Median nerve (brachial-artery puncture)
   b. Posterior tibial nerve
   c. Femoral nerve
5. Extensor tendon sheath injury, resulting in "false cortical thumb"[10]
6. Inaccuracy of blood gas estimated owing to[11-16]
   a. Excessive heparinization of syringe (falsely low PCO_2 and pH)[14,15]
   b. Hypothermic or hyperthermic infant (Nomogram should be used to correct the resulting body temperature.)[16]
   c. Gas bubbles in syringe
      (1) Spuriously high PO_2
      (2) Spuriously low PCO_2
   d. Excessive delay in processing (See Chap. 14, E, Sampling for Capillary Blood-Gas Estimation.[8])

References

1. WUNDERLICH B, REYNOLDS RN: Arterial blood sampling in babies. Am J Dis Child 123:446, 1972
2. SMITH AD: Arterial blood sampling in neonates. Lancet 1:254, 1975
3. SHAW JC: Arterial sampling from the radial artery in premature and full-term infants. Lancet ii:389, 1968
4. STINE MJ, HARRIS H: Validity of arterial hematocrits in newborns. Am J Dis Child 142:66, 1988
5. WALL PM, KUHNS LR: Percutaneous arterial sampling using transillumination. Pediatrics 59:1032, 1977
6. ALLUE X: Letter to the Editor: Blood sampling from scalp arteries. Pediatrics 53:583, 1974
7. SCHLUETER MA, JOHNSON BB, SUDMAN DA, et al: Blood sampling from scalp arteries in infants. Pediatrics 51:120, 1973
8. NELSON DL, HABLE KA, MATSEN JM: Proteus mirabilis osteomyelitis in two neonates following needle puncture. Successful treatment with ampicillin. Am J Dis Child 125:109, 1973
9. PAPE KE, ARMSTRONG DL, FITZHARDINGE PM: Peripheral median nerve damage secondary to brachial arterial blood gas sampling. J Pediatr 93:852, 1978
10. SKOGLAND RR, GILES EJ: The false cortical thumb. Am J Dis Child 140:375, 1986
11. ADAMS AP, MORGAN-HUGHES JO, SYKES MK: pH and blood gas analysis. Methods of measurement and sources of error using electrode systems. Anaesthesia 22:575, 1967
12. FAN LL, DELLINGER KT, MILLS AL: Potential errors in neonatal blood gas measurements. J Pediatr 97:650, 1980
13. HANSON JE, SIMMONS DH: A systematic error in the determination of blood PCO_2. Am Rev Respir Dis 115:1061, 1977
14. ACCURSO FJ, BAILEY DL, COTTON EK: Effect of syringe heparinization technique on arterial blood gas determination. Pediatr Res 14:588, 1980
15. BRADLEY JG: Errors in the measurement of blood PCO_2 due to dilution of the sample with heparin solution. Br J Anaesth 44:231, 1972
16. DELMAN GR, NUNN JF: Normograms for correction of blood PO_2, PCO_2, pH and base excess for time and temperature. J Appl Physiol 21:1484, 1966

14 Capillary Blood Sampling

Billie Lou Short

A. INDICATIONS[1-8]

1. Microsample for routine laboratory analysis
2. Capillary blood-gas analysis
3. Micro blood culture

B. CONTRAINDICATIONS

1. Infant in shock
2. Compromised blood flow to extremity
3. Local edema
4. Local infection
5. Severe polycythemia (venous hematocrit above 70%)
6. Monitoring capillary PO_2 when value above 60 mm Hg.[6,8,9] Hyperoxia can be missed.

C. PRECAUTIONS

1. Avoid anteromedial aspect of heel.
2. Do not use temperature above 40°C (104°F) to warm heel. Pack should feel warm, not hot, to touch.[10,11]

   Warming of the heel does not improve blood-gas values, but may increase blood flow; therefore, some consider warming optional.

3. Do not use scalpel blade.
4. Never use lancet longer than 2.5 mm.[12-14] Lancets now made with a depth of 1 mm are safer.
5. Avoid covering site with adhesive bandage—may cause skin maceration.
6. Recognize that
   a. Capillary hematocrit and blood gases may not reflect arterial levels in first 3 hours of life (venous stasis).[7]
   b. Skin preparation with alcohol may alter blood-sugar value obtained with Dextrostix (Ames)

when result is read by optical electrical method (reflectometer).[15]
   c. Although pH and PCO_2 correlate with arterial blood gases, PO_2 does not correlate well, especially when PO_2 is >60 mm Hg. Hyperoxia can be missed.[8,16-18]

D. EQUIPMENT

Sterile
1. Lancet, tip not longer than 2.5 mm
2. Alcohol swab (70%)
3. 2 × 2 gauze squares

Unsterile
1. Containers for blood collection
2. Warm compress to warm heel if necessary (optional)

Special Equipment for Capillary Blood Culture by Modified Method of Jennings et al[19-22]
1. Surgical gloves
2. Iodophor preparation
3. 18- and 20-gauge venipuncture needles
4. Tuberculin syringe flushed with 1:10,000 heparin and heparin expelled
5. Blood culture bottle or tube with 3- to 5-ml of medium

   Optimal ratio of sample to medium is 1:10.

Special Equipment for Capillary Blood-Gas Sampling
All equipment is unsterile.

1. Collection tubes.
2. Sealing wax or caps
3. Mixing bars
4. Magnet
5. Container with ice

E. TECHNIQUE

Heel Sampling[12,13]

1. Warm heel by wrapping in wet towel or diaper at 39°C to 40°C.[2] Towel should feel warm to touch.
   a. Temperature above 40°C may cause burns.
   b. Warming time should be approximately 5 minutes.
   c. Can be optional, although it may increase blood flow to the area
2. Select puncture site (Fig. 14-1).
3. Cleanse with alcohol; allow to dry.
4. Grasp heel firmly at arch and ankle (Fig. 14-2).
5. Puncture heel with one continuous, deliberate motion.
   a. Perpendicular to skin
   b. Depth not to exceed 2.5 mm
6. Avoid excessive squeezing or "milking," which may cause hemolysis and which activates hemostasis.
7. Wipe off first drop with dry gauze.
8. Apply pressure as far away from puncture site as possible.
9. Draw blood into tubes by capillary action as drops form. Intermittent pressure with forefinger may aid blood flow.
10. Seal capillary tubes with wax to depth of 4 mm or cap securely.
11. Press dry gauze to site, and hold foot above heart level until bleeding stops.

Sampling from Digital Artery[15,23,24]

1. Use lateral surface, distal phalanx of 2nd, 3rd, or 4th finger to avoid bone and cartilage.
2. Lancet for finger should be less than 1.5 mm.
3. Follow technique as for heel sampling.

Capillary Sampling for Blood Culture[19–23]

1. Technique similar to routine capillary sampling, except as specified.
2. Prepare skin with Iodophor and allow to dry.
3. Aspirate beads of blood through 18-gauge venipuncture needle into heparinized syringe without touching needle to skin.
4. Obtain approximately 0.15 ml of blood for each blood culture bottle.
5. Inject blood into culture bottles.

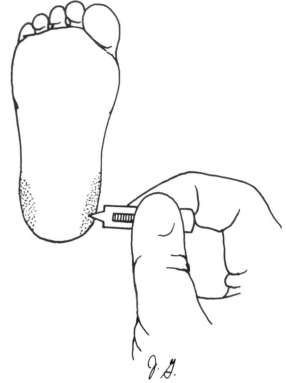

FIG. 14-1
Capillary sampling from the heel. Stippled areas indicate correct sites for sampling.

FIG. 14-2
Foot and heel restrained correctly for capillary sampling. Gloves should be worn.

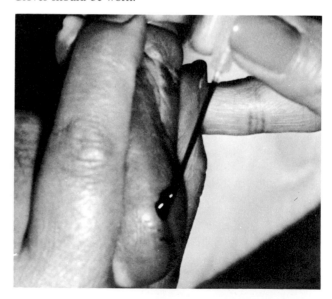

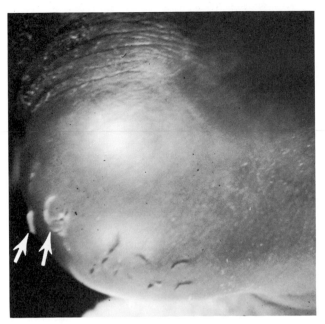

FIG. 14-3
Infection resulting from capillary sampling by heel stick. Swollen, shiny skin over area of cellulitis. Arrows indicate pus extruding from site of multiple punctures.

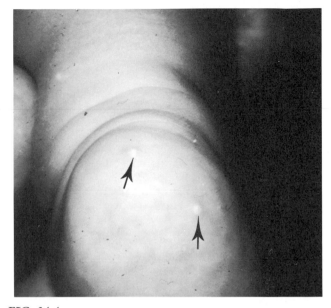

FIG. 14-4
Arrows indicate calcified subcutaneous nodules resulting from capillary sampling by heel stick in the newborn period. Infant was 6 months old at time of photograph.

Sampling for Capillary Blood-Gas Estimation[2,4,6,8,17,18,24–26]

Sampling techniques are the same as for heel sampling.

1. Hold heel at body level (horizontal) to avoid venous stasis.
2. Fill tubes from anticoagulant end (red marker).
3. Hold tubes horizontal; allow filling as long as there is enough blood to cover tip without bubbles.
4. Discard tube if air is introduced.
5. Seal one end with wax to depth 4 mm after filling or cap.
6. Mix blood to ensure anticoagulation.
   a. Most samples can be mixed by rocking the tube back and forth three to four times and do not require the iron filament.
   b. Use iron-mixing filament if desired.
      (1) Introduce the iron filament and seal other end to depth of 2 mm.
      (2) Use magnet to move filament within tube, mixing blood and anticoagulant.
7. Immerse sealed sample in ice-water mixture.
8. Analyze promptly.
   a. pH stable about 2 hours at 0°C.
   b. pH decreases after 20 minutes at room temperature.
   c. PO_2 unreliable after 30 minutes at 0°C.
   d. Chance of clotting increases with time.

F. COMPLICATIONS

1. Inaccuracy of blood-gas estimation—causes
   a. Circulatory stasis
   b. Contamination with air (lowers PCO_2 and raises PO_2)
   c. Delay in analysis
   d. Inadequate or excessive anticoagulation
2. Cellulitis (Fig. 14-3)
3. Osteomyelitis of calcaneus.
4. Abscess formation
5. Calcified nodules, usually disappearing by 18 to 30 months (Fig. 14-4)[11,27,28]
6. Tissue loss and scarring of heel
7. Amputation of finger tip
8. Injury to digital nerve
9. Erroneously high Dextrostix values[1,16]
10. Overestimating potassium concentration
11. Underestimating PO_2

References

1. KAPLAN SA, YUCEOGLU AM, STRAUSS J: Chemical microanalysis: Analysis of capillary and venous blood. Pediatrics 24:270, 1959
2. BANNISTER A: Comparison of arterial and arterialized capillary blood in infants with respiratory distress. Arch Dis Child 44:726, 1969
3. FIORINI A: A complication of capillary glucose monitoring. Br Med J 293:597, 1896
4. GLASGOW JFT, FLYNN DM, SAWYER PR: A comparison of descending aortic and "arterialized" capillary blood in the sick newborn. Can Med Assoc J 106:660, 1972
5. HOLT RJ, FRANKCOMBE CH, NEWMAN RL: Capillary blood cultures. Arch Dis Child 49:318, 1974
6. HUNT CE: Capillary blood sampling in the infant: Usefulness and limitations of two methods of sampling, compared with arterial blood. Pediatrics 51:501, 1973
7. KOCH G, WENDEL H: Comparison of pH, carbon dioxide tension, standard bicarbonate and oxygen tension in capillary blood and in arterial blood during the neonatal period. Acta Paediatr Scand 56:10, 1967
8. McLAIN BI, EVANS J, DEAN PRF: Comparison of capillary and arterial blood gas measurements in neonates. Arch Dis Child 63:743, 1988
9. GARG K: Arterialized capillary blood. Can Med Assoc J 107:16, 1972
10. BLUMENFELD TA, HETELENDY WG, FORD SH: Simultaneously obtained skin-puncture serum, skin-puncture plasma, and venous serum compared, and effects of warming the skin before puncture. Clin Chem 23:1705, 1977
11. MEITES S: Skin-puncture and blood-collecting technique for infants: Update and problems. Clin Chem 34(9):189, 1988
12. BLUMENFELD TA, TURL GK, BLANC WA: Recommended site and depth of newborn heel stick punctures based on anatomical measurements and histopathology. Pediatr Res 12:444, 1978
13. FENTON LF, BERTIE B, GAINES J, CIPRIANA J: A superior method for obtaining blood from the heel of the newborn infant. Clin Pediatr 16:815, 1977
14. REINER CB, MEITES S, HAYES JR: Optimal sites and depths for skin puncture of infants and children as assessed from anatomical measurements. Clin Chem 36(3):547, 1990
15. KARNA P, POLAND RL: Monitoring critically ill newborn infants with digital capillary blood samples: An alternative. J Pediatr 92:270, 1978
16. SEXSON WR, GRAZAITIS DM: Erroneously high Dextrostix values caused by isopropyl alcohol. Pediatr Res 14:611, 1980
17. KNELSON JH, AVERY ME: Capillary PO_2 in neonates. Pediatrics 43:638, 1969
18. STEFAN L, LESCHIN A, GRAY K: Capillary PO_2 in neonates. Pediatrics 43:637, 1969
19. FISCHER GW, CRUMRINE MH, JENNINGS PB: Experimental *Escherichia coli* sepsis in rabbits. J Pediatr 85:117, 1974
20. JENNINGS PB, DIXON RS, McCARTHY MK, METTLER PR: A modified peripheral capillary blood culture sampling technique. Pediatrics 57:966, 1976
21. KNUDSON RP, ALDEN ER: Neonatal heelstick blood culture. Pediatrics 65:505, 1980
22. MANGURTEN HH, LeBEAU LJ: Diagnosis of neonatal bacteremia by a microblood culture technique. J Pediatr 90:990, 1977
23. CORBERT AJS, BURNARD ED: Oxygen tension measurements on digital blood in the newborn. Pediatrics 46:780, 1970
24. DUC CV, COMARASAMY N: Digital arterial oxygen tension as a guide to oxygen therapy in the newborn. Biol Neonate 24:134, 1974
25. FOLGER G, KOURI P, SABBAH H: Arterialized capillary blood sampling in the neonate. A reappraisal. Heart Lung 9:521, 1980
26. GANDY G, GRANN L, CUNNINGHAM N, et al: The validity of pH and PCO_2 measurements in capillary samples in sick and healthy newborn infants. Pediatrics 34:192, 1964
27. LILEN LD, HARRIS VJ, RAMAMURTHY RS, PILDES RS: Neonatal osteomyelitis of the calcaneus: Complication of heel puncture. J Pediatr 88:478, 1976
28. SELL EJ, HANSEN RC, STRUCK-PIERCE S: Calcified nodules on the heel: A complication of neonatal intensive care. J Pediatr 96:473, 1980

15 Management of Vascular Spasm, Thrombosis, and Infiltrates

Garth Asay

Spasm and thrombosis may result from vascular manipulation, catheters, trauma, polycythemia, sepsis, or as an idiopathic event.[1] Arterial spasm is transient, usually lasting less than 4 hours from onset. Any arterial region may be affected.

Spasm

A. ASSESSMENT

1. Extremity
   a. Compare with opposite extremity
   b. Appearance
      (1) Blue color in toes or fingers
      (2) White color distal to spasm
      (3) Pale or mottled
      (4) Decreased movement
   c. Cool to the touch
   d. Abnormal pulse
      (1) Palpation: absent or diminished
      (2) Doppler ultrasound: flattened
      (3) Oxymetry: "search" alarm
2. Central
   a. Renal artery
      (1) Hypertension
      (2) Hematuria
         (a) Occult
         (b) Gross
      (3) Oliguria
   b. Aorta
      (1) Diminished pulses to lower extremities
      (2) Systemic hypertension
      (3) Bowel ischemia
         (a) Hematochezia
         (b) Decreased motility and distention
         (c) Perforation

B. MANAGEMENT

1. Extremity
   a. Warm contralateral extremity (reflex vasodilation)
   b. If necessary, restore circulating volume with blood, albumin, or plasma.
   c. Maintain limb in horizontal position.
   d. Maintain neutral thermal environment for affected extremity, i.e., keep heat lamps off area.
   e. Wrap other extremities with elastic bandages to increase their vascular resistance and encourage flow to affected extremity.
   f. Consider removing catheter.

      Catheter may be removed at any point in the management. Continually assess the need for keeping the catheter in place (i.e., the benefits of arterial access and treatment through the line vs. the risk of thrombosis and further complications.)

   g. Give tolazoline (0.25–0.5 mg/kg) intra-arterially (UAC or peripheral) or intravenously.
      (1) Constrictively wrap all unaffected extremities first.
      (2) Maintain good circulatory volume.
      (3) Monitor for hypotension and be prepared to treat it immediately.
2. Central
   a. Evaluate and restore circulating volume as necessary.
   b. If not previously removed, remove catheter.
   c. Treat hypertension.
      (1) Use vasodilators or β-blockers.
      (2) Limit use of diuretics because hypovolemia may potentiate thrombus formation.

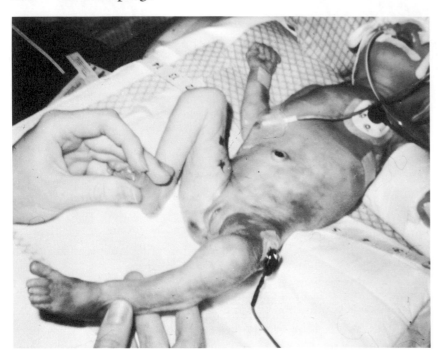

FIG. 15-1
Complication of UAC. Clot at bifurcation of aorta. Darker areas indicate compromised areas of skin. There is skin loss at tip of the right big toe. The infant showed generalized skin mottling related to severe hypertension owing to thrombotic compromise of right renal arterial blood flow.

Arterial Thrombosis

The presence of arterial thrombosis is likely if management of spasm proves unsuccessful or if symptoms persist longer than 4 hours. Signs of thrombosis may be absent initially, with development of more serious symptoms within hours to days (Fig. 15-1).

A. ASSESSMENT

1. Blood pressure
   a. Systemic hypertension
   b. Decreased blood pressure in affected extremities
2. Weak or absent pulses
3. Symptoms of congestive heart failure
   a. Tachypnea
   b. Poor feeding
   c. Poor perfusion
   d. Edema
   e. Enlarged liver
4. Thrombocytopenia
5. Diagnostic imaging
   a. Real-time ultrasonography
      (1) Portable
      (2) Noninvasive
      (3) Monitors progress over time
   b. Contrast angiography to visualize clot
      (1) Gives best definition of thrombosis
      (2) Requires infusion of radiocontrast material that may be hypertonic or give undesired increase in vascular volume
   c. Radionuclide flow study: flow interrupted

B. ACUTE MANAGEMENT

1. If not previously done, follow the management steps for arterial spasm.
2. Thrombolytic therapy
   a. Urokinase: fibrinolytic agent

   Urokinase and streptokinase have both been used successfully and safely as fibrinolytic agents in the neonate. Urokinase, unlike streptokinase, is non-antigenic and produces a direct activation of plasminogen with a linear dose-effect relationship. Close clinical observation and serial investigation with noninvasive techniques such as real-time ultrasound and Doppler studies are useful to document the response to therapy.[11]

(1) Use urokinase, 1500 to 6000 IU/kg hourly, by continuous intravenous (or intra-arterial) infusion until clot resolves.[1,12]

(2) Assess flow every 4 to 8 hours during fibrinolytic therapy, and, if there is no improvement in flow, double the infusion rate.

Doses up to 10,000 to 16,000 IU/kg hourly are usually tolerated.[7,10]

(3) During administration, monitor and maintain coagulation studies as follows
   (a) Fibrinogen ≥100 to 200 mg/dl
   (b) Fibrin split products ≤10 to 40 μg/ml

During thrombolytic therapy with urokinase, the prothrombin time (Normal = 14 to 20) and partial thromboplastin time (Normal = 35 to 55) are usually unaffected.

Baseline laboratory testing should be performed prior to therapy. Repeat testing should be performed 3 to 4 hours after initiation of fibrinolytic therapy and one to three times daily thereafter to maintain values in the above range.[11]

b. Heparin

Can be used as an adjunct therapy during or following thrombolytic therapy but hemorrhagic symptoms are more likely than when using urokinase alone.

(1) Bolus: intravenous infusion of 25 to 100 U/kg over the first hour[7,8]
(2) Maintenance: 15 to 25 U/kg/hr IV
(3) Coagulation studies
   (a) PT ≤ 14 to 18 seconds
   (b) PTT > 55 seconds (usually 1.5 to 2 times baseline)

c. Tissue plasminogen activator (tPA) dosage: 0.5 mg/kg hourly over 3 hours[5,6]

tPA is still investigational. It binds strongly and specifically to fibrin and allows for preferential, efficient activation of fibrin-bound plasminogen.

3. Involve surgical consultant concomitent with thrombolytic therapy.

Although surgical intervention is rarely warranted as initial therapy in neonates, the complications of thrombolytic therapy may require immediate surgical attention. Microvascular sur-gery and thrombectomy may be clinically indicated as a potential life-saving measure in cases where deterioration is progressive.[2] However, the outcome for conservative medical management is generally good and the indications for surgery should be evaluated on an individual basis (e.g., bowel perforation or uncontrolled hypertension).

C. FOLLOWUP MANAGEMENT OF AFFECTED EXTREMITY

1. Maintain limb in the horizontal position.
2. Protect from trauma.
3. Maintain neutral thermal environment.
4. Avoid drawing blood from or placing IVs in compromised extremity.
5. Keep compromised tissue dry, sterile, and exposed.

D. CONTRAINDICATIONS TO THROMBOLYTIC THERAPY

1. Active bleeding including pulmonary, gastrointestinal, or intracranial[9]
2. Recent major surgery[9]

   Minor surgery sites (e.g., thoracotomy tube, venous cutdown) may require local therapy if bleeding occurs.

Venous Thrombosis

Venous thrombosis is most often associated with central venous catheters. Small vessels with low blood flow are also presenting sites of involvement. A thrombus may be present for days prior to detection. Central sites may include vena cavae, renal veins, and portal and hepatic veins.

A. ASSESSMENT

In contrast to arterial thrombosis, signs and symptoms of venous thrombosis may be subtle or absent.

1. Insidious edema of head, neck, or extremities often with bluish discoloration
2. Unexplained thrombocytopenia (clot consumption)
3. End-organ dysfunction (Table 15-1)

B. MANAGEMENT

Diagnostic and therapeutic options were outlined previously in the section Arterial Thrombosis. Treatment is usually conservative until revascularization occurs.

Catheter Thrombosis

Thrombosis of a central catheter with resulting occlusion may occur without directly attributable systemic symptoms.

A. ASSESSMENT

1. Dampened monitor waveform
2. Inability to aspirate blood through catheter
3. Obstruction of catheter

B. MANAGEMENT

1. Remove catheter if no longer medically critical.
2. If maintenance of catheter is essential, attempt clot dissolution
   a. Using strict sterile technique, instill into the catheter urokinase diluted to 5000 IU/ml in a volume equal to the internal volume of the catheter (usually 0.2–0.4 ml for umbilical catheters).
   b. Leave in contact with the thrombus for 5 to 10 minutes.
   c. Aspirate every 5 minutes until the clot is clear.
   d. If the catheter is not patent after 30 minutes, repeat the procedure.[4]

Intravenous Infiltration

A. ASSESSMENT

1. Self limited
   a. Small area of local involvement
   b. Minimal swelling
   c. Mild pale or bluish discoloration
2. Requires further therapeutic intervention
   a. Local subcutaneous swelling
      (1) Tense, overlying skin
      (2) Central cutaneous blanching
      (3) Absent capillary refilling after digital pressure
   b. Blistering

B. MANAGEMENT

1. Initiate early for greatest efficacy.
2. Remove catheter.
3. Relieve any constricting bands that may be acting as a tourniquet (e.g., armboard restraint).
4. Cleanse area with sterile saline.
5. Elevate area.
6. If mild involvement, keep area clean and dry.
7. If area is blanched and tense, inject hyaluronidase[13] locally
   a. Cleanse area with iodophor prep and allow to dry.
   b. Prepare 1 ml hyaluronidase (150 IU/ml) in a syringe with a 25-guage needle.
   c. Using sterile technique, inject a small amount of the hyaluronidase subcutaneously at the edge of the infiltrate.
   d. Continue making small injections in a circular pattern around the perimeter of the infiltration, evenly distributing the entire amount of hyaluronidase. Direct injection to periphery, rather than into center of affected area.

   A good response is indicated by immediate relief of blanching, followed by a more gradual resolution of swelling.

8. Alternative therapy[3]
   a. Cleanse area with iodophor and allow to dry.
   b. Using sterile technique and a 20- to 22-guage needle, make multiple perforations of the superficial layers of skin over the area of greatest swelling.
   c. Gently squeeze the infiltrated fluid out of the subcutaneous tissue through the puncture sites.
9. Following either method, apply continuous saline soaks at room temperature over the involved area to aid drainage until pressure is relieved in infiltrated area.
10. Apply local therapy as appropriate for burns if there is deep blistering or loss of skin.
11. Request surgical evaluation if scarring or deeper involvement appears likely.

    Intravenous infiltrations may be deeper than initially suspected. If there is involvement of muscle or anticipated deep scarring of the skin, surgical management with debridement and skin grafting may be indicated.

TABLE 15-1
Trouble Shooting Vascular Problems

Problem	Symptoms	Treatment
Aortic thrombosis	Diminished pulses in lower extremities	Remove catheter
	Renal compromise oliguira rising creatinine	Confirm diagnosis Doppler ultrasound radiologic flow study
	Poor distal perfusion	Attention to compromised extremities
	Hypertension	Antihypertensives
	Congestive heart failure	Thrombolytic therapy fibrinolytics heparin
	Bowel ischemia/perforation	Surgical thrombectomy if symptoms are severe
Renal artery thrombosis	Systemic hypertension	Renal ultrasound
	Hematuria	Creatinine, plasma renin, UA
	History of UAC	Urinalysis
	Oliguria	Antihypertensives
Peripheral artery thrombosis	Skin discoloration blue or white	Remove catheter Keep horizontal, dry, warm
	Absent or decreased pulse	Maintain adequate circulating volume
	Decreased skin temperature	Constrictive wrap on opposite extremity
		Low dose systemic tolazoline
UVC associated thrombosis	Portal vein thrombosis or hepatic necrosis may develop without visible signs. jaundice hepatomegaly	Remove catheter Confirm diagnosis ultrasound flow study Thrombolytic or heparin therapy Surgical thrombectomy
Renal vein thrombosis	Classic triad gross hematuria thrombocytopenia enlarged kidney	Renal ultrasound Heparin Thrombolytics
Isolated catheter occlusion (no systemic symptoms)	Dampened monitor waveform inability to aspirate blood inability to infuse through line	Urokinase (5000 U/kg) Leave in place for 10 minutes; aspirate; repeat if needed

References

1. Manco-Johnson M: Diagnosis and management of thromboses in the perinatal period. Sem Perinatol 14:393, 1990
2. Schmidt B, Zipursky A: Thrombotic disease in newborn infants. Clin Perinatol 11:461, 1984
3. Bagnall H, Gomperts E, Atkinson J: Continuous infusion of low-dose urokinase in the treatment of central venous catheter thrombosis in infants and children. Pediatrics 83:963, 1989
4. Weinberg G, Brion Luc, Vega-Richf C: Dangers of arterial catheters in critically ill neonates (letter). Pediatrics 85:627, 1990
5. Reznik V, Anderson J, Griswold W, et al: Successful fibrinolytic treatment of arterial thrombosis and hypertension in a cocaine-exposed neonate. Pediatrics 84:735, 1989
6. McDonald M, Hathaway W: Anticoagulant therapy by continuous heparinization in newborn and older infants. J Pediatr 101:451, 1982
7. Kennedy L, Drummond W, Knight M, et al: Successful treatment of neonatal aortic thrombosis with tissue plasminogen activator. J Pediatr 116:798, 1990
8. Levy M, Benson L, Burrows P, et al: Tissue plasminogen activator for the treatment of thromboembolism in infants and children. J Pediatr 118:467, 1991
9. Bhat R, Fisher E, Doshi U, et al: Neonatal abdominal aortic thrombosis. Crit Care Med 9:858, 1981
10. Olsen M, Blumer J, Gauderer M, Izant R: Streptokinase dissolution of a right atrial thrombus. J Pediatr Surg 20:19, 1985
11. Hurtubise M, Bottino J, Lawson M, McCredie K: Restoring patency of occluded central venous catheters. Arch Surg 115:212, 1980
12. Zenk K, Dungy C, Greene G: Nafcillin extravasation injury. Am J Dis Child 135:1113, 1981
13. Chandavasu O, Garrow D, Valda V, et al: A new method for the prevention of skin sloughs and necrosis secondary to intravenous infiltration. Am J Perinatol 3:4, 1986

Part 4
Miscellaneous Sampling

16 Lumbar Puncture

S. Lee Marban

A. INDICATIONS

1. To diagnose central nervous system (CNS) infection (meningitis, encephalitis)[1,2]

   Routine inclusion of lumbar puncture (LP) in the initial sepsis evaluation of newborn infants (1 to 7 days of life) has been questioned.[3–5] Meningitis occurs less frequently in this population than in older infants, and meningitis without bacteremia is very unlikely. Also, the procedure may be poorly tolerated by newborns with cardiopulmonary compromise.[6–8] An LP is indicated if early bacteremia is documented, or if signs of CNS involvement are present (seizures or coma). An LP is also indicated in assessment for infection in the later neonatal period.

2. To monitor efficacy of antimicrobial therapy in the presence of CNS infection[9] by examining cerebrospinal fluid (CSF) cell count, microbiology, and drug levels
3. To diagnose subarachnoid hemorrhage
4. To diagnose CNS involvement with leukemia
5. To drain CSF in communicating hydrocephalus associated with intraventricular hemorrhage[10–12]

   Efficacy of serial LPs in temporary amelioration or long-term improvement of post-hemorrhagic hydrocephalus is controversial.[13–16] The actual removal of fluid may be less important than the establishment of dural openings for leakage and decompression of CSF into the adjacent tissues. Potential risks of repeated LPs[17,18] must be weighed against possible benefit.

6. To inject chemotherapeutic agents
7. To instill contrast material for myelography

B. CONTRAINDICATIONS

1. Bleeding diathesis
2. Infection at or near puncture site
3. Lumbosacral anomalies

4. Increased intracranial pressure[19]
   a. Unilateral mass (tumor or hematoma)
   b. Posterior fossa tumor
   c. Noncommunicating hydrocephalus
5. Respiratory instability when the procedure may cause added compromise

C. EQUIPMENT

All equipment is sterile, except face mask. Prepackaged lumbar puncture kits are available.

   False-positive gram stain due to nonviable organisms in prepackaged specimen containers has been reported.[20]

1. Gloves and mask
2. Cup with iodophor antiseptic solution
3. Gauze swabs
4. Towels or transparent aperture drape
5. Spinal needle with short bevel and stylet, 22-gauge × 1½ inches
6. Three or more specimen tubes with caps
7. Adhesive bandage

D. PRECAUTIONS

1. Monitor vital signs, ensure an adequate airway, and be aware of potential for aspiration with abdominal compression.
2. Use strict aseptic technique as for a major procedure. See Chapter 4.
3. Always use a stylet to avoid development of intraspinal epidermoid tumor.[21,22]

   Incidence of traumatic LP is not reduced by use of needle without stylet.[23]

4. If infant has significant respiratory compromise, avoid fully flexed lateral decubitus position.[6–8]
5. To prevent traumatic tap caused by over penetration, insert needle slowly while removing stylet at intervals to detect CSF as soon as subdural space is entered.

109

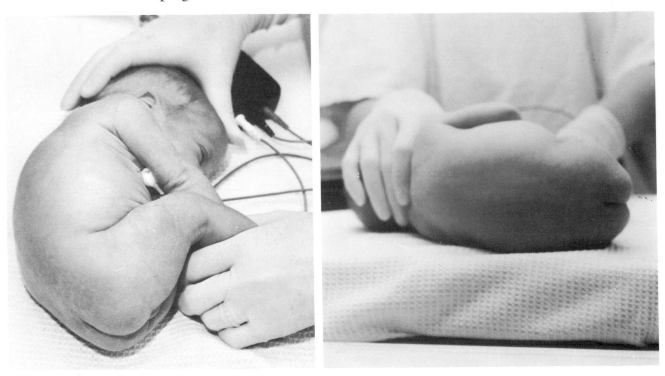

FIG. 16-1
Restraining infant for lumbar puncture in the lateral recumbant position. Neck need not be flexed.

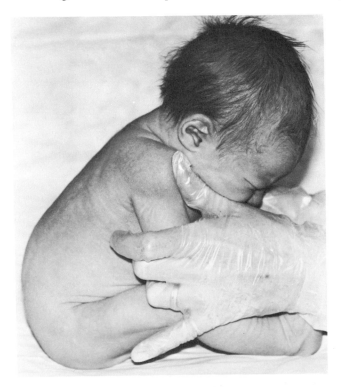

FIG. 16-2
Restraining infant for lumbar puncture in the sitting position.

FIG. 16-3
(*A*) Externally palpable anatomic landmarks.
(*B*) Vertebral bodies removed to show anatomy of spinal cord in lumbosacral area in relation to external landmarks.

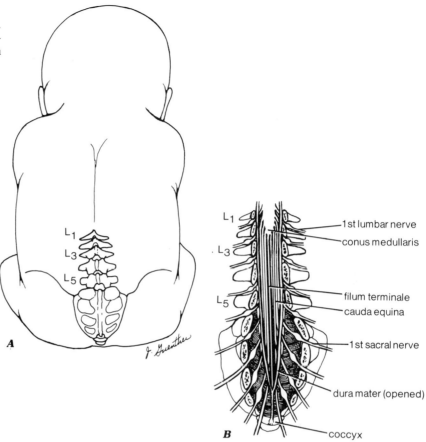

A

L₁
L₃
L₅

B

1st lumbar nerve
conus medullaris
filum terminale
cauda equina
1st sacral nerve
dura mater (opened)
coccyx

L₁
L₃
L₅

6. Palpate landmarks accurately to prevent puncture above L2-L3 interspace.

E. TECHNIQUE[24–26]

1. Have assistant restrain infant in lateral decubitus or sitting position, with spine flexed (Figs. 16-1 and 16-2). Neck need not be fully flexed.
2. Palpate interspace that falls immediately above or below line drawn between iliac crests in the L3-L4 or L4-L5 interspace (Fig. 16-3).
3. Prepare as for major procedure (see Chapter 4). Wash hands thoroughly. Put on mask and sterile gloves.
4. Clean lumbar area three times with antiseptic.
   a. Begin at desired interspace and wash in enlarging circles to include iliac crests.
   b. Allow antiseptic to dry, or blot excess with sterile gauze.

5. Drape, leaving puncture site and infant's face exposed. Transparent aperture drape is recommended because it does not obstruct the view of patient.

   Local anesthesia is generally not used in neonates. Use of lidocaine injection does not reduce physiologic instability during the procedure.[27] See Chapter 5 for local anesthetic techniques.

6. Insert needle into desired interspace (Fig. 16-4).
   a. Aim slightly cephalad to avoid vertebral bodies (Fig. 16-5).
   b. If resistance is met, withdraw needle slightly and redirect more cephalad.
   c. Hold a finger on vertebral process above interspace to aid in locating puncture site if infant moves.
7. Advance needle slowly to a depth of 1 cm to 1.5 cm in term infant, less in preterm infant.
   a. Remove stylet frequently to check for fluid.

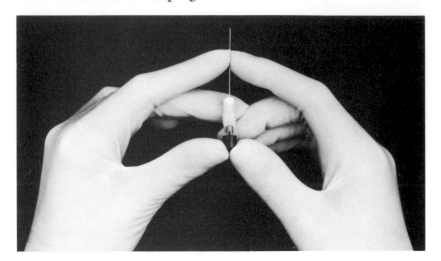

FIG. 16-4
Holding spinal needle in two hands for maximal stabilization.

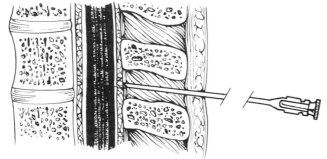

FIG. 16-5
Inserting spinal needle in slightly cephalad direction to avoid vertebral bodies.

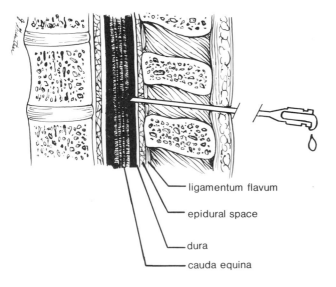

FIG. 16-6
Needle has penetrated the dura, and stylet has been removed to allow free flow of spinal fluid.

ligamentum flavum

epidural space

dura

cauda equina

b. Anticipate change in resistance, which may be felt as needle passes through ligamentum flavum and dura (Fig. 16-6). This is often more difficult to appreciate in young infant than in older child.

c. Wait for fluid after removing stylet, because flow may be slow.

d. Try one interspace above or below if no fluid is obtained, using new needle for each attempt.

8. Collect CSF for diagnostic studies. Accurate opening pressure measurement is possible in a quiet infant.

a. Collect 1 ml of CSF in each of 3 to 4 tubes.

b. Send first sample for bacterial culture.

c. Send last sample for cell count unless fluid becomes visibly more bloody during tap.

d. Send remainder for desired chemical and microbiologic studies.

e. Look for clearing of fluid in successive collections in event of traumatic tap.

9. For myelography or instillation of chemotherapeutic agents, it is not necessary to remove spinal fluid.

10. For treatment of hydrocephalus, remove CSF until flow ceases (up to 10 minutes).

11. Remove needle and place adhesive bandage over puncture site.

F. COMPLICATIONS

1. Sudden intracranial decompression with herniation of cerebral tissue through foramen magnum

2. Cardiopulmonary arrest

3. Hypoxemia from knee-chest position[6–8]

4. Aspiration

5. Infection
   a. Meningitis from LP performed during bacteremia[28–30]
   b. Spinal abscess[31]
   c. Epidural abscess[32]
   d. Vertebral osteomyelitis[32]

6. Bleeding
   a. Spinal epidural hematoma[33]
   b. Spinal or intracranial subdural hematoma[34,35]
   c. Spinal or intracranial subarachnoid hematoma[35,36]
   d. Rupture of intracranial aneurysm[35]

7. Intraspinal epidermoid tumor from epithelial tissue introduced into spinal canal[21,22]

8. Spinal cord puncture and nerve damage if puncture site is above L2.

9. Sixth nerve palsy caused by removal of excessive CSF with resulting traction on nerve[37]

10. Deformity of lumbar spine secondary to acute spondylitis[38]

11. Contamination of CSF sample with blood from puncture of epidural venous plexus on posterior surface of vertebral body[23,25]

References

1. KJELDSBERG CR, KREIG AF: Cerebrospinal fluid and other body fluids. In Henry JB (ed): Clinical Diagnosis and Management by Laboratory Methods, 17th Ed. Philadelphia, WB Saunders, 1984, 459

2. GORELICK PB, BILLER J: Lumbar puncture: Techniques, indications, and complications. Postgrad Med J 79:257, 1986

3. ELDADAH M, FRENKEL LD, HIATT IM, HEGYI T: Evaluation of routine lumbar punctures in newborn infants with respiratory distress syndrome. Pediatr Infect Dis J 6:243, 1987

4. HENDRICKS-MUNOZ KD, SHAPIRO DL: The role of the lumbar puncture in the admission sepsis evaluation of the premature infant. J Perinatol 10:60, 1990

5. SCHWERSENSKI J, McINTYRE L, BAUER CR: Lumbar puncture frequency and cerebrospinal fluid analysis in the neonate. Am J Dis Child 145:54, 1991

6. SPAHR RC, MacDONALD HM, MUELLER-HEUBACH E: Knee-chest position and neonatal oxygenation and blood pressure. Am J Dis Child 135:79, 1981

7. WEISMAN LE, MERENSTEIN GB, STEENBARGER JR: The effect of lumbar puncture position in sick neonates. Am J Dis Child 137:1077, 1983

8. GLEASON CA, MARTIN RJ, ANDERSON JV, et al: Optimal position for a spinal tap in preterm infants. Pediatrics 71:31, 1983

9. LEBEL MH, McCRACKEN GH: Delayed cerebrospinal fluid sterilization and adverse outcome of bacterial meningitis in infants and children. Pediatrics 83:161, 1989

10. GOLDSTEIN GW, CHAPLIN ER, MAITLAND J: Transient hydrocephalus in premature infants: treatment by lumbar punctures. Lancet i:512, 1976

11. PAPILE L-A, BURSTEIN J, BURSTEIN R, et al: Posthemorrhagic hydrocephalus in low-birth weight infants: Treatment by serial lumbar punctures. J Pediatr 97:273, 1980

12. KREUSSER KL, TARBY TJ, KOVNAR E, et al: Serial lumbar punctures for at least temporary amelioration of neonatal posthemorrhagic hydrocephalus. Pediatrics 75:719, 1985

13. MANTOVANI JF, PASTERNAK JF, MATHEW OP, et al: Failure of daily lumbar punctures to prevent the development of hydrocephalus following intraventricular hemorrhage. J Pediatr 97:278, 1980

14. ANWAR M, KADAN S, HIATT IM, HEGYI T: Serial lumbar punctures in prevention of post-hemorrhagic hydrocephalus in preterm infants. J Pediatr 107:446, 1985

15. DYKES FD, DUNBAR B, LAZARRA A, AHMANN PA: Posthemorrhagic hydrocephalus in high-risk preterm infants: Natural history, management, and long-term outcome. J Pediatr 114:611, 1989

16. Ventriculomegaly Trial Group. Randomized trial of early tapping in neonatal posthemorrhagic ventricular dilatation. Arch Dis Child 65:3, 1990

17. MACMAHON P, COOKE RWI: Hyponatremia caused by repeated cerebrospinal fluid drainage in posthemorrhagic hydrocephalus. Arch Dis Child 58:385, 1983

18. SMITH KM, DEDDISH RB, OGATA ES: Meningitis associated with serial lumbar punctures and posthemorrhagic hydrocephalus. J Pediatr 109:1057, 1986

19. BELL W, MCCORMICK W: Increased Intracranial Pressure. Philadelphia, WB Saunders, 1978, 42

20. WEINSTEIN RA, BAUER FW, HOFFMAN RD, et al: Factitious meningitis: Diagnostic error due to nonviable bacteria in commercial lumbar puncture trays. JAMA 233:878, 1975

21. SHAYWITZ BA: Epidermoid spinal cord tumors and previous lumbar punctures. J Pediatr 80:638, 1972

22. BATNITZKY S, KEUCHER TR, MEALEY J, CAMPBELL RL: Iatrogenic intraspinal epidermoid tumors. JAMA 237:148, 1977

23. SCHREINER RL, KLEIMAN MB: Incidence and effect of traumatic lumbar puncture in the neonate. Dev Med Child Neurol 21:483, 1979

24. HUGHES WT, BUESCHER ES: Pediatric Procedures, 2nd Ed. Philadelphia, WB Saunders, 1980, 178

25. BONADIO WA: Interpreting the traumatic lumbar puncture. Contemporary Pediatrics 6:109, 1989

26. SWAIMAN KF: Pediatric Neurology. Baltimore, CV Mosby, 1989, 105

27. PORTER FL, MILLER JP, COLE FS, MARSHALL RE: A controlled clinical trial of local anesthesia for lumbar punctures in newborns. Pediatrics 88:663, 1991

28. ENG RHK, SELIGMAN SJ: Lumbar puncture-induced meningitis. JAMA 245:1456, 1981

29. TEELE DW, DASHEFSKY B, RAKUSAN T, KLEIN JO: Meningitis after lumbar puncture in children with bacteremia. N Eng J Med 305:1079, 1981

30. FEDER HM, ADELMAN AM, PUGNO PA, DALLMAN JJ: Meningitis following normal lumbar punctures. J Fam Pract 20:437, 1985

31. RIFAAT M, EL-SHAFEI I, SAMRA K, SOROUR O: Intramedullary spinal abscess following spinal puncture. J Neurosurg 38:366, 1973

32. BERGMAN I, WALD ER, MEYER JD, PAINTER MJ: Epidural abscess and vertebral osteomyelitis following serial lumbar punctures. Pediatrics 72:476, 1983

33. DULAC O, AICARDI J, LEPINTRE J, JARRIAU P: Hematome epi-dural intra-rachidien apres ponction lombaire. Arch Fr Pediatr 32:77, 1975

34. SPANU G, BERLANDA P, RODRIGUEZ Y, BAENA R: Spinal subdural haematoma: A rare complication of lumbar puncture. Neurochirurgia 31:157, 1988

35. HART IK, BONE I, HADLEY DM: Development of neurological problems after lumbar puncture. Br Med J 296:51, 1988

36. BLADE J, GASTON F, MONTSERRAT E, et al: Spinal subarachnoid hematoma after lumbar puncture causing reversible paraplegia in acute leukemia. J Neurosurg 58:438, 1983

37. BRYCE-SMITH R, MACINTOSH RR: Sixth-nerve palsy after lumbar puncture and spinal analgesia. Br Med J 1:275, 1951

38. LINTERMANS JP, SEYHNAEUE V: Spondolytic deformity of the lumbar spine and previous lumbar punctures. Pediatr Radiol 5:181, 1977

17 Subdural Tap

S. Lee Marban

A. INDICATIONS[1-3]

1. To diagnose acute convexity subdural collection
2. To sample convexity subdural collection for hematologic, microbiologic, and biochemical studies
3. To drain convexity subdural collection to reduce increased intracranial pressure and to prevent development of craniocerebral disproportion

A subdural tap can be performed on any infant whose coronal sutures are sufficiently open to allow passage of a needle. For diagnosis of acute subdural fluid collection, computerized tomography is preferred if patient can be moved to a radiology suite.

B. CONTRAINDICATIONS

1. General instability when risk exceeds benefit
2. Bleeding diathesis
3. Infection over puncture site
4. Repeated taps when infant is asymptomatic and head is not growing rapidly[2]

C. EQUIPMENT

All equipment is sterile except safety razor and face mask.

1. Gloves and face mask
2. Cup with iodophor antiseptic solution
3. Gauze swabs
4. Drapes or surgical towel
5. Two short bevel needles, 19- to 22-gauge × 1 inch, with stylets
6. Specimen tubes with caps
7. Adhesive bandage (optional)
8. Safety razor

D. PRECAUTIONS

1. Use strict aseptic technique as for major procedure. (See Chapter 4.)

2. Insert needle as far laterally as possible and at least 1 cm from midline to avoid puncturing sagittal sinus. Do not direct needle medially during insertion.
3. Allow fluid to drain spontaneously. Do not aspirate.
4. Remove needle if there is not a definite alteration of resistance on dural entry after penetration to approximately 0.5 to 1 cm.
5. Secure base of needle at all times to avoid inadvertent movement of needle tip.
6. If frequent taps are required, vary puncture site slightly to prevent fistula formation.
7. Following procedure, apply sufficient pressure to scalp to prevent subgaleal fluid collection.

E. TECHNIQUE[4,5]

1. Place infant supine, with crown of head at table edge.
2. Have assistant restrain infant and steady infant's head (Fig. 17-1).

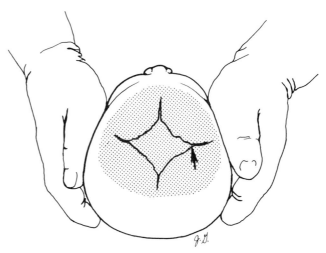

FIG. 17-1
Position and restraint for subdural tap. Stippling demonstrates area to be prepared for procedure. Arrow indicates site for needle puncture.

3. Shave head over a wide area surrounding anterior fontanelle (Fig. 17-1).
4. Locate junction of coronal sutures and fontanelle.
5. Put on mask. Wash hands and put on sterile gloves.
6. Clean fontanelle and surrounding area three times with antiseptic. (See Chapter 4 for aseptic preparation for major procedure.)
   a. Begin at fontanelle, and wash in enlarging circles.
   b. Allow antiseptic to dry. Blot excess with sterile gauze.
7. Place sterile towel under infant's head.
8. Locate coronal suture by palpation at lateral corner of anterior fontanelle.
9. Insert needle slowly through coronal suture, just lateral to its junction with anterior fontanelle (see Fig. 17-1).
   a. Hold needle perpendicular to skin surface.
   b. Grasp needle shaft with thumb and index finger, bracing hand against infant's head to main-

tain control of needle during insertion (Fig. 17-2).
10. Advance until "pop" is felt. Remove stylet (Fig. 17-2).
11. Allow fluid to drain spontaneously into sterile tubes until flow ceases.
12. If no fluid appears, remove needle slowly. Do not reinsert on same side.
13. Repeat procedure on opposite side with a new, sterile needle.
14. After removing needle, apply firm pressure to puncture site with sterile gauze.
15. Dress with small adhesive bandage if necessary.

F. COMPLICATIONS[4-6]

1. Subdural bleeding
   a. From laceration of superior sagittal sinus or smaller vessel
   b. From removal of excessive fluid

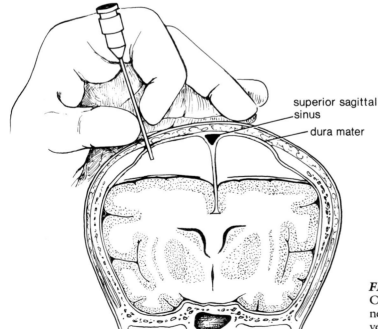

FIG. 17-2
Coronal section anatomic drawing showing subdural needle penetrating the dura in patient with bilateral convexity subdural fluid collections. Operator's fingers are placed for maximal stabilization of the needle.

2. Infection
3. Trauma to underlying cortex caused by inserting needle too far
4. Fistula formation after repeated taps
5. Subgaleal fluid accumulation

References

1. RABE EF: Subdural effusions in infants. Pediatr Clin North Am 14:831, 1967

2. VOLPE JJ: Neurology of the Newborn, 2nd Ed. Philadelphia, WB Saunders, 1987, 289
3. CURLESS RG: Subdural empyema in infant meningitis: Diagnosis, therapy, and prognosis. Childs Nerv Syst 1:211, 1985
4. ROSMAN NP: Subdural and ventricular taps. In Reece RM (ed): Manual of Emergency Pediatrics, 2nd Ed. Philadelphia, WB Saunders, 1978, 670
5. HUGHES WT, BUESCHER ES: Pediatric Procedures, 2nd Ed. Philadelphia, WB Saunders, 1980, 187
6. McDONALD JV: Hemorrhage as a complication of subdural puncture. Neurology 8:722, 1958

18 Suprapubic Bladder Aspiration

S. Lee Marban

A. INDICATIONS

To obtain urine for culture[1–8]

B. CONTRAINDICATIONS

1. Empty bladder due to recent void or dehydration

   A full bladder is essential for success of the procedure and avoidance of complications.

2. Skin infection over puncture site
3. Distention or enlargement of abdominal viscera (e.g., dilated loops of bowel, massive hepatomegaly)
4. Genitourinary anomaly with enlargement of pelvic structures (e.g., ovarian cyst, distention of vagina or uterus)
5. Bleeding diathesis

C. EQUIPMENT

All equipment is sterile (except transillumination light).

1. Gloves
2. Gauze sponges and cup with antiseptic solution, or
3. Prepared antiseptic-impregnated swabs
4. 3-ml syringe
5. 23-gauge × 1½-inch needle, or 23-gauge scalp-vein set

   Needle size from 25-gauge to 21-gauge may be used, but the needle must be 1 to 1½-inches in length.[1,3,5,7–11]

6. Transillumination light (optional)

D. PRECAUTIONS

1. Use strict aseptic technique.
2. Delay procedure if infant has urinated in last hour.

   If infant is systemically ill, do not delay antibiotic therapy for further urine production.

3. Correct bleeding diathesis before procedure. (Consider catheterization as alternative.)
4. Be certain of landmarks. Do not insert needle over pubic bone or off midline.

E. TECHNIQUE[1,3,7,8]

1. Have assistant restrain infant in supine, frog-leg position.
2. To avoid reflex micturition, ask assistant to
   a. Place tip of little finger in anus of female infant and apply pressure anteriorly, or
   b. Pinch base of penis gently in male infant.[1,2,8]
3. Determine presence of urine in bladder.
   a. Verify that diaper has been dry for at least 1 hour.
   b. Palpate or percuss bladder.
   c. Transilluminate (if there is no excess pubic fat or edema).[12]
4. Locate landmarks. Palpate top of pubic bone. The site for needle insertion is 1 to 2 cm above the symphysis pubis, in the midline (Fig. 18-1).
5. Wash hands and put on gloves.
6. Clean suprapubic area (including area over pubic bone) three times with antiseptic solution. Blot dry with sterile gauze.
7. Palpate symphysis pubis and insert needle 1 to 2 cm above symphysis in the midline (Fig. 18-2).
   a. Maintain needle perpendicular to table.
   b. Advance needle 2 to 3 cm. A slight decrease in resistance may be felt when the bladder is penetrated.
8. Aspirate gently.
   a. Withdraw needle if no urine is obtained.
   b. Do not probe with needle or attempt to redirect it to obtain urine.
   c. Wait at least 1 hour before repeating procedure.
9. Withdraw needle. Apply gentle pressure over puncture site with sterile gauze to stop any bleeding.

FIG. 18-1
The bladder in the neonate, with immediate anatomical relations. Asterisk (*) indicates approximate site for needle insertion.

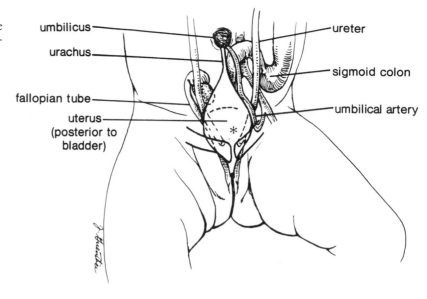

FIG. 18-2
(*A*) Insertion of needle 1 to 2 cm above symphysis pubis. (*B*) Midline sagittal section to emphasize the intraabdominal position of the full bladder in the neonate and its posterior anatomical relations.

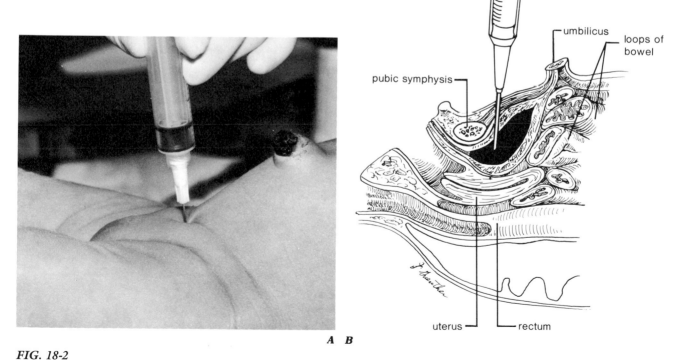

A   B

10. Remove needle and place sterile cap on syringe, or transfer urine to sterile container to send for culture.

F. COMPLICATIONS

1. Bleeding
   a. Transient microscopic hematuria[4,8]
   b. Gross hematuria[3,5,6,11,13,14]
   c. Abdominal wall hematoma[15]
   d. Bladder wall hematoma[5,16]
   e. Pelvic hematoma[17]
2. Infection
   a. Abdominal wall abscess[10,18]
   b. Sepsis[19,20]
   c. Osteomyelitis of pubic bone[21]
3. Perforation
   a. Bowel[10,20,22,23]
   b. Pelvic organ[22]

References

1. HUGHES WT, BUESCHER ES: Pediatric Procedures, 2nd Ed. Philadelphia, WB Saunders, 1980, 287
2. PRYLES CV: Percutaneous bladder aspiration and other methods of urine collection for bacteriologic study. Pediatrics 36:128, 1965
3. NELSON JD, PETERS PC: Suprapubic aspiration of urine in premature and term infants. Pediatrics 36:132, 1965
4. BAILEY RR, LITTLE PJ: Suprapubic bladder aspiration in diagnosis of urinary infection. Br Med J 1:293, 1969
5. SACCHAROW L, PRYLES CV: Further experience with the use of percutaneous suprapubic aspiration of the urinary bladder. Pediatrics 43:1018, 1969
6. SHANNON FT, SEPP E, ROSE GR: The diagnosis of bacteriuria by bladder puncture in infancy and childhood. Aust Paediatr J 5:97, 1969
7. ABBOTT GD, SHANNON FT: How to aspirate urine suprapubically in infants and children. Clin Pediatr 9:277, 1970
8. STEVENS DC, SCHREINER RL, GRESHAM EL: Suprapubic bladder aspiration in the neonate. Perinatology/Neonatology 5:47, 1981
9. ARONSON AS, GUSTAFSON B, SVENNINGSEN NW: Combined suprapubic aspiration and clean-voided urine examination in infants and children. Acta Paed Scand 62:396, 1973
10. POLNAY, L, FRASER AM, LEWIS JM: Complications of suprapubic bladder aspiration. Arch Dis Child 50:80, 1975
11. CARLSON KP, PULLON DHH: Bladder hemorrhage following transcutaneous bladder aspiration. Pediatrics 60:765, 1977
12. BUCK JR, WEINTRAUB WH, CORAN AG, et al: Fiberoptic transillumination: A new tool for the pediatric surgeon. J Pediatr Surg 12:451, 1977
13. LANIER B, DAESCHNER CW: Serious complication of suprapubic aspiration of the urinary bladder. J Pediatr 79:711, 1971
14. ROCKOFF AS: Hemorrhage after suprapubic bladder aspiration. J Pediatr 89:327, 1976
15. KUNZ HH, SIEBERTH HG, FREIBERG J, et al: Zur Bedeutung der Blasenpunktion fur den sicheren Nachweis einer Bakteriurie. Deutsche Medizinische Wochenschrift 100:2252, 1975
16. MORELL RE, DURITZ G, OLTORF C: Suprapubic aspiration associated with hematoma. Pediatrics 69:455, 1982
17. MANDELL J, STEVENS P: Supravesical hematoma following suprapubic urine aspiration. J Urol 119:286, 1978
18. UHARI M, REMES M: Suprapubic abcess—A complication of suprapubic bladder aspiration. Arch Dis Child 52:985, 1977
19. MUSTONEN A, UHARI M: Is there bacteremia after suprapubic aspiration in children with urinary tract infection? J Urol 119:822, 1978
20. PASS RF, WALDO FB: Anaerobic bacteremia following suprapubic bladder aspiration. J Pediatr 94:748, 1979
21. KALAGER T, DIGRANES A: Unusual complication after suprapubic bladder puncture. Br Med J 1:91, 1979
22. WEATHERS WT, WENZEL JE: Suprapubic aspiration: Perforation of a viscus other than the bladder. Am J Dis Child 117:590, 1969
23. SCHREINER RL, SKAFISH P: Complications of suprapubic bladder aspiration. Am J Dis Child 132:98, 1978

19 Bladder Catheterization

S. Lee Marban

A. INDICATIONS

1. To obtain urine for culture, particularly when suprapubic collection is contraindicated and when clean-catch specimen is unsatisfactory[1,2]
2. To precisely monitor urinary output[1]
3. To quantify bladder residual[2,3]
4. To relieve urinary retention (e.g., in neurogenic bladder)[4–6]
5. To perform cystography[2,7]

B. CONTRAINDICATIONS

In the presence of bleeding diathesis, risk–benefit considerations are important.

C. EQUIPMENT

All equipment is sterile.

1. Gloves
2. Gauze sponges and cup with antiseptic solution (not containing alcohol), or
3. Prepared antiseptic impregnated swabs
4. Towels for draping
5. Surgical lubricant
6. Cotton-tipped applicators
7. 5 Fr infant feeding tube
8. Container for specimen collection

D. PRECAUTIONS

1. Use strict aseptic technique.
2. Use adequate illumination.
3. Avoid vigorous irrigation of perineum in preparation for catheterization. This may introduce infection into the urinary tract.
4. Avoid separating labia minora too widely to prevent tear of fourchette.
5. Use catheter of smallest diameter (5 Fr) to avoid traumatic complications.
6. Do not force catheter. If catheter does not pass easily, suspect obstruction and abandon procedure.
7. To avoid coiling and knotting, insert catheter only as far as necessary to obtain urine.
8. If urine is not obtained in female infant, recheck location of catheter by visual inspection or by radiographic examination. It may have passed through introitus into vagina.
9. Remove catheter as soon as possible to avoid infectious complications.
10. If catheter can not be removed easily, do not force. Consult urology; it may be knotted.

E. TECHNIQUE

Male Infant[1,7]

1. Set up equipment, and squeeze small amount of lubricant onto sterile field.
2. Restrain infant supine in frog-leg position.
3. Wash hands and put on gloves.
4. Stabilize shaft of penis with nondominant hand. This hand is now considered contaminated.
5. If infant is uncircumcised, gently retract foreskin just enough to expose meatus.

   The young male infant has physiologic phimosis and foreskin usually cannot be fully retracted.[7]

6. Apply gentle pressure on penis to avoid reflex micturition.
7. Using free hand for rest of procedure, clean glans three times with antiseptic solution. Begin at meatus and work outward and down shaft of penis. Blot dry with sterile gauze.
8. Drape sterile towels across lower abdomen and across infant's legs.

121

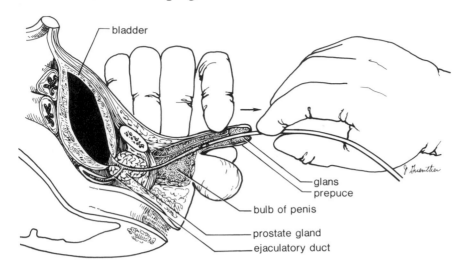

FIG. 19-1
Anatomic drawing demonstrating bladder catheterization in the male.

bladder

glans
prepuce
bulb of penis
prostate gland
ejaculatory duct

→ direction of gentle traction on penis

9. Place wide end of feeding tube into specimen container.
10. Lubricate tip of feeding tube copiously.
11. Move specimen container and feeding tube onto sterile drape between infant's legs.
12. Gently insert feeding tube through meatus only until urine is seen in tube (Fig. 19-1).
   a. Do not insert extra tubing length in attempt to stabilize indwelling catheter. This will increase risk of knotting.[15–18]
   b. During insertion, apply gentle caudal traction on penile shaft to prevent kinking of urethra (Fig. 19-1).
   c. If resistance is met at external sphincter, hold catheter in place with minimal pressure. Generally, spasm will relax after several minutes, allowing easy passage of catheter.[1,7] If not, suspect obstruction and abandon procedure.
   d. Do not move catheter in and out. This will increase risk of urethral trauma.
   e. If there is phimosis or tightly adherent foreskin, attempt to line up preputial ring and meatus.[7] If meatus cannot be visualized, insert catheter through preputial ring in slightly inferior direction. If there is any question about catheter position, abandon procedure.
13. Collect specimen for culture.
14. If catheter is to remain indwelling, connect feeding tube immediately to a closed sterile system for urine collection. Tape tube securely to inner thigh.
15. If catheter is to be removed, gently withdraw it when urine flow ceases.

Female Infant[1,2,7,8]
1. Follow steps 1 through 3 of technique for male infant.
2. Retract labia minora
   a. Use sterile gauze sponges with nondominant hand, or
   b. Have assistant retract labia with two cotton-tipped applicators (Fig. 19-2).
3. Using free hand for rest of procedure, cleanse area between labia minora three times with antiseptic solution.
   a. Swab in anterior to posterior direction to avoid drawing fecal material into field.[1]
   b. Blot dry with sterile gauze.
4. Follow steps 8 through 11 of technique for male infant.
5. Visualize meatus (Fig. 19-2).
   a. Most prominent structure is vaginal introitus. Urethral meatus lies immediately anterior (between clitoris and introitus).
   b. Meatus may be obscured by introital fold. Gently push fold down with cotton-tipped applicator.[2]

FIG. 19-2
External genitalia in the female. Retraction of labia majora and minora with cotton-tipped applicators. Arrow indicates urethral meatus.

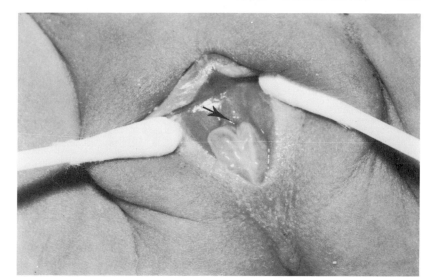

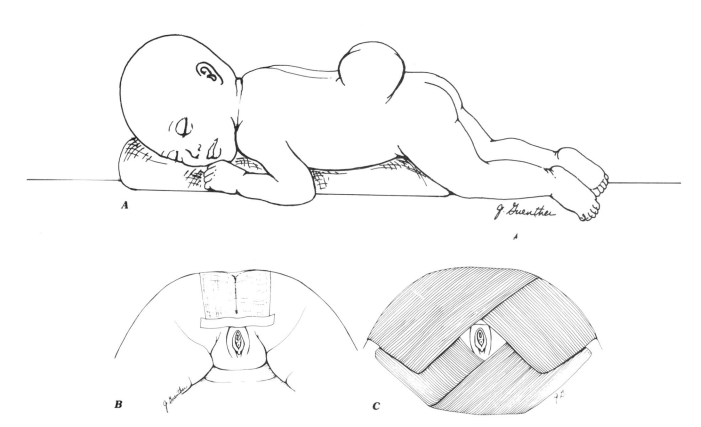

FIG. 19-3
(*A*) Position of infant for prone catheterization. (*B*) Placement of gauze pad over anus. (*C*) Placement of drapes. (Adapted from Campbell J: Catheterizing prone female infants: How can you see what you're doing? MCN 4:376, 1979. Based on drawing by NL Gahan.)

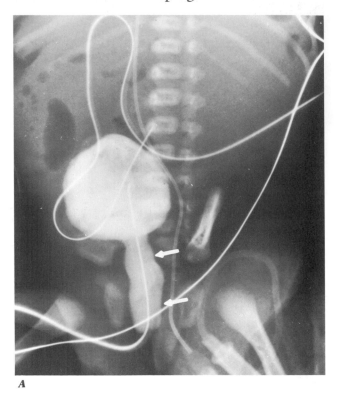

A

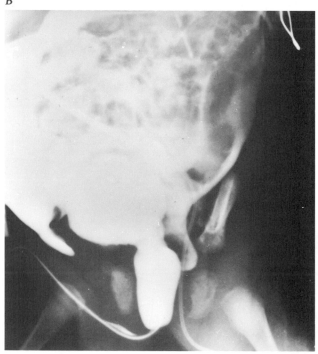

B

c. If meatus is not visible, infant may have female hypospadias (meatus is on roof of vagina, just inside introitus).[7] Urethra must be catheterized blindly, which may require curved tip catheter or urologic assistance.

6. Gently insert catheter only until urine appears in tube. Do not insert extra tubing.

7. Follow steps 13 through 15 of technique for male infant.

Female Infant in Prone Position[9]

This technique is useful in an infant who cannot be placed supine (e.g., one with large myelomeningocele).

1. Position infant prone on folded blanket so head and trunk are elevated about 3 inches above knees and lower legs. Hips should be flexed with knees abducted (Fig. 19-3A).

2. Place gauze pad over anus and secure with tape across buttocks, to avoid contamination of perineum from reflex bowel evacuation (Fig. 19-3B).

3. Follow procedure for female catheterization above. Place sterile drapes as shown in Fig. 19-3C.

F. COMPLICATIONS

1. Mechanical
   a. Catheter malposition[7,11]
   b. Catheter knot[15–18]
2. Trauma
   a. Urethral erosion or tear[11]
   b. Urethral false passage[11,12]
   c. Perforation of urethra or bladder (Fig. 19-4)[11,13]
   d. Tear of fourchette[11]
   e. Urethral stricture[14]
   f. Urinary retention secondary to urethral edema[11]
3. Infection[10,11]
   a. Urethritis
   b. Epididymitis
   c. Cystitis
   d. Pyelonephritis
   e. Sepsis

FIG. 19-4
(*A*) Cystogram showing dilated posterior urethra (arrows) secondary to posterior urethral valves. (*B*) Subsequent film shows perforation of the bladder, with free contrast material in the peritoneal cavity.

References

1. HUGHES WT, BUESCHER ES: Pediatric Procedure, 2nd Ed. Philadelphia: WB Saunders, 1980, 283
2. REDMAN JF, BISSADA NK: Direct bladder catheterization in infant females and young girls. Clin Pediatr 15:1060, 1976
3. MAINPRIZE TC, DRUTZ HP: Accuracy of total bladder volume and residual urine measurements: Comparison between real-time ultrasonography and catheterization. Am J Obstet Gynecol 1960:1013, 1989
4. BORZYSKOWSKI M, MUNDY AR: The management of the neuropathic bladder in childhood. Pediatr Nephrol 2:56, 1988
5. JOSEPH DB, BAUER SB, COLODNY AH, et al: Clean intermittent catheterization of infants with neurogenic bladder. Pediatrics 84:78, 1989
6. BASKIN LS, KOGAN BA, BENARD F: Treatment of infants with neurogenic bladder dysfunction using anticholinergic drugs and intermittent catheterisation. Br J Urol 66:532, 1990
7. BEN-AMI T, LEBOWITZ RL: Pediatric uroradiology. In Retik AB, Cukier J, (eds): Pediatric Urology. Baltimore, Williams and Wilkins, 1986, 32
8. REDMAN JF: Techniques of genital examination and bladder catheterization in female children. Urol Clin North Am 17:1, 1990
9. CAMBELL J: Catheterizing prone female infants: How can you see what you're doing? American Journal of Maternal Child Nursing 4:376, 1979
10. TURCK M, GOFFE B, PETERSDORF RG: The urethral catheter and urinary tract infection. J Urol 88:834, 1962
11. McALISTER WH, CACCIARELLI A, SHACKELFORD GD: Complications associated with cystography in children. Radiology 111:167, 1974
12. KOLEILAT N, SIDI AA, GONZALEZ R: Urethral false passage as a complication of intermittent catheterization. J Urol 142:1216, 1989
13. HUGHES JP, GAMBEE J, EDWARDS C: Perforation of the bladder: A complication of long-dwelling Foley catheter. J Urol 109:237, 1973
14. EDWARDS LE, LOCK R, POWELL C, JONES P: Postcatheterisation urethral strictures. A clinical and experimental study. Br J Urol 55:53, 1983
15. SUGAR EC, FIRLIT CF: Knot in urethral catheter due to improper catheterization technique. Urology 22:673, 1983
16. KLEIN EA, WOOD DP, KAY R: Retained straight catheter: Complications of clean intermittent catheterization. J Urol 135:780, 1986
17. KANENGISER S, JUSTER F, KOGAN S, RUDDY R: Knotting of a bladder catheter. Pediatr Emerg Care 5:37, 1989
18. ANDERSON MH: Urethral catheter knots. Pediatrics 85:852, 1990

20 *Tympanocentesis*

S. Lee Marban

A. INDICATIONS

1. To confirm diagnosis of otitis media in infant who presents with signs of sepsis and abnormal tympanic movement on pneumomassage[1-5]

   The normal newborn tympanic membrane is relatively dull and white, often without a light reflex[6] (see Color Fig. 20-1 at the beginning of this book). Otitis media is diagnosed primarily by decreased mobility of the drum, with or without erythema.[6] Symptoms are more systemic than localized.[7,8]

2. To identify specific causative organisms[1,4,6-10]
   a. In hospitalized neonate, where more unusual causative organisms may be present
   b. In infant with onset while on antibiotics
   c. When there is unsatisfactory response to antimicrobial therapy

B. CONTRAINDICATIONS

Inability to clearly visualize tympanic membrane and its landmarks

C. EQUIPMENT

All equipment is sterile (except ear curette)

1. Gloves
2. Cotton-tipped culture swabs and appropriate culture medium
3. Cup containing 70% ethyl alcohol
4. Gauze sponges
5. Puncturing device (Fig. 20-1)
   a. 18-gauge to 22-gauge × 3½-inch spinal needle,[6-8,10-12] without stylet, or
   b. Intravenous cannula-stylet device for alternative method[13] (see below)
6. Otoscope with open operating head and speculum (Use largest speculum that will fit into external auditory meatus.)
7. Suction trap (Fig. 20-1)
   a. 3-ml syringe, or
   b. 30-inch IV extension tubing attached to plunger-free tuberculin syringe by catheter adapter[12]

   If catheter adapter is not available, male adapter end of tubing can be wrapped with ½-inch cloth tape to ensure snug fit into syringe.

8. Blunt ear curette

D. PRECAUTIONS

1. Be sure of landmarks on tympanic membrane (TM). Clean external auditory canal (EAC) adequately to ensure good visualization.
2. Have assistant restrain infant securely.
3. Advance needle only as far as required to obtain fluid (just beyond point of puncture of TM).
4. Avoid procedure if blue color is noted behind TM. Blue discoloration may be due to defect in bony floor of tympanic cavity which allows jugular bulb to enter middle ear.[10,11]
5. Avoid superior portion of TM to prevent injury to middle ear structures.[10,11]
6. Avoid margin of TM and handle of malleus. Puncture at these sites may result in development of cholesteatoma.[10]

E. TECHNIQUE

1. Immobilize infant.
2. Obtain culture from EAC for comparison with culture from middle ear. This may help distinguish between contaminant and true pathogen in middle ear fluid.
3. Clean EAC of vernix, cerumen, and debris with ear curette.

FIG. 20-1
Equipment for aspiration of middle ear. Bent spinal needle is attached directly to 3-ml syringe (top), or to 30-inch IV extension tubing attached to tuberculin syringe by catheter adapter (bottom).

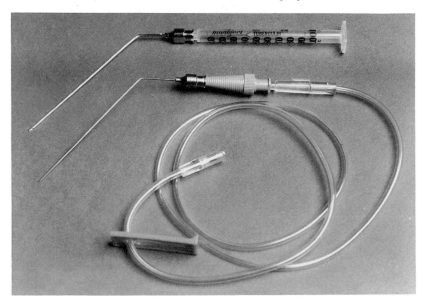

4. Ensure good visualization of TM and identify landmarks[6] (Fig. 20-2; also see Color Fig. 20-1 at beginning of this book).
   a. In neonates, TM is angled more sharply than in adult and may be more difficult to see. Upward traction on pinna will straighten EAC and allow better visualization.
   b. Tympanocentesis should be performed only in anterior–inferior or posterior–inferior quadrant of TM.

5. Instill 70% alcohol into EAC for 60 seconds.

   Caution: No information is available regarding risk of antiseptic burns to EAC in neonates. Antisepsis is considered unnecessary by some authors.[8,10]

6. Remove alcohol by tilting head to allow drainage or by blotting with gauze wick. Allow EAC to dry completely.
7. Wash hands and put on sterile gloves.

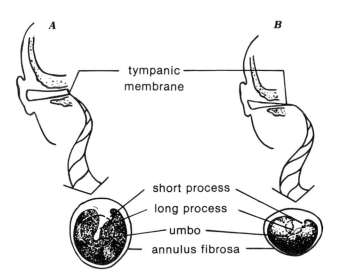

FIG. 20-2
Tympanic membrane in the adult (*A*) and infant (*B*). The portion of the tympanic membrane that may be visualized through the speculum at one time is within the dotted line.

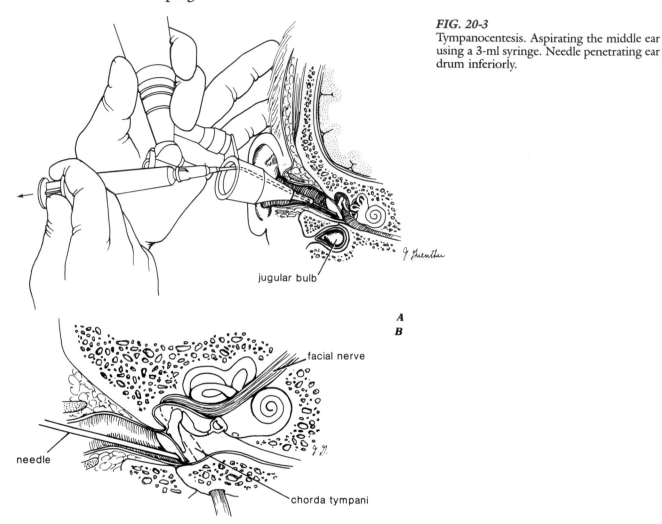

FIG. 20-3
Tympanocentesis. Aspirating the middle ear using a 3-ml syringe. Needle penetrating ear drum inferiorly.

jugular bulb

A
B

facial nerve

needle

chorda tympani

8. Bend spinal needle to 30 to 45 degree angle at a point two-thirds distance from tip.
9. Attach suction device to needle (Fig. 20-1).
    a. 3-ml syringe, or
    b. 30-inch IV extension tubing attached to plunger-free tuberculin syringe with catheter adapter or tape (see Equipment, above).
10. Insert otoscope. Advance needle through operating head into EAC. Puncture TM inferiorly as shown in Fig. 20-3.
11. Apply negative pressure to aspirate effusion by
    a. Pulling back gently on plunger of 3-ml syringe, or

    b. Applying oral negative pressure to IV extension tubing.
12. Withdraw needle and culture aspirate on appropriate medium.
    a. If fluid is visible in syringe, remove needle and expel fluid directly into culture medium. With tuberculin syringe method, reinsert sterile plunger to expel fluid.
    b. If fluid is not visible, remove syringe from needle and use cotton-tipped culture swab to remove fluid from hub of needle.[13] Send swab for culture.

Alternate Technique[14]

1. Prepare patient as described in steps 1 through 4 of general technique above. Preparation of EAC with alcohol is unnecessary because contamination of needle is prevented by cannula.
2. Wash hands and put on sterile gloves.
3. Bend needle of IV cannula-stylet set to 30 to 45 degree angle as described in general technique.
4. Slip cannula forward over bent needle to cover bevel (Fig. 20-4).
5. Attach 3-ml syringe.
6. Advance needle and cannula through operating head of otoscope to TM.
7. Retract cannula and perforate TM with needle.
8. Aspirate and culture fluid as described in general technique.

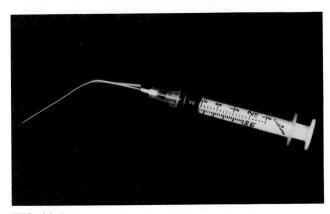

FIG. 20-4
Apparatus for alternative technique. Note plastic cannula advanced over needle tip.

F. COMPLICATIONS[10,11,15]

1. Damage to underlying structures from puncture of TM at incorrect site or excessive penetration
   a. Hearing loss from injury to ossicles
   b. Facial paralysis from facial nerve injury
   c. Ipsilateral impairment of taste from severance of chorda tympani
2. Hemorrhage
   a. Trauma to highly vascular EAC
   b. Perforation of jugular bulb
   c. Laceration of carotid artery
3. Cholesteatoma (ingrowth of epithelium from puncture of TM at margin or at handle of malleus)

References

1. TEELE DW, PELTON SI, KLEIN JO: Bacteriology of acute otitis media unresponsive to initial antimicrobial therapy. J Pediatr 98:537, 1981
2. BLUESTONE CD: Treatment of otitis media with effusion. Scand J Infect Dis (Suppl)39:26, 1983
3. BLUESTONE CD: Surgical management of otitis media. Pediatr Infect Dis 3:392, 1984
4. CARLIN SA, MARCHANT CD, SHURIN PA, et al: Early recurrences of otitis media: Reinfection or relapse? J Pediatr 110:20, 1987
5. ARRIAGA MA, BLUESTONE CD, STOOL SE: The role of tympanocentesis in the management of infants with sepsis. Laryngoscope 99:1048, 1989
6. BALKANY TJ, BERMAN SA, SIMMONS MA, JAFEK BW: Middle ear effusions in neonates. Laryngoscope 88:398, 1978
7. BLAND RD: Otitis media in the first six weeks of life: Diagnosis, bacteriology and management. Pediatrics 49:187, 1972
8. TETZLAFF TR, ASHWORTH C, NELSON JD: Otitis media in children less than twelve weeks of age. Pediatrics 59:827, 1977
9. SHURIN P, HOWIE V, PELTON S, et al: Bacterial etiology of otitis media during the first six weeks of life. J Pediatr 92:893, 1978
10. SCHWARTZ RH: Myringotomy: A neglected office procedure. Am Fam Physician 20:102, 1979
11. HUGHES WT, BUESCHER ES: Pediatric Procedures, 2nd Ed. Philadelphia, WB Saunders, 1980, 196
12. GUARISCO JL, GRUNDFAST KM: A simple device for tympanocentesis in infants and children. Laryngoscope 98:244, 1988
13. JANEKE JB: A hint for myringotomies in acute otitis media. South African Medical Journal 49:171, 1975
14. BROOK I: Otitis media in children: A prospective study of aerobic and anaerobic bacteriology. Laryngoscope 89:992, 1979
15. BLUESTONE CD, KLEIN JO: Intratemporal complications and sequelae of otitis media. In Bluestone CD, Stool SE (eds): Pediatric Otolaryngology, 2nd Ed. Philadelphia, WB Saunders, 1990, 452

21   Bone Marrow Aspiration

Mhairi G. MacDonald

A. INDICATIONS

1. Evaluation of hematologic disorders[1-5]
   a. Severe, persistent anemia
   b. Aplastic states, including monocellular types of bone marrow depression
   c. To differentiate leukemoid reaction from suspected leukemia
2. Evaluation of suspected storage disease (e.g., Neimann–Pick disease)[6]
3. Detection of metastatic tumor cells[7,8]
4. Culture, e.g., for fungal disease and disseminated tuberculosis
5. Cytogenic studies.[9,10] Allows chromosomal analysis (even after transfusion of donor blood) within 3 to 4 hours when mitotic figures present

B. CONTRAINDICATIONS

1. Sampling from sternum is absolutely contraindicated because of danger of damage to intrathoracic and mediastinal organs.
2. Risk/benefit should be considered carefully in presence of coexistent coagulopathy, such as hemophilia.

C. EQUIPMENT*

Sterile
1. Surgical gloves
2. Cup with antiseptic solution
3. Gauze squares
4. Transparent aperture drape
5. 0.5% lidocaine HCl without epinephrine in 2-ml syringe with 25-gauge venipuncture needle

6. 18-gauge bone marrow needle, approximately 3 cm long, with short, sharp bevel and fitted with adjustable metal guard (Fig. 21-1)

   Bone marrow aspiration has been successfully performed in preterm infants as young as 23 weeks gestational age using an Osgood bone marrow needle: 9-gauge, $1/2$ inch (personal communication, Robert D. Christenson, MD).†

7. Two 10-ml syringes with Luer–Lok‡

Unsterile
1. Small sandbag to aid in stabilizing limb
2. Clean glass slides and coverglasses
3. Other items, as indicated
   a. Wintrobe sedimentation tube for preparation for buffy-coat examination
   b. Wright's stain, Giemsa stain
   c. Acidified Zenker's solution for fixation of clot
   d. Appropriate culture media

D. PRECAUTIONS

1. Avoid sternal puncture.
2. Correct coagulopathy as far as possible prior to procedure.
3. Sandbags alone are not sufficient to stabilize limb (see E, Technique). Apply stabilizing counterpressure *directly* opposite site of penetration to avoid bone fracture.
4. Use maximum of 2 ml lidocaine. Aspirate before injection to avoid intravascular injection.
5. Be aware that less pressure is required to insert bone marrow needle than in older children.
6. Apply adequate pressure to control bleeding after procedure.

---

*A bone marrow aspiration kit that contains all equipment necessary, including a disposable Illinois bone marrow needle, is commercially available. Kormed Inc., 2510 Northland Drive, St. Paul, Minnesota 55120

†Popper and Sons, Inc., New Hyde Park, NY 10040

‡All available anticoagulants introduce some artifactual change in marrow specimen. It is our practice not to prepare the syringe routinely with anticoagulant unless performing a buffy-coat analysis.

E. TECHNIQUE

Tibia (Fig. 21-2)[1,11,12]

1. Use triangular area at proximal end of medial surface of tibia, approximately 1 cm medial and 1 cm distal to tibial tuberosity.
2. Have assistant restrain infant in supine position.
3. Place small sandbag directly beneath puncture site.
4. Prepare and drape as for major procedure (see Chap. 4).
5. Raise small, dermal bleb with lidocaine.
6. Wait 1 to 2 minutes.
7. Reintroduce venipuncture needle at center of bleb and infiltrate subcutaneous tissue as needle is slowly advanced.
8. Inject further small volume of lidocaine when needle reaches bone. (Tip of needle should be inserted into bone for subperiosteal injection.)
9. Place tip of forefinger on venipuncture needle to mark depth of penetration prior to removal.
10. Wait 2 to 3 minutes.
11. Adjust guard on shaft of bone marrow needle. Allow distance for penetration, which is 2 to 3 mm further than depth of penetration of venipuncture needle.
12. Check that bevel of bone marrow needle obturator is flush with bevel of needle.
13. Have an assistant support infant's limb *directly opposite* site of marrow puncture. (Alternatively, the

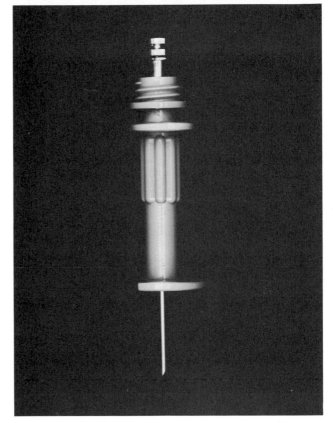

FIG. 21-1
Lateral view of disposable Illinois bone marrow needle.

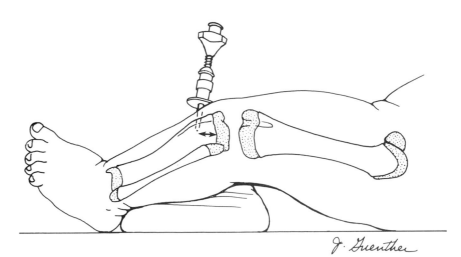

FIG. 21-2
Bone marrow aspiration from tibia. Arrow indicates distance of 1 cm.

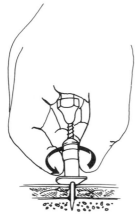

FIG. 21-3
Passing needle into bone with circular motion.

FIG. 21-4
Forcible withdrawal of plunger to obtain bone marrow aspirate.

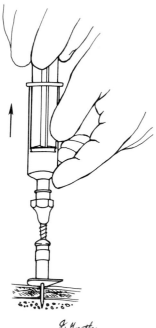

operator's nondominant hand can be used for support. However, this hand cannot be reintroduced into the sterile field.)

14. Hold needle between thumb and forefinger of dominant hand, with hub held against thenar eminence to provide control (Fig. 21-3).

15. Introduce needle at angle of 45 to 60 degrees to skin, directed caudally.

16. Pass needle into marrow cavity with slow, steady, circular motion.

17. Continue to advance needle until *firmly* fixed in bone (does not sway when touched).

18. Remove obturator from needle, and attach firmly to 10-ml syringe.

19. Withdraw plunger forcefully until drop of marrow appears in the syringe (Fig. 21-4).

> A drop of marrow is sufficient. Excessive suction may dilute sample.

20. Rotate, advance or retract needle if no marrow is obtained initially.

21. Remove syringe and place sample on slide (see *F*, Preparation of Marrow Smear).

22. Attach second syringe, rotate needle by 90 degrees, and repeat procedure if marrow is required for additional studies.

> If buffy-coat and volumetric studies are required, the sample should be collected in a syringe washed with EDTA anticoagulant and placed in a Wintrobe sedimentation tube for centrifugation.

23. Remove needle and apply pressure over site for 5 minutes or until there is hemostasis.

FIG. 21-5
Bone marrow aspiration from the femur. Arrow indicates distance of 1 to 2 cm.

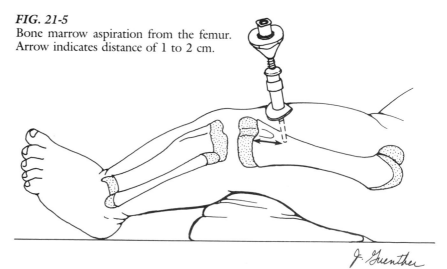

Femur (Fig. 21-5)

1. Use site in distal one third, midline anteriorly, 1 to 2 cm above lateral condyle.
2. Prepare site as for tibia.
3. Introduce bone marrow needle directed cephalad at a 60-degree angle to femur.
4. Complete procedure as for tibia.

Posterior Iliac Crest (Fig. 21-6)[13]

1. Have assistant restrain infant in lateral recumbent position, with hips flexed.
2. Locate site
   a. Superior and lateral to intergluteal cleft
   b. Inferomedial to crest of ilium
3. Prepare site as for tibia.
   a. Prepare skin area from sacrococcygeal junction in posterior midline to level of 2nd lumbar vertebra superiorly and over superior iliac spine anteriorly.
   b. Mark position of posterior iliac spine prior to administering local anesthetic, because bony landmarks may be lost.
4. Introduce needle (see Fig. 21-6).
   a. At midpoint of posterior iliac crest immediately superior to posterior superior iliac spine
   b. In line toward anterior-superior iliac spine, which may be palpated through drapes with free hand
5. Complete procedure as for tibia.

F. PREPARATION OF MARROW SMEAR

1. Clean slides with filter paper or 95% alcohol to remove all fingerprints.
2. Have assistant prepare smear as soon as sample is obtained.

Method A: Slide Method

1. Place drop of marrow on one end of slide (a), and set at 45-degree angle to allow blood to drip off (marrow particles will adhere to slide) (see Fig. 21-7 A).
2. Place second ("spreader") slide (b) on slide at a 45-degree angle, and allow marrow sample to adhere and diffuse laterally, almost to edges of spreader slide (see Fig. 21-7 B).
3. Place spreader slide with adherent marrow on third slide (c), and push forward with smooth movement to make homogeneous film with feather edge (see Fig. 21-7 C and D).

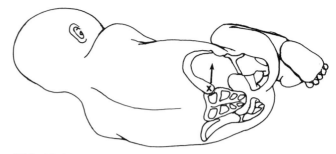

FIG. 21-6
Position for bone marrow aspiration from the posterior iliac crest. (*X*, site of needle entry; *arrow*, direction of needle penetration.

FIG. 21-7
Preparation of a bone marrow smear. (*A*) Marrow sample on angled slide. (*B*) Marrow particles adhering to end of spreader—slide *b*. (*C* and *D*) Making marrow smear on slide *c*.

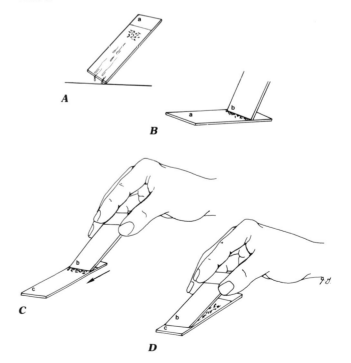

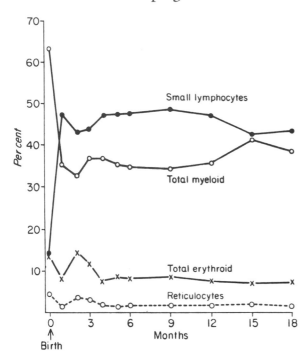

FIG. 21-8
Changes in mean percent incidence of small lymphocytes, myeloid cells, and erythroblasts in bone marrow of normal infants. Blood reticulocytes are shown for comparison with the erythroid changes in the marrow. The mean values for month 0 (birth) were obtained during the first 4 days after birth. (Rosse C, Kraemer MJ, Dillon TL, et al: Bone marrow cell populations of normal infants: The predominance of lymphocytes. J Lab Clin Med 89:1233, 1977. Reprinted with permission.)

4. Allow to air dry before staining (see Fig. 21-8, bone marrow cell populations in normal infants[3]).

Method B: Coverglass Method[11]

1. Hold coverglass by its corner in left hand.
2. Place small drop of marrow at center of coverglass.
3. Hold second coverglass in right hand.
4. Approximate two slides over each other, and allow marrow to spread evenly between two surfaces.
5. Separate coverglasses with sliding maneuver before fluid reaches edges.
6. Allow preparation to air dry before staining (see Fig. 21-8, bone marrow cell populations in normal infants[3]).

G. PROCESSING MARROW FROM SECOND "DRAW"[14–16]

According to examination required:

1. Allow marrow to clot in syringe, and squirt into Zenker's solution for tissue section and histologic review, or
2. Place anticoagulated specimen in Wintrobe tube for centrifugation for volumetric analysis (Fig. 21-9), or
3. Examine slides microscopically prior to staining if patient thought to have lipid storage disease, or
4. Place marrow obtained for chromosomal analysis in tissue-culture medium, or
5. Place marrow for culture into appropriate medium.

H. COMPLICATIONS

1. Subperiosteal bleeding[17]
2. Injury to blood vessels[13]
3. Limb fracture[13]
4. Cellulitis or osteomyelitis[1,18]
5. Sternal penetration[19,20]
   a. Pneumothorax
   b. Mediastinitis
   c. Pneumomediastinum
   d. Pericardial hemorrhage or tamponade
   e. Hemothorax[1]
6. Bone changes on x-ray film
   a. Lytic lesions[17]
   b. Exostoses[21]
   c. Subperiosteal calcification (secondary to hematoma)[20]
7. Respiratory compromise due to positioning

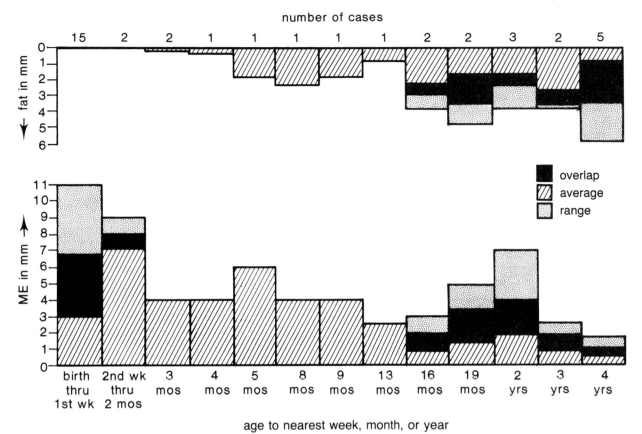

FIG. 21-9
Tibial aspirations. Influence of age on myeloid (ME) and fat values. (Sturgeon P: Volumetric and microscopic pattern of bone marrow in normal infants and children. Pediatrics 7:584, 1951. Copyright © American Academy of Pediatrics, 1951)

References

1. Downing V: Bone marrow examination in children. Pediatr Clin North Am 2:243, 1955
2. Oski F: Neonatal hematology: The erythrocyte and its disorders. In Nathan DC, Oski F (eds): Hematology in Infancy and Childhood, 3rd ed, pp 25–27. Philadelphia, WB Saunders, 1987
3. Rosse C, Kraemer MJ, Dillon TL, et al: Bone marrow cell populations of normal infants: The predominance of lymphocytes. J Lab Clin Med 89:1225, 1977
4. Pease G: Bone marrow findings in disorders of the hemopoietic system: A review. Am J Clin Pathol 25:654, 1955
5. Smith C: Bone marrow examination in blood disorders of infants and children. Med Clin North Am 31:525, 1947
6. Sloan H, Breslow J: Foam cells. In Nathan D, Oski F (eds): Hematology of Infancy and Childhood. Philadelphia, WB Saunders, 1974, p 760
7. Delta B, Pinkel D: Bone marrow aspiration in children with malignant tumors. J Pediatr 64:542, 1964
8. Mackay B, Massae S, King O, Butler J: Diagnosis of neuroblastoma by electron microscopy of bone marrow aspirates. Pediatrics 56:1045, 1975
9. Golomb HM, Vardiman JW, Rowley JD et al: Correlation of clinical findings with Quinacrine-banded chromosomes in 90 adults with acute non-lymphocytic leukemia. N Eng J Med 299:613, 1978
10. Page B, Coulter J: Bone marrow aspirations for chromosome analysis in newborn. Br Med J 1:1455, 1978
11. Propp S: An improved technique of bone marrow aspiration. Blood 6:585, 1951

12. STURGEON P: Volumetric and microscopic pattern of bone marrow in normal infants and children. Pediatrics 7:577, 1951

13. MILLER D: Normal values and examination of the blood: Perinatal period, infancy, childhood, and adolescence. In Miller D, Pearson H, Baehner R, McMillan C (eds): Smith's Blood Diseases of Infancy and Childhood, pp 20–21. St Louis, CV Mosby, 1978

14. FONG TP, OKAFOR LA, SCHMITZ TH ET AL: An evaluation of cellularity in various types of bone marrow specimens. Am J Clin Pathol 72:812, 1979

15. GRUPPO R, LAMPKIN B, GRANGER S: Bone marrow cellularity determination comparison of the biopsy, aspirate, and buffy coat. Blood 49:29, 1977

16. JACOBS P, KAHN L: Marrow buffy coat and biopsy. Lancet 2:684, 1978

17. MCNUTT D, FUDENBERG H: Bone-marrow biopsy and osteoporosis. N Engl J Med 1:46, 1972

18. SHAH M, WATANAKUNAKORN C: *Staphylococcal aureus* sternal osteomyelitis complicating bone marrow aspiration. South Med J 71:348, 1978

19. KATO K: Sternal marrow puncture in infants and children. Am J Dis Child 54:209, 1937

20. BAKIR F: Fatal sternal puncture. Diseases of the Chest 44:435, 1963

21. MURPHY W: Exostosis after iliac bone marrow biopsy. AJR 129:1114, 1977

22 Punch Skin Biopsy

Marilea Kay Miller

A. INDICATIONS

1. Diagnosis of skin lesions[1-8]
2. Electron and light microscopic identification of certain hereditary and metabolic disorders[9-15]
3. Genetic, enzymatic, or morphologic studies on established fibroblast strains[16]

B. TYPES OF SKIN BIOPSY[6,10,17]

1. Punch skin biopsy is appropriate when full thickness is unnecessary
   a. Provides alternative to scraping, vaporizing, or cauterizing small lesions
   b. Allows pathologic evaluation and rapid diagnosis of certain conditions
2. Surgical excision by trained dermatologist or surgeon is preferable when
   a. It is important to examine junction between lesion and normal skin
   b. Lesions are atrophic, sclerotic, very elevated, or have large bulli
   c. It is important to acquire adequate, full thickness of skin
   d. It is planned to remove an entire, large lesion

C. CONTRAINDICATIONS

Bleeding disorder when risk outweighs benefits

D. EQUIPMENT

Sterile

1. Towel or tray to form sterile area
2. 70% alcohol or other suitable antiseptic agent
3. 4 × 4 gauze squares
4. Lidocaine HCL 1% without epinephrine in 1-ml tuberculin syringe with 27- or 30-gauge needle (Use epinephrine-free local anesthesia to avoid distorting skin vascularity.)
5. Blunt tissue forceps
6. Fine, curved scissors or no. 15 scalpel blade
7. Sharp 3 or 4 mm punch* (see Fig. 22-1)

   Skin biopsy has been performed on the fetus[11,18] and may be done postmortem on stillborn or recently deceased infants to produce fibroblast cultures for karyotype. Under the latter circumstances, punch or excisional biopsy from the freshest appearing, least macerated skin area(s) is appropriate.

8. 5-0 silk or nylon suture with small curved needle on needle holder, or Steristrip
9. Adhesive bandage

*Disposable punches ranging from 2 mm to 8 mm are available from Acuderm inc., 5370 N.W. 35 Terrace, Ft. Lauderdale, FL 33309, phone 1-800-327-0015.

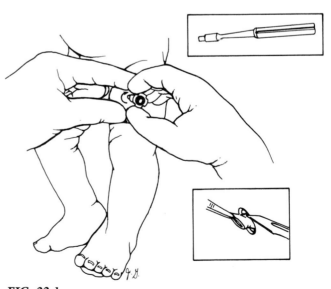

FIG. 22-1
Punch skin biopsy. (*Inset, top*) Disposable biopsy punch. (*Inset, bottom*) Cutting the dermal pedicle.

TABLE 22-1
Punch Biopsy Preservatives and Transport Media

Purpose	Fixation Technique/ Transport Media
Light microscopy	10% formalin
Electron microscopy	Glutaraldehyde 3% (chilled and neutral buffered)
Immunofluorescent studies	Michel's solution or quick freezing
Frozen sections	Liquid nitrogen
Fibroblast culture	Viral transport media or aerobic, nonradioactive blood culture media

Unsterile
1. Razor
2. Specific tissue fixative(s) and transport media (Table 22-1)

E. PRECAUTIONS

1. Avoid sites, if possible, where a small scar would potentially be cosmetically disfiguring
   a. Tip, bridge, and columella of nose
   b. Eyelids
   c. Lip margins
   d. Nipples
   e. Fingers or toes
   f. Areas overlying joints
   g. Lower leg below the knee
2. Avoid very small punch (2 mm or less), because this limits ability to interpret pathologic findings.
3. Avoid multiple applications to one site.
4. Be gentle, to avoid separating epidermis from dermis.
5. Check biopsy site for signs of infection until healing occurs.
6. Avoid freezing tissue for electron microscopy because cellular detail will then be destroyed (see Table 22-1).
7. Avoid placing biopsy specimen in or on saline because artifactual hydropic degeneration of basal cells and subepidermal bulli formation may occur.

F. TECHNIQUE[6,8,17,19,20]

See Figure 22-1.

1. Restrain and position patient
2. Choose site for biopsy.
   a. For melanocytic or keratinocytic nevi, choose more mature areas.
   b. When malignancy is suspected, take multiple biopsies of both early and fully developed lesions.
   c. For large, chronic lesions, obtain specimen from periphery, and include some normal skin.
   d. For diffuse eruptions, choose site that displays early, typical efflorescence.
   e. For acute eruptions and bullous disease, choose entire small early lesion, taking care to keep roof intact.
   f. For discrete small lesions, try to leave 1 to 2 mm margins of normal skin around the lesions.
   g. Avoid excoriated lesions.
3. Shave skin, if necessary.
4. Prepare as for minor procedure (see Chap. 4).
5. Inject 0.25 to 0.5 ml lidocaine intradermally beneath the lesion.
6. Wait 5 minutes.
7. Stretch skin surrounding lesion taut.
8. Carefully place punch over the lesion and twist in rotary back and forth cutting motion until subcutaneous fat is obtained. Biopsy should include epidermis, full thickness of dermis, and some subcutaneous fat.
9. Remove punch.
10. Use blunt forceps in one hand to transfix or grasp and elevate the biopsy.
11. Use scalpel blade or scissors in the other hand to transect or cut the punch specimen at its base as deep into the fat tissue as possible.
12. Place specimen in container with appropriate preservative or transport media.
13. Label container with patient name, date, and exact site of biopsy.
14. Control bleeding at site of biopsy with gentle pressure on sterile 4 × 4 gauze square.
15. If no suture is placed, expect healing by primary epithelialization in 7 to 14 days, with a resulting small white area a few millimeters in diameter if the biopsy extended to the dermis–subcutaneous fat interface. A similar scar will be seen, but healing occurs by secondary intention and takes slightly longer, if excision extends well into the subcutaneous fat.

16. If suture or steristrips are placed, leave for 5 days on face and for 12 days on trunk, limbs, or scalp.

G. COMPLICATIONS[6]

1. Infection
2. Unsightly scarring or keloid formation (rare)
3. Excessive bleeding (rare, except in patient with coagulation defect)

References

1. FRETZIN D: Biopsy in vesiculobullous disorders. Cutis 20:639, 1977
2. GRAHAM J, BARR R: Papulosquamous eruptions: Usefulness of biopsy in establishing diagnosis. Cutis 20:629, 1977
3. HAZELRIGG D, JARRATT M: Diagnosis of scabies. South Med J 68:549, 1975
4. MONTES L: How useful is a biopsy in a case of suspected fungal infection? Cutis 20:665, 1977
5. ROSES D, ACKERMAN A, HARRIS M, ET AL: Assessment of biopsy technique and histopathologic interpretations of primary cutaneous malignant melanoma. Ann Surg 189:294, 1979
6. SOLOMON L, ESTERLY N: Diagnostic procedures. In Solomon L, Esterly N (eds): Neonatal Dermatology, Philadelphia, WB Saunders, 1973, p 29
7. SOLTANI K, PACERNICK L, LORINCZ A: Lupus erythematosus-like lesions in newborn infants. Arch Dermatol 110:435, 1974
8. THOMPSON J, TEMPLE W, LAFRENIERE R, ET AL: Punch biopsy for diagnosis of pigmented skin lesions. Am Fam Physician 37:123, 1988
9. CARPENTER S, KARPATI G, ANDERMANN F: Specific involvement of muscle, nerve and skin in late infantile and juvenile amaurotic idiocy. Neurology 22:170, 1972
10. FARRELL D, SUMI S: Skin punch biopsy in the diagnosis of juvenile neuronal ceroid-lipofuscinosis. Arch Neurol 34:39, 1977
11. FLEISHER L, LONGHI R, TALLAN H, ET AL: Homocystinuria: Investigations of cystathionine synthase in cultured fetal cells and the prenatal determination of genetic status. J Pediatr 89:677, 1974
12. MARTIN J, CEUTERICK C: Morphological study of skin biopsy specimens: A contribution to the diagnosis of metabolic disorders with involvement of the nervous system. J Neurol Neurosurg Psychiatry 41:232, 1978
13. MARTIN J, JACOBS K: Skin biopsy as a contribution to diagnosis in late infantile amaurotic idiocy with curvilinear bodies. Eur Neurol 10:281, 1973
14. O'BRIEN J, BERNET J, VEATH M, PAA D: Lysosomal storage disorders: Diagnosis by ultrastructural examination of skin biopsy specimens. Arch Neurol 32:592, 1975
15. SPICER S, GARVIN A, WOHLTMANN H, SIMSON J: The ultrastructure of the skin in patients with mucopolysaccharidoses. Lab Invest 31:488, 1974
16. COOPER JT, GOLDSTEIN S: Skin biopsy and successful fibroblast culture. Lancet 2:673, 1973
17. ARNDT KA: Operative procedures. In Arndt KA (ed): Manual of Dermatologic Therapeutics. Boston, Little, Brown & Co, 1978, p 223
18. GOLBUS M, SAGEBIEL R, FILLY R, ET AL: Prenatal diagnosis of ichthyosiform erythroderma (epidermolytic hyperkeratosis) by fetal skin biopsy. N Engl J Med 302:93, 1980
19. ACKERMAN AB: Biopsy: Why, where, when, how. J Dermatol Surg 1:21, 1975
20. RUIZ-MALDONADO R, PARISH LC, BEARE JM: Therapeutic aspects of pediatric dermatology. In Ruiz-Maldonado R, Parish LC, Beare JM (eds): Textbook of Pediatric Dermatology. Philadelphia, Grune & Stratton, 1989, p 50

Part 5
Vascular Access

23 Peripheral Intravenous (IV) Line Placement

Mhairi G. MacDonald
Martin Raymond Eichelberger

Percutaneous Method

A. INDICATIONS

To provide partial or total fluid or nutritional requirements when provision via the gastrointestinal tract is not possible.

B. EQUIPMENT

Sterile

1. 70% alcohol swabs (or other antiseptic—see Chap. 4)
2. Appropriate needle (minimum 23-gauge for blood transfusion)
   a. 21- to 27-gauge butterfly needle
   b. 21- to 24-gauge over-the-needle cannula device
3. Connection for cannula
4. 2 × 2 gauze squares
5. Cotton balls
6. Isotonic saline in 3-ml syringe
7. Heparinized flush solution (heparin 1 to 2 U/ml in 0.25 to 0.5N saline) for heparin lock

Unsterile

1. Tourniquet
2. Procedure light
3. Materials for restraint (see Chap. 3)
4. Safety razor
5. Transilluminator (optional)
6. Warm compress to warm limb if necessary (e.g., disposable diaper, see D5)
7. Transparent, disposable medicine cup or small paper cup (optional)
8. Scissors

9. Roll of 0.5- to 1-inch porous adhesive tape, transparent tape, or semipermeable transparent dressings[1-6]
   a. If using tape, use the minimum amount necessary on fragile premature skin.
   b. Transparent tape or dressing will facilitate observation of IV site.
   c. Precut self-adhesive taping devices are available from Veni-Gard Jr.*

C. PRECAUTIONS

1. Avoid areas adjacent to superficial skin loss or infection.
2. Avoid vessels across joints, because immobilization is more difficult.
3. Take care to differentiate veins from arteries.
   a. Palpate for arterial pulsation.
   b. Note effect of vessel occlusion.
      (1) Limb vessel: arteries collapse; veins fill
      (2) Scalp vessel: arteries fill from below; veins fill from above
   c. Note color of blood obtained.
   d. Look for blanching of skin over vessel when fluid is infused (arterial spasm).
4. If limb requires warming prior to procedure, do not exceed 40°C (104°F). Pad should feel warm, *not* hot to touch.

   Always ensure that water is mixed (in tap or container) to desired temperature, before wetting pad. Sequential use of hot and cold sources can lead to uneven heating of the pad.

*Consolidated Medical Equipment Inc., 310 Broad Street, Utica, NY 13501

5. Shave adequate area of head to permit stabilization of the IV.
6. Apply tourniquet correctly (see D7 and Chap. 12).
   a. Minimize time applied.
   b. Avoid use in areas with compromised circulation.
   c. Avoid use for scalp vessels—tends to increase vessel fragility.
7. When using peripheral scalp veins, avoid sites beyond the hair line.
8. We do not recommend the use of nitroglycerin to dilate the vein, as described by Hecker et al[7] or Vaksman et al[8] because of the potential for side-effects and apparent lack of effectiveness in the neonate.[9,10]
9. Be aware that it has been reported that bacterial contamination, phlebitis, and septicemia are more common with use of plastic cannulae.[11–15]
10. Be alert for signs of phlebitis or infiltration.
    a. Inspect site hourly.
    b. Discontinue IV immediately at any sign of local inflammation or cannula malfunction.
    c. Consider changing IV site every 72 hours to avoid complications.[16,17] Rotation of IV site prior to onset of complications allows reuse of veins within 4 to 7 days.
11. Arrange tape dressing at IV site to allow adequate inspection or use transparent sterile dressing over site of skin entry.[18]

    Leibovici was unable to show a positive impact of a daily change of the dressing, as compared to change every 72 hours, on the incidence of infusion phlebitis.[19] Maki et al recommended not removing the transparent dressing until the catheter/needle is removed.[4]

12. Consider use of protective skin preparation in small premature infants, to prevent skin trauma on removal of tape or dressing.*
    a. Forms tough, protective coating, which bonds to skin
    b. Does not require removal when changing dressing

---

*For example, Skin Prep protective dressing wipes. United Division of Howmedica, Inc., 11775 Starkey Road, Largo, FL 33543

13. Write date, time, and needle/cannula size on piece of tape secured to site.
14. Loop IV tubing and tape onto forearm, to take tension off the IV device.

D. TECHNIQUE

1. Prepare as for minor procedure (see Chap. 4).
2. Use transillumination to visualize vessel if needed (see Chap. 11).
3. Select vessel for cannulation. The following is the suggested order of preference (see Fig. 12-1).
   a. Back of hand—dorsal venous plexus
   b. Forearm—median antebrachial, accessory cephalic veins
   c. Scalp veins—supratrochlear, superficial temporal, posterior auricular
   d. Foot—dorsal venous plexus
   e. Acutecubital fossa—basilic or cubital veins
   f. Ankle—small saphenous, great saphenous veins
4. Shave area if using scalp vein.
5. Warm limb with warm compress, if necessary (rarely needed) for approximately 5 minutes.
6. Restrain extremity on IV board (see Chap. 3).
7. Apply tourniquet if anatomical site indicates.
   a. Place as close to venipuncture site as possible.
   b. Tighten until peripheral pulsation stops.
   c. Release partially until arterial pulse is fully palpable.
8. Prepare skin area with antiseptic. Allow to dry.
9. Attach syringe to needle/cannula and test patency by forcing small amount of saline through.
10. Detach syringe.
11. Select straight segment of vein or confluence of two tributaries.
12. Grasp needle between thumb and first finger. For butterfly needle, grasp plastic wings (Fig. 23-1).
13. Anchor vein with index finger of free hand, and stretch skin overlying it. This maneuver may also be used to produce distention of scalp veins.
14. Hold needle parallel to vessel, in direction of blood flow.
15. Introduce needle through skin, a few millimeters distal to point of entry into vessel (see Chap. 12).
16. Introduce needle gently into vessel until blood appears in tubing of scalp-vein needle, or in cannula on withdrawal of stylet.

When using a very small vessel, or in an infant with poor peripheral circulation, blood may not appear immediately in tubing. *Wait.* If in doubt, inject a small amount of saline after releasing tourniquet.

17. Remove stylet. Do not advance needle further, because back wall of vessel may be pierced.
18. Advance cannula as far as possible.

    Injecting a small amount of blood or flush solution into the vein prior to advancing the cannula may assist cannulation (Fig. 23-2).[20]

19. Remove tourniquet.
20. Infuse small amount of saline gently to confirm intravascular position.
21. Anchor needle or cannula as shown in Figures 23-3 and 23-4.
22. Attach IV tubing and secure to skin. (Tubing of butterfly needle should be secured to skin lateral to needle.)

E. CONVERSION OF PERIPHERAL IV LINE TO A HEPARIN LOCK

1. Wash hands and put on gloves.
2. Clean IV tubing and catheter connection with antiseptic solution.
3. Stop intravenous infusion and remove IV tubing from hub of IV needle or cannula.
4. Seal hub with a sterile, plug or T-connector system (e.g., Argyle intermittent infusion plug* or Burron spin-lock port extension set† that has been primed with the required quantity of heparinized saline).

   As an improvisation, a stopcock with two dead heads may be used. However, at least 3 ml of flush solution is necessary to flush all parts of a stopcock. This increases the margin for error, with possible fluid overload in very small premature infants.

5. Clean plug with antiseptic and inject 0.4 to 0.8 ml heparinized saline solution through plug to flush blood from needle or cannula.
6. Clean plug with antiseptic prior to every use.

*Sherwood Medical Company, St. Louis, MO 63103
†Burron Medical Inc., Bethlehem, PA 18018

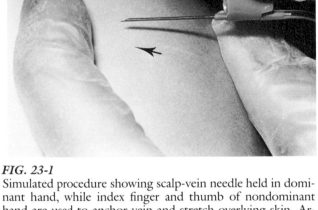

FIG. 23-1
Simulated procedure showing scalp-vein needle held in dominant hand, while index finger and thumb of nondominant hand are used to anchor vein and stretch overlying skin. Arrow indicates direction of blood flow.

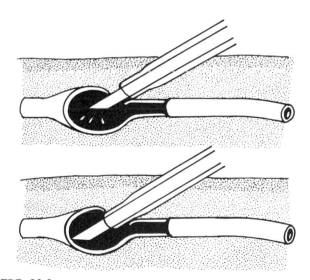

FIG. 23-2
Injecting a small amount of blood or flush solution will distend wall of vein and facilitate cannulation. (Redrawn from Filston HC, Johnson DG: Percutaneous venous cannulation in neonates: A method for catheter insertion without "cutdown." Pediatrics 48, No. 6:896, 1971. Copyright © American Academy of Pediatrics, 1971)

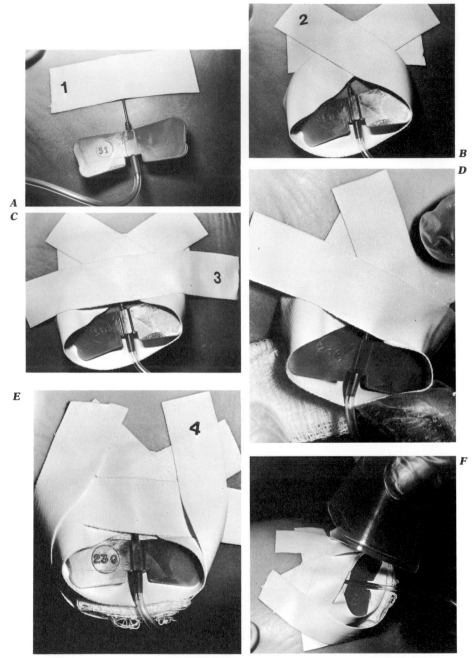

FIG. 23-3
(*A through C*) Method for securing scalp vein needle with adhesive tape. Apply tapes in order, as numbered 1 to 3. (*D*) Place gauze square to elevate needle slightly from skin. (*E*) Secure gauze in place with tape number 4. (*F*) Protect IV site with transparent medicine cup, with section of rim contoured anteriorly. (Alternatively, use small paper cup with the bottom removed.) Make sure not to obscure point of skin entry with tape.

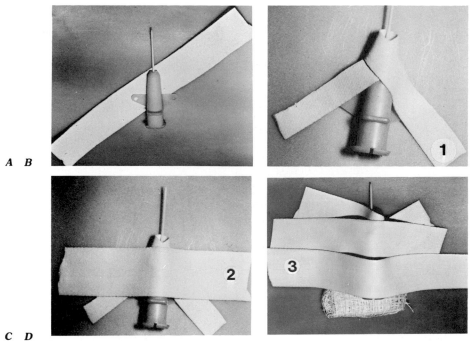

A   B

C   D

FIG. 23-4
Method for securing peripheral intravenous cannula with adhesive tape. (*A*) Place tape 1 behind cannula as shown, with adhesive side up. (*B*) Fold tape 1 anteriorly across the catheter-hub junction. (*C*) Place tape 2 as shown. (*D*) Fold 2 × 2 gauze pad in half and slip under hub to prevent pressure on skin. Hold in place with tape 3. The area of skin entry can be dressed with semipermeable sterile transparent dressing. Avoid obscuring with opaque dressing.

7. Refill heparin lock with heparinized flush solution after every IV infusion. (Flush routinely every 6 to 12 hours, depending on frequency of use.)

F. COMPLICATIONS[21]

1. Phlebitis[16,17]
2. Infection[22–24]

There is an increase in the incidence of both phlebitis and infection when a needle remains in place longer than 72 hours[17] and is heavily manipulated.[25] Also with film-type dressings.[1–6]

Batton and associates failed to confirm a difference in the incidence of infection when 25-gauge needles were compared with 24-gauge Teflon cannulas. However, the Teflon cannulas remained functional three times as long as steel needles with no apparent increase in complications.[16]

Alpan et al found that heparinization of the intravenous infusate (1 U/ml) significantly reduced the incidence of phlebitis and doubled the duration of patency.[26]

When lines are used for parenteral nutrition, the coinfusion of a lipid solution with the hyperosmolar TPN solution prolongs the life of the vein.[27,28]

3. Hematoma
4. Venospasm
5. Embolization of clot with forcible flushing
6. Air embolus
7. Infiltration of subcutaneous tissue with IV solution (For management of this complication see Chap. 15.)

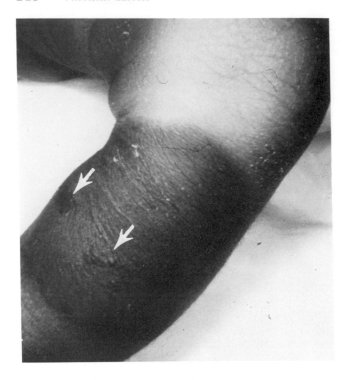

FIG. 23-5
Result of infusion of lidocaine into subcutaneous tissues of lower limb. Arrows indicate areas of blistering.

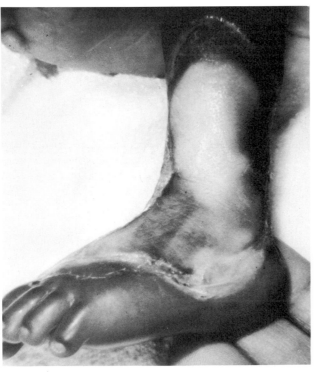

A

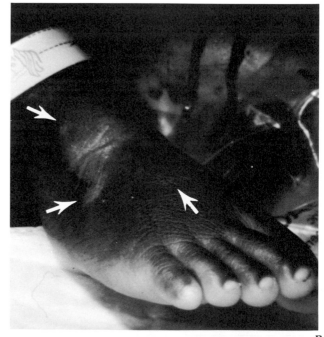

B

FIG. 23-6
(*A*) Extensive deep skin slough that required grafting, caused by IV infiltration. (*B*) Follow-up on a case similar to that shown in *A*. Area of scarring and muscle loss (indicated by arrows) was associated with foot drop.

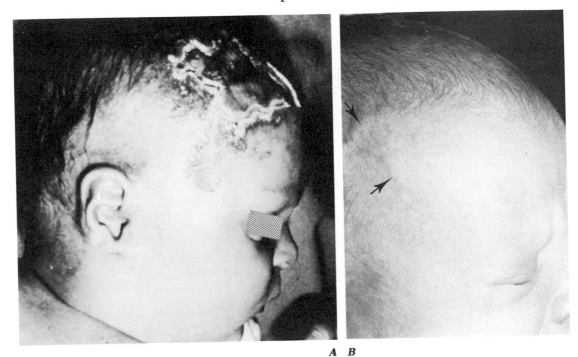

A B

FIG. 23-7
(*A*) Skin slough on scalp caused by inadvertent infusion into the frontal branch of the temporary artery, indicated by arrows in *B*.

a. Superficial blistering (Fig. 23-5)
b. Deep slough, which may require skin graft (Fig. 23-6)
c. Calcification of subcutaneous tissue due to infiltration of calcium-containing solution.

Note that there may be some extravasation into adjacent tissues even though blood can be aspirated from the needle/cannula.

8. Accidental injection or infusion into artery with anteriospasm and possible tissue necrosis (Fig. 23-7)
9. Ischemia or gangrene of lower extremity, complicating infusion into saphenous vein. Mechanism unclear.[24]
10. Burn from
    a. Transilluminator (Fig. 23-8; also see Chap. 11)
    b. Compress used to warm limb prior to procedure
11. Hypernatremia, fluid overload, or heparinization of infant due to improper flushing technique or solution.

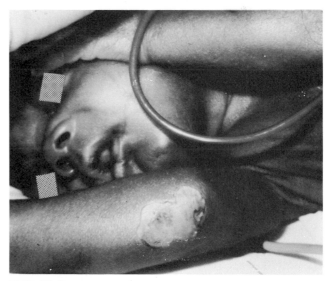

FIG. 23-8
Burn from transilluminator used to locate vein in antecubital fossa.

Cutdown Method

The method described has the advantage of avoiding incision of vessel prior to introduction of catheter.

> This is an important advantage in the very small infant in whom it is difficult to avoid excessive venotomy and transection of the vein.

A. INDICATIONS

1. To provide route for peripheral intravenous therapy when percutaneous method is not possible
2. To provide more stable and reliable IV line in situations where even brief cessation of therapy might compromise infant
3. To provide emergency IV therapy to infants in shock

B. CONTRAINDICATIONS

1. Risk/benefit should be weighed carefully in presence of bleeding diathesis.
2. Should not be used as routine procedure for starting IVs when percutaneous method is technically difficult but not impossible.

C. EQUIPMENT

Sterile

1. Gown and gloves
2. Cup with antiseptic solution (e.g., an iodophor)
3. Sterile aperture drape
4. 0.5% lidocaine HCl in 2-ml syringe
5. Two 25-gauge venipuncture needles
6. Two curved mosquito hemostats
7. 22-gauge cannula with needle stylet
8. T-connector for cannula
9. Heparinized saline (for heparin lock. See Percutaneous Method)
10. Half-strength normal saline in a 5-ml syringe
11. 5-0 nylon suture
12. 5-0 nylon suture on small, curved needle
13. Needle holder
14. No. 11 scalpel blade and handle
15. Semipermeable, sterile transparent dressing

Unsterile

1. Materials for restraint (see Chap. 3)
2. Transilluminator (cover with sterile plastic glove to maintain sterile field; see Chap. 11)
3. Roll of 0.5- to 1-inch porous adhesive tape

D. PRECAUTIONS

1. Aspirate prior to injection of lidocaine to prevent inadvertent intravascular infusion.
2. Take care not to make initial skin incision too deep, to avoid severing underlying vein.
3. Avoid infusing extremely irritating or hypertonic solutions.

E. TECHNIQUE

Anatomical Considerations: The great saphenous vein is constant in its anatomical position, just anterior to the medial malleolus. It is the only structure of importance in this area.

The cutdown procedure is facilitated by the fact that the vein lies on tough periosteum and has sufficient elasticity to allow withdrawal through a small incision without the danger of rupture.

1. Restrain foot in equinovalgus position.
2. Palpate medial malleolus, and locate point of incision 1 cm anterior and 1 cm superior to malleolus (Fig. 23-9).
3. Scrub, put on mask, gown, and gloves, and prepare area of incision, as for major procedure (see Chap. 4).
4. Drape area.
5. Mark line of incision by scratching skin with hypodermic needle prior to infiltration with local anesthetic.
6. Infiltrate skin along line of incision with 0.5 to 1 ml of lidocaine, then extend infiltration into subcutaneous tissue.
7. Wait 5 minutes for anesthesia.
8. Make 1-cm transverse incision through skin, down to superficial subcutaneous fat.

   > A vertical, rather than a transverse, incision is optional. The former has the advantage in that it offers the opportunity to extend the incision cephalad, should the posterior wall of the vein be perforated on the initial attempt at cannulation. However, it has the disadvantage that it may be made too lateral or medial to the vein.

9. Introduce curved hemostat into incision, with tip down. Spread blades of hemostat parallel to vein to dissect tissue down to periosteum. Continue this step until adequate visualization of vein is achieved (Fig. 23-10).
10. Reintroduce curved hemostat into incision, with

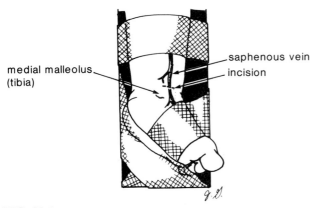

FIG. 23-9
Position of restraint for cutdown on the great saphenous vein at the ankle, indicating site of incision.

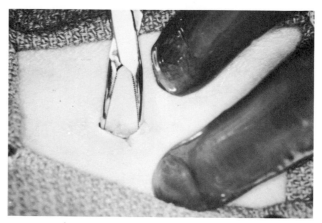

FIG. 23-10
Blades of curved hemostat are spread parallel to vein to dissect the subcutaneous connective tissue down to the periosteum.

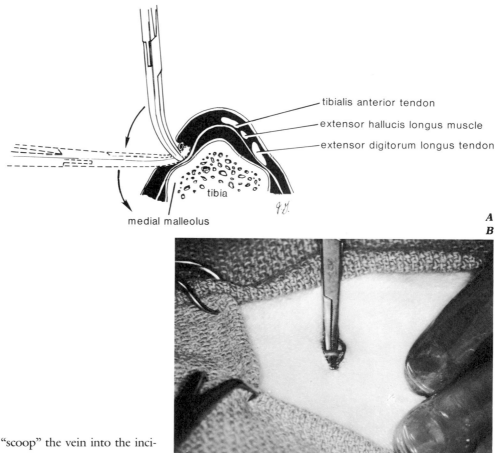

FIG. 23-11
A curved hemostat is used to "scoop" the vein into the incision.

FIG. 23-12
The hemostat has been carefully opened and the subcutaneous connective tissue spread, leaving the vein surface clean. A ligature is placed between the blades of the hemostat.

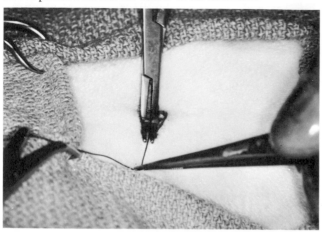

tip down, and pass down to periosteum. With a "scooping" motion, through approximately 180 degrees, isolate vein, and draw into incision (Fig. 23-11).

11. Open hemostat carefully. Spread subcutaneous tissue, leaving vein surface clean.
12. Place 5-0 nylon suture loosely around vein and clamp at end of suture with hemostat, to allow for distal control of vessel (Fig. 23-12). (Do not tie ligature.)
13. Place ligature with clamp across extended index finger and inside palm of nondominant hand, retracting it in an upward and caudad direction (Fig. 23-13).
14. Introduce cannula/stylet into vein at a 45-degree angle, with bevel down. Once vein has been entered, angle cannula parallel to vein (Fig. 23-14).
15. Advance cannula into vein, while withdrawing inner needle stylet.
16. Advance cannula up to hub and infuse small volume of saline flush solution to confirm intravenous position.

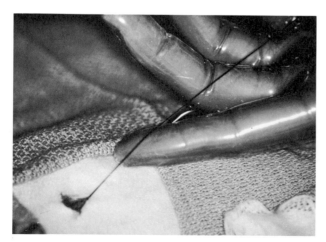

FIG. 23-13
Outward and caudad traction is exerted on the suture.

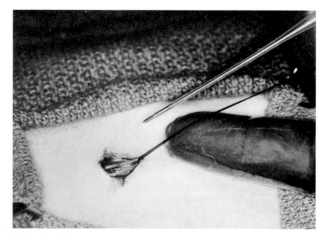

FIG. 23-14
Introducing the cannula into the vein.

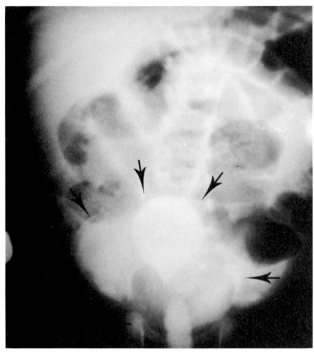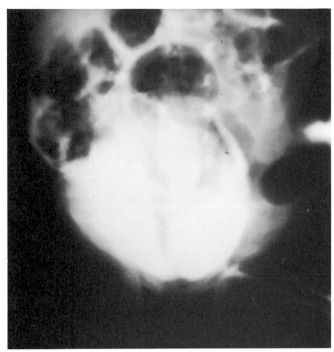

A   B

FIG. 23-15
Cystogram in infant who had not urinated for more than 24 hours despite "adequate" intravenous fluids. (*A*) The bladder appears normal, but there is a "mass-effect" displacing the intestines in approximate area indicated by arrows. (*B*) Radiographic contrast material, injected through a long catheter introduced into the femoral vein via the great saphenous vein, has extravasated into the abdominal cavity.

17. Remove traction suture and close skin incision with one or two simple 5-0 nylon sutures.
18. Attach cannula to infusion tubing and regulate IV.
19. Secure cannula to skin as shown in Figure 23-4.

F. COMPLICATIONS

1. Same for percutaneous IV
2. Inadvertent infusion of local anesthetic into artery or vein
3. Severance of vein owing to excessively deep initial incision
4. Infiltration of intravenous infusion into body cavity (Fig. 23-15)

   This is a complication related to placement of very long catheters. When infusion of an extremely irritating or hypertonic solution is required, the catheter is preferably inserted into the central venous system (see Chaps. 28 to 30).

5. Varicose veins secondary to postinfusion phlebitis[29]

References

1. HOFFMAN KK, WESTEN SA, KAISER DL: Bacterial colonization and phlebitis-associated risk with polyurethane film for peripheral intravenous site dressings. Am J Infect Control 16:101, 1988
2. WILLE JC, BLUSSÉ E, VanOvd ABLAS A: A comparison of four film-type dressings by their antimicrobial effect on the flora of the skin. J Hosp Infect 14:153, 1989
3. VERNON HJ, LANE AT, WISCHERATER LJ, ET AL: Semipermeable dressing and transepidermal water loss in premature infants. Pediatrics 86:357, 1990
4. MAKI DG, RINGER M: Evaluation of dressing regimens for prevention of infection with peripheral intravenous catheters. JAMA 258:3396, 1987
5. CRAVEN DE, LICHTENBERG DA, KUNCHES LM, ET AL: A randomized study comparing a transparent polyurethane dressing to a dry gauze dressing for peripheral intravenous sites. Infect Control 6:361, 1985
6. HOLLAND KT, HARNBY D, PEEL B: A comparison of the in vivo antibacterial effects of "Op-Site", "Tegaderm" and "Ensure" dressings. J Hosp Infect 6:299, 1985
7. HECKER JR, LEWIS GBM, STANLEY H: Nitroglycerin ointment as an aid to venepuncture. Lancet 1:332, 1983

8. VAKSMANN G, REY G, BREVERE G-M, ET AL: Nitroglycerin ointment as an aid to venous cannulation in children. J Pediatr 111:89, 1987

9. MAYNARD EC, OH W: Topical nitroglycerin ointment as an aid to insertion of peripheral venous catheters in neonates. J Pediatr 114:474, 1989

10. GURAN P, BEAL G, BRION N, ADVENIER C: Topical nitroglycerin as an aid to insertion of peripheral venous catheters in neonates (Letter). J Pediatr 115:1025, 1989

11. BENTLY DW, LEPPER MA: Septicemia related to indwelling venous catheters. JAMA 206:1749, 1968

12. BOLASNY BL, MARTIN CE, CONKLE DM: Careful technique with plastic intravenous catheters. Surg Gynecol Obstet 132:1030, 1971

13. CORSO JA, AGOSTINELLA R, BRANDISS MW: Maintenance of venous polyethylene catheters to reduce risk of infection. JAMA 210:2075, 1969

14. DRUSKIN MS, SIEGAL PD: Bacterial contamination of indwelling intravenous polyethylene catheters. JAMA 185:966, 1963

15. FEKETY FR, THOBURN R: Nature and prevention of intravenous catheter infection. John Hopkins Medical Journal 121:134, 1967

16. BATTON DG, MAISLES JM, APPELBAUM JM: Use of intravenous cannulas in premature infants: A controlled study. Pediatrics 70:487, 1982

17. LOWENBRAUN S, YOUNG V, KENTOUR D, SERPICK AA: Infection from intravenous "scalp-vein" needles in a susceptible population. JAMA 212:451, 1970

18. DOWNING JW, CHARLES KK: Intravenous cannula fixing and dressing—comparison between the use of transparent polyurethane dressing and conventional technique. South African Medical Journal 721:191, 1987

19. LEIBOVICI C: Daily change of an antiseptic dressing does not prevent infusion phlebitis: A controlled trial. Am J Infect Control 17:23, 1989

20. FILSTON HC, JOHNSON DG: Percutaneous venous cannulation in neonates: A method for catheter insertion without "cut-down." Pediatrics 48:896, 1971

21. JOHNSON RV, DONN SM: Life span of intravenous cannulas in a neonatal intensive care unit. Am J Dis Child 142:968, 1988

22. HILDEBRAND WL, SCHREINER RL, YACKO MS, ET AL: Placing a needle in an infant's scalp vein. Am Fam Physician 21:139, 1980

23. LLOYD-STILL JD, PETER G, LOVEJOY FH: Infected "scalp-vein" needles. JAMA 213:1496, 1970

24. MCNAIR TJ, DUDLEY HAF: The local complications of intravenous therapy. Lancet 2:365, 1959

25. CRONIN WA, GERMANSON TP, DONOWITZ LG: Intravascular cannula colonization and related blood stream infection in critically ill neonates. Infect Control Hosp Epidemiol 11:301, 1990

26. ALPAN G, EYAL F, SPRINGER C, ET AL: Heparinization of alimentation solutions administered through peripheral veins in premature infants: A controlled study. Pediatrics 74:375, 1984

27. PINEAULT M, CHESSEX P, PLEDBOEUF B, BISAILLON S: Beneficial effect of coinfusing a lipid emulsion on venous patency. J Parenter Enter Nutr 13:637, 1989

28. PHELPS SJ, LOCHRANE EB: Effect of the continuous administration of fat emulsion on the infiltration rate of intravenous lines in infants receiving peripheral parenteral nutrition solutions. J Parenter Enter Nutr 13:628, 1989

29. SHUSTER S, LAKS H: Varicose veins following ankle cutdowns. J Pediatr Surg 8:245, 1973

24 Umbilical Artery Catheterization

Mhairi G. MacDonald

A. INDICATIONS

Catheter should remain in place only as long as primary indications exist, with the exception of secondary indication number 3.

Primary

1. Frequent or continuous (see Chap. 9, umbilical artery oximeter) measurement of lower aortic blood gases for oxygen tension (Po_2) or oxygen content (percent saturation)
2. Continuous monitoring of arterial blood pressure
3. Angiography
4. Resuscitation (use of umbilical venous line may be first choice)

Secondary

1. Infusion of maintenance glucose-electrolyte solutions or medications
2. Exchange transfusion
3. To provide vital infusions[1] and a port for frequent blood sampling in the very low birth weight infant

B. CONTRAINDICATIONS

1. Evidence of local vascular compromise in lower limbs or buttock areas
2. Peritonitis
3. Necrotizing enterocolitis
4. Omphalitis
5. Omphalocele

C. EQUIPMENT

Several standardized graphs for premeasurement of catheter length to be inserted are available (Figs. 24-1, 24-2, 24-3).

Sterile

1. Sterile gown and gloves
2. Cup with antiseptic solution
3. Surgical drape with central aperture (transparent drape recommended)
4. Catheter
   a. Single hole
      (1) Reduces surfaces for potential thrombus formation
      (2) Recorded pressure tracing will change when hole is occluded.
   b. Made of flexible material that does not kink as it follows the curves of vessels
   c. Relatively rigid walls with frequency characteristics suitable for accurate measurement of intravascular pressure
   d. Small capacity (minimum volume of blood to be withdrawn to clear catheter prior to blood sampling)
   e. Radiopaque

   The need to visualize the catheter position on x-ray outweighs the theoretical risk of increased thrombogenicity related to a radiopaque strip.[2]

   f. Smooth, rounded tip[2,3]—nonthrombogenic material[4]

   The ideal catheter is not yet available. Silastic catheters are theoretically less thrombogenic but are more difficult to insert because of their lack of rigidity. Introduction of hydrophilic stiffening polymers into the silastic material has the potential to remove this disadvantage but is still in the research phase. Catheters constructed of polyurethane with heparin bonded to the surface have theoretical advantages, but their effectiveness in reducing the incidence of thrombosis formation has not been demonstrated.[5]

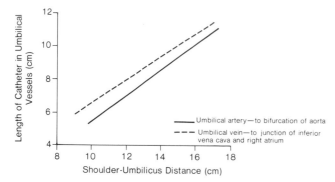

FIG. 24-1
Graph for determination of length of catheter to be inserted for appropriate low aortic or venous placement. Length of catheter is measured from umbilical ring. Length of umbilical stump must be added. The shoulder umbilicus distance is the perpendicular distance between parallel horizontal lines at the level of the umbilicus and through the distal ends of the clavicles. (Adapted from the data of Dunn P: Localisation of the umbilical catheter by postmortem measurement. Arch Dis Child (Robinson R, Meadow R [eds]) 41:69, 1966)

Use of heparinized flush solution is common practice. Rajani and others have shown that using a heparinized solution containing 1 unit heparin/ml for flushing the umbilical arterial line prolonged catheter life by reducing the incidence of fibrin thrombus formation in the catheter lumen.[7,8] However, the incidence of platelet thrombi on the *outside* of the catheter and associated thromboembolic phenomena were not affected. Horgan et al[9] found that the use of 1 U/ml heparin did not reduce the incidence of UAC-related thrombi, but did lower the incidence of their sequelae. Butt et al[10] could demonstrate no significant benefit associated with increasing the rate of infusion from 1 to 2 ml/hr (heparin 1 U/ml) and Bosque et al[11] showed that continuous infusion of heparin 1 U/ml is more effective than intermittent infusion in maintaining patency of the UAC. The excess of bleeding problems reported by Hall and associates may be related to the more concentrated solution of heparin used (3.3 U/ml).[12]

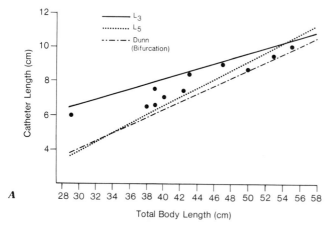

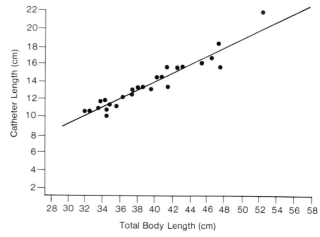

FIG. 24-2
(*A*) Graph for distance of catheter insertion from the umbilical ring for L3, L5, and aortic bifurcation. Large dots (●) represent catheters positioned at L4. (Rosenfeld W, Estrada R, Jhaveri R, et al: Evaluation of graphs for insertion of umbilical artery catheters below the diaphragm. J Pediatr 98:628, 1981) (*B*) Graph for catheter insertion to level of T8 using total body length. (Rosenfeld W, Biagtan J, Schaeffer H, et al: Evaluation of graphs for insertion of umbilical artery catheters below the diaphragm. J Pediatr 98:628, 1981)

g. 5 Fr gauge for infants > 1200 g
h. 3.5 Fr gauge for infants < 1200 g
5. Scissors for cutting catheter
6. Blunt needle adapter (if using catheter without hub)
   a. No. 18 for 5 Fr catheter
   b. No. 20 for 3.5 Fr catheter
7. Three way stopcock with Luer-Lok
8. 10-ml syringe
9. 0.25 to 0.5N saline flush solution (saline with heparin, 1 to 2 U/ml)

> In very small premature infants, hypernatremia may result from receiving excess sodium in flush solutions. We recommend using 0.25N rather than more concentrated saline solutions.[6]

10. Tape measure
11. 20-cm narrow umbilical tie
12. No. 11 scalpel blade and holder
13. 4 × 4 gauze sponges
14. Two curved mosquito hemostats
15. Toothed iris forceps
16. Two curved, nontoothed iris forceps
17. 2% lidocaine HC1 without epinephrine
18. 3-ml syringe and needle to draw up lidocaine
19. Small needle holder
20. 4-0 silk suture on small, curved needle
21. Suture scissors

Unsterile
1. Cap and mask
2. Wooden tongue depressor

D. PRECAUTIONS

1. Avoid use of feeding tubes as catheters (associated with higher incidence of thrombosis).[13]
2. Fold drapes so as not to obscure infant's face and upper chest.
3. Take time and care to dilate lumen of artery before attempting to insert catheter.
4. Catheter should not be forced past an obstruction.
5. *Never* advance catheter once placed and secured.
6. Loosen umbilicus at tie on completion of procedure and x-ray confirmation of position.
7. Avoid covering the umbilicus with dressing. Dressing may delay recognition of bleeding or catheter displacement.

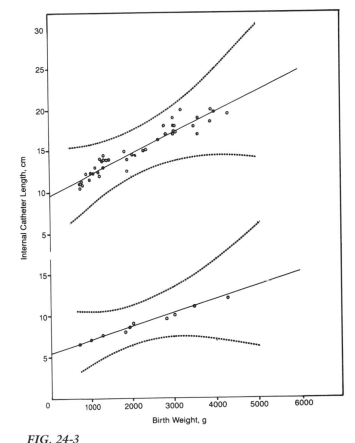

FIG. 24-3
Estimates of insertional length of umbilical catheters (umbilical artery catheter tip inserted between T-6 and T-10; umbilical vein catheter tip inserted above diaphragm in inferior vena cava near right atrium) based on birth weight (BW) (with 95% confidence intervals). Modified estimating equations utilizing BW are as follows: umbilical artery length = 2.5 × BW + 9.7 (top graph) and umbilical vein length = 1.5 × BW + 5.6 (bottom graph), where BW is measured in kilograms and lengths in centimeters. (Shukla H, Ferrara A: Am J Dis Child 140:787, 1986)

8. Always obtain radiographic or ultrasound[14,15] confirmation of catheter position. If doubt remains, obtain a lateral x-ray study.[16,17]
9. Be certain catheter is secure, and examine frequently when infant placed in prone position, because hemorrhage may go unrecognized.
10. Take care not to allow air to enter catheter. Always have catheter fluid-filled and attached to closed

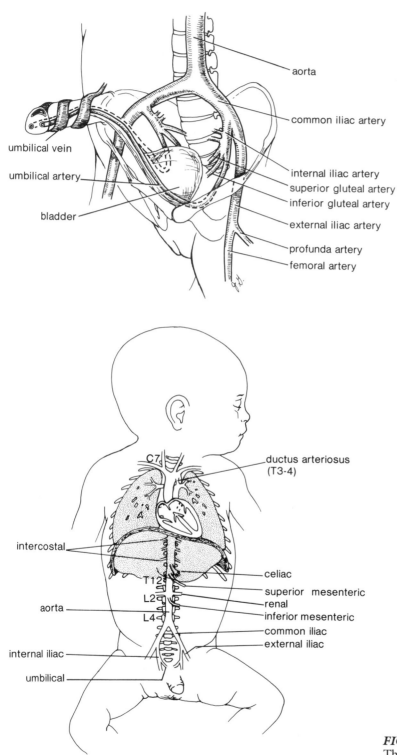

aorta

common iliac artery

umbilical vein

umbilical artery

internal iliac artery

superior gluteal artery

inferior gluteal artery

external iliac artery

bladder

profunda artery

femoral artery

FIG. 24-4
Anatomical relations of the umbilical arteries, showing relationship with major arteries supplying buttocks and lower limb.

C7

ductus arteriosus (T3-4)

intercostal

celiac

T12

superior mesenteric

L2

renal

aorta

inferior mesenteric

L4

common iliac

external iliac

internal iliac

umbilical

FIG. 24-5
The aorta and branches.

stopcock prior to insertion. Check for air bubbles in catheter before flushing or starting infusion.

11. When removing catheter, cut suture at skin, not on catheter, to avoid catheter transection.

E. TECHNIQUE

Anatomical Note: The umbilical arteries are the direct continuation of the internal iliac arteries. Their diameters at their origins are 2 to 3 mm. As they approach the umbilicus, their lumina become small and the walls thicken significantly. In a fullterm infant, each artery is approximately 7.0 cm long (Fig. 24-4).

A catheter introduced into the umbilical artery will usually pass into the aorta from the internal iliac artery. Occasionally, it will pass into the femoral artery via the external iliac artery or into one of the gluteal arteries. The latter two sites are unsuitable for sampling, pressure measurement, or infusion.

1. Choose either of two positions (Fig. 24-5).

High position is associated with fewer episodes of blanching and cyanosis of the lower extremities.[18] However, hypertension may be more common with high catheter position,[19] and Schick et al have reported an increased risk of intraventricular hemorrhage associated with high positioning of the UAC.[20]

a. *Low position*[21-23]: level of lumbar vertebrae 3 to 4 (Fig. 24-6)
   (1) Catheter tip is below major aortic branches, such as renal mesenteric arteries.
   (2) In most newborns, this position coincides with aortic bifurcation at upper end of fourth vertebra.
b. *High position*[13,18,24]: level of thoracic vertebrae 6 to 9 (Fig. 24-7) Catheter tip is above origin of celiac axis.

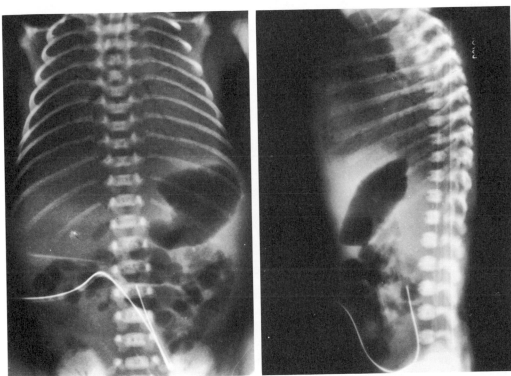

A   B

FIG. 24-6
AP (*A*) and lateral (*B*) radiographs showing optimal low position of an umbilical artery catheter. Catheter tip is at the level of the superior margin of the fourth lumbar vertebral body, which in newborns usually corresponds to the aortic bifurcation.

FIG. 24-7
Umbilical arterial catheter in satisfactory high position at the level of the ninth thoracic vertebral body on AP (*A*) and lateral (*B*) projections.

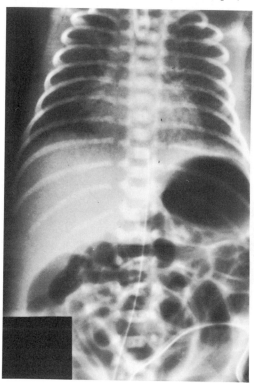 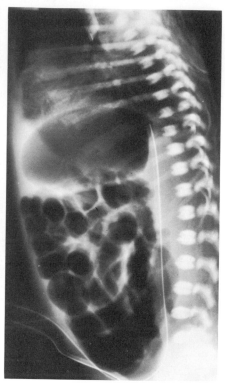

A   B

2. Make external measurements necessary to estimate length of catheter to be inserted (see Figs. 24-1 to 24-3).[25-31]

3. Prepare as for major procedure (see Chap. 4).

4. Attach stopcock to hub of catheter and fill system with flush solution. Turn stopcock "off" to catheter.

   If catheter does not have a hub, cut flared end of catheter with scissors and insert blunt-needle adapter of appropriate size. This will reduce catheter deadspace.

5. Place sterile gauze around umbilical stump and elevate out of sterile field, or have ungloved assistant grasp cord by cord clamp or forceps and pull cord vertically out of sterile field.

6. Prepare cord and surrounding skin with antiseptic solution to radius of approximately 5 cm.

7. Drape area surrounding cord.

8. Place umbilical tape around umbilicus, and tie loosely with single knot.
   a. Tighten only enough to prevent bleeding and place, if possible, around Wharton's jelly rather than skin.
   b. It may be necessary to loosen tie when inserting catheter.

9. Cut cord horizontally with scalpel (Fig. 24-8).
   a. Approximately 1 to 1.5 cm from skin
   b. Avoiding tangential slice

   Bloom et al have described an alternate approach to the artery with lateral arteriotomy.[32] To perform this method 3 to 4 cm of cord must be preserved because the cord must be rolled over a Kelly clamp 180 degrees.[32,33]

   (1) Clamp across end of cord with mosquito hemostat in nondominant hand and pull firmly towards the infant's head.

(2) Roll cord 180 degrees over hemostat toward abdominal wall.

(3) Identify arteries in superior right and left lateral aspects of cord.

(4) Approximately 1 cm from abdominal wall incise Wharton's jelly down to arterial wall, using the No. 11 scalpel blade.

(5) Incise artery through half of circumference. If necessary, dilate lumen with iris forceps.

(6) Insert catheter into lumen of artery, directed in a caudad direction, for predetermined distance.

10. Control bleeding by gentle tension on umbilical tape.

11. Blot surface of cord stump with gauze swab. Avoid rubbing because this damages tissue and obscures anatomy.

12. Identify cord vessels (Fig. 24-9).

   a. Vein is easiest to identify as large, thin-walled, sometimes gaping vessel. It is most frequently situated at the 12 o'clock position at the base of the umbilical stump.

   b. Arteries are smaller, thick-walled, and white and may protrude slightly from cut surface.

   c. Omphalomesenteric duct is rarely present.

13. Grasp cord stump, using toothed forceps, at point close to (but not on) artery to be catheterized. If available, it may be helpful to have an assistant scrub and

   a. Apply two curved mosquito hemostats to Wharton's jelly on opposite sides of cord, away from vessel to be cannulated

   b. Apply traction to stabilize cord stump

14. Introduce one of points of curved iris forceps into lumen of artery and probe gently to depth of 0.5 cm.

15. Remove forceps and bring points together before introducing them once more into lumen.

16. Probe gently to depth of 1 cm (up to the curved "shoulder" of forceps), keeping points together.

17. Allow points to spring apart, and maintain forceps in this position for 15 to 30 seconds to dilate vessel (Fig. 24-10).

   Time spent in ensuring dilatation prior to catheter insertion increases likelihood of success.

18. Release cord and set aside toothed forceps, while keeping curved forceps within artery.

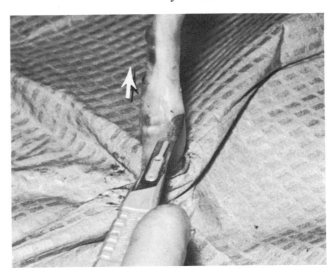

FIG. 24-8
Traction is being placed on cord in direction of arrow. Operator is about to make horizontal cut across cord.

FIG. 24-9
The vessels of the umbilical cord. Thin-walled vein at 12 o'clock position is indicated by nontoothed forceps. Blood is oozing from an umbilical artery. The second artery is partially obscured and indicated by arrow.

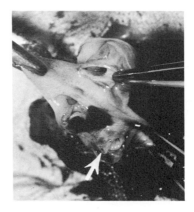

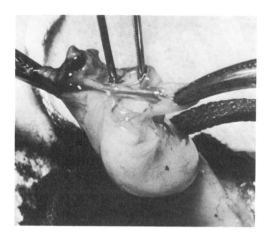

FIG. 24-10
Points of iris forceps have been allowed to spring apart in order to dilate the lumen of the artery.

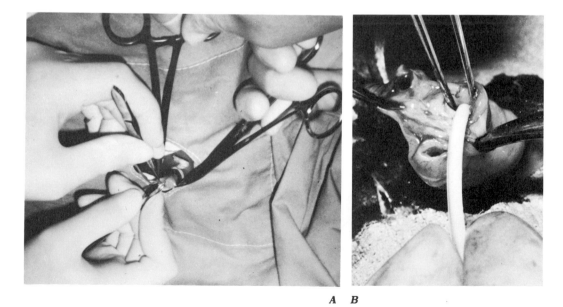

A   B

FIG. 24-11
Inserting the catheter into the artery between prongs of dilating forceps. Note that the umbilical tape has been tied around the skin of the umbilicus; this should be loosened once the catheter is secured in place.

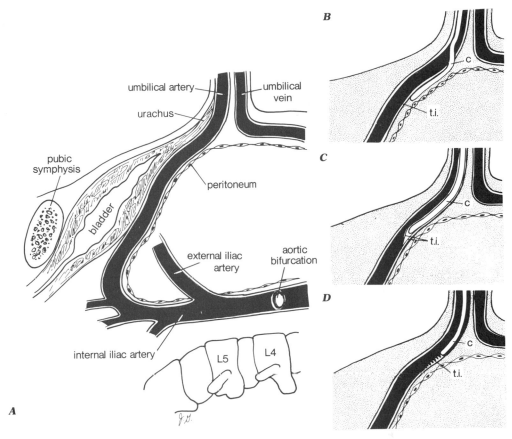

FIG. 24-12
Some reasons for failure of umbilical artery catheterization. (*A*) Sagittal midline section to show normal anatomy of umbilical artery. (*B*) Catheter (C) has perforated umbilical artery within anulus umbilicalis and is dissecting perivascularly and external to peritoneum. (*C*) Catheter (C) has ruptured through tunica intima (t.i.) and dissected into subintimal space. (*D*) Catheter (C) invaginating tunica intima (t.i.) after stripping it from a more distal point. (Adapted from Clark JM, Jung AL: Umbilical artery catheterization by a cut down procedure. Pediatrics [Neonatology Suppl] 59:1036, 1977. Copyright © American Academy of Pediatrics, 1977)

19. Grasp catheter 1 cm from tip, between free thumb and forefinger, or with curved iris forceps.
20. Insert catheter into lumen of artery, between prongs of dilating forceps (Fig. 24-11).
21. Remove curved forceps, having passed catheter approximately 2 cm into vessel with a firm, steady motion. Grasp cord again with toothed tissue forceps and pull gently toward head of infant. This mild traction will facilitate passage of catheter at angle between cord and abdominal wall.
22. After passing the catheter approximately 5 cm, as-

pirate to verify intraluminal position. Clear blood by injecting 0.5 ml of flush solution.

The catheter may now be used to measure blood gases.

23. Take appropriate action if insertion is complicated (Fig. 24-12).
    a. Resistance before tip reaches abdominal wall (< 3 cm from surface of abdominal stump)
       (1) Loosen umbilical tape.
       (2) Redilate artery.

b. "Popping" sensation rather than "relaxation"
  (1) Catheter may have exited lumen and created false channel.
  (2) Remove and use second artery.
  (3) If unsuccessful, draw 0.5 ml lidocaine from vial. Reinsert tip of catheter approximately 2 cm into UAC and drip lidocaine into vessel. Apply *constant gentle* pressure until vessel dilates.
c. Backflow of blood, particularly around vessel
  (1) Tighten umbilical tape.
  (2) Catheter may be in false channel with extravascular bleeding.
d. Resistance is encountered at anterior abdominal wall or sharp turn in vessel as it angles around bladder toward internal iliac artery (approximately 6 to 8 cm from surface of umbilical stump in 2- to 4-kg neonate).
  (1) Apply gentle but steady pressure for 30 to 60 seconds.
  (2) Position infant on side with same side elevated as artery being catheterized. Flex hip.
  (3) Instill lidocaine as for 23 b (3).

Do not force catheter!

e. Easy insertion, but no blood return
  (1) Catheter is outside vessel in false channel.
  (2) Remove and observe infant carefully for evidence of complication.
24. Place marker tape on catheter with base of tape flush with surface of cord, so that displacement of the catheter may be readily recognized.
25. *Remove umbilical tape* and place purse-string suture around base of the cord (not through skin or vessels). Three bites into cord (with needle facing away from catheter) are sufficient to include all three vessels within suture.

   If desired, form marker tape into bilateral wings and sew the tails of the purse string suture through the wings to anchor the catheter in a symmetrical fashion. This is a useful method in very small premature infants because it avoids sticking tape to the abdominal wall.[34] Or, remove needle and wrap ends of suture in opposite direction around catheter for about 3 cm, and tie, taking care not to kink catheter.

26. Secure catheter temporarily by looping over upper abdomen and taping.
27. Obtain x-ray film or ultrasound (see D 8) to check catheter position.
   a. Catheter tip above T_6 or between T_{11} and L_2
     (1) Measure distance between actual and appropriate position on x-ray film.
     (2) Withdraw equal length of catheter.
     (3) Repeat x-ray study.
     (4) Note procedure in chart.
   b. Catheter tip below L_5
     (1) Remove catheter.
     (2) Never advance catheter once in situ, because this will introduce length of contaminated catheter into vessel.
28. If desired secure catheter with tape bridge (Fig. 36-16)
29. Continue routine cord care with triple dye or other agent of choice.
30. Stabilize catheter, stopcock, and syringe, using tongue depressor (optional).
   a. Reduces risk of air embolus if syringe maintained in vertical position
   b. Prevents accidental disconnection of catheter system

F. CARE OF INDWELLING CATHETER

For setup and maintenance of arterial pressure transducer see Chapter 8.

1. Keep catheter free of blood to prevent clot formation.
   a. Flush catheter with 0.5 ml of flush solution, slowly over at least 5 seconds each time blood sample is drawn.
   b. Infuse IV solution continuously through catheter between samples to prevent retrograde flow.
   c. Note amounts of blood removed and IV fluid/flush solution infused, and add to fluid-balance record.
2. Watch for indications of clot formation.
   a. Decrease in amplitude of pulse pressure on blood pressure tracing
   b. Difficulty withdrawing blood samples
3. Take appropriate action if clot forms.
   a. Do not attempt to flush clot forcibly.
   b. Remove catheter. Replace only if critical line.

4. Avoid enteral feedings with catheter in situ if possible. Increased risk of mesenteric thromboembolism has been suggested.[35]

G. OBTAINING BLOOD SAMPLES FROM CATHETER

(With emphasis on aseptic technique and minimizing stress to the vessel)

Equipment

1. Gloves
2. Alcohol swabs
3. Rubber-tipped clamps or disposable IV tubing clamps
4. Syringe of 0.6 ml flushing solution
5. 3-ml syringe for cleaning line
6. Syringe for blood sample
7. Ice, if necessary for sample preservation
8. Appropriate requisition slips and labels

Technique

1. Wash hands and put on gloves.
2. Form sterile field.
3. Clean the connection site of the stopcock/catheter using an alcohol swab.
4. Clamp the umbilical catheter.
5. Connect the 3-ml syringe, release the clamp, and *slowly* draw back 2 to 3 ml of fluid over 1 minute to clear the line. Reclamp the catheter. Remove syringe and place on sterile field.

   Data published by Brown et al[36] indicates that, for 3.5 and 5 Fr catheters, accurate measurements of pH, sodium, and potassium can be obtained after withdrawal of 1 ml of blood. However, if blood glucose values are desired, a minimum of 3 ml from a 3.5 Fr and 4 ml from a 5 Fr catheter must be withdrawn.

6. Attach sampling syringe. Release clamp and draw back specimen desired. Reclamp the catheter.
7. Reattach the syringe containing the fluid and blood cleared from the line.
   a. Clear the connection of air.
   b. *Slowly replace the fluid and blood cleared from the line and remove the syringe.*
8. Attach the syringe of flushing solution to the stopcock, clear air from connection, and *slowly* flush line.

9. Clean the stopcock connection with alcohol.
10. Record all blood removed and volume of flush used on infant's daily record sheet.

H. REMOVAL OF UMBILICAL ARTERY CATHETER

Indications

1. No further clinical indication
2. Need for less frequent direct PO_2 measurements
3. Sufficient stabilization of blood pressure to allow intermittent monitoring
4. Hypertension
5. Hematuria not due to other recognizable cause
6. Catheter-related sepsis
7. Catheter-related vascular compromise
8. Onset of platelet consumption coagulopathy
9. Peritonitis
10. Necrotizing enterocolitis
11. Omphalitis

Technique

1. Leave umbilical tie loose around cord stump as precaution against excessive bleeding.

   Reinsertion of purse-string suture through dried Wharton's jelly is preferable if

   a. Umbilical tape must be tied on skin, rather than Wharton's jelly
   b. Catheter has been in situ for longer than 48 hours, because artery may have lost ability to spasm

2. Withdraw catheter slowly and evenly, until approximately 5 cm remain in vessel, tightening purse-string suture or umbilical tie.
3. Discontinue infusion.
4. Pull remainder of catheter out of the vessel at rate of 1 cm/min (to allow vasospasm). If there is bleeding, apply lateral pressure to the cord by compressing between thumb and first finger.

I. COMPLICATIONS[37-42]

Catheterization of the umbilical artery is probably always associated with some degree of reversible damage to the arterial intima.[43,44]

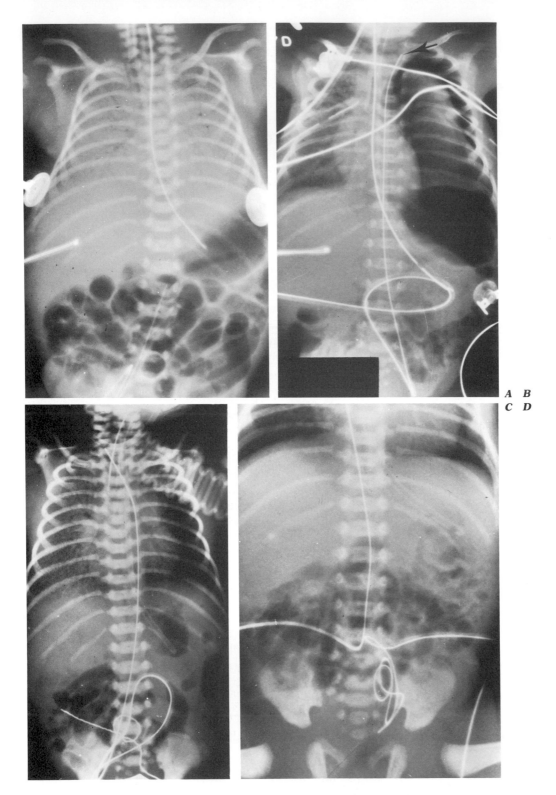

A B
C D

FIG. 24-13
Various umbilical artery catheter (UAC) malpositions. (*A*) Unacceptable position at L-2 because of the proximity of the renal arteries. (*B*) UAC in a left brachycephalic artery. (*C*) UAC in a right brachycephalic artery. (*D*) UAC in a pelvic artery.

1. Malpositioned catheter (Figs. 24-13 to 24-15)[35,45,46]
   a. Vessel perforation[45,47,48]
   b. Refractory hypoglycemia with catheter tip opposite celiac axis[49-51]
   c. Peritoneal perforation[52]
   d. False aneurysm[53-58]
   e. Movement of catheter tip position due to changes in abdominal circumference.
   f. Sciatic nerve palsy[59,60]
   g. Misdirection of catheter into internal or external iliac artery (see Figs. 24-13D and 24-16)[43]

   Schreiber et al have described a double arterial catheter technique to correct this problem.[43]

2. Vascular accident
   a. Thrombosis (Fig. 24-17)[20,21,61-64]
   b. Embolism/infarction (Fig. 24-16)[17,34,65-68]
   c. Vasospasm[17,69-73]
   d. Loss of extremity (Fig. 24-18)[71]
   e. Hypertension (Fig. 24-19)[18,74-80]
   f. Paraplegia[81-86]
   g. Congestive heart failure (aortic thrombosis)[85]
   h. Air embolism (Fig. 24-20)

3. Equipment-related
   a. Breaks in catheter and transection of catheter[7,45,70,82,85-88]
   b. Plasticizer in tissues[47]
   c. Electrical hazard[70]
      (1) Improper grounding of electronic equipment
      (2) Conduction of current through fluid-filled catheter
   d. Intravascular knot in catheter[89]

4. Other
   a. Hemorrhage (including that related to catheter loss or disconnection and over heparinization)[37,65,70,90-92]
   b. Infection[25,65,66,93-101]

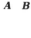 *A B*

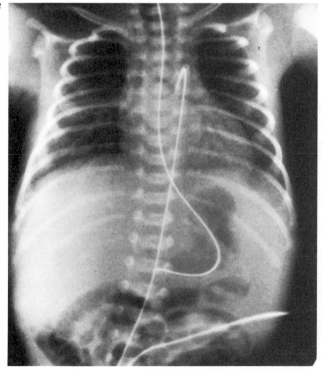 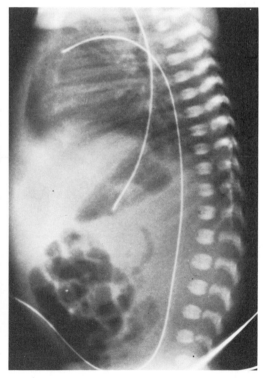

FIG. 24-14
AP (*A*) and lateral (*B*) radiographs demonstrating passage of an umbilical artery catheter into the pulmonary artery via a patent ductus arteriosus.

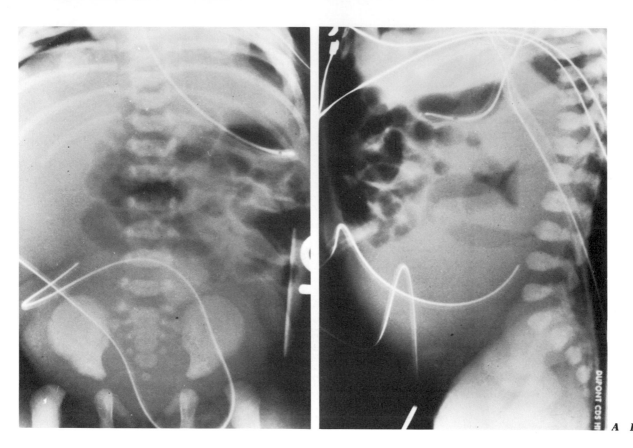

A B

FIG. 24-15
Effect of abdominal mass simulating catheter misplacement. AP (*A*) and lateral (*B*) films, which show remarkable displacement of an umbilical artery catheter by a giant hematocolpos in a 1-day-old infant.

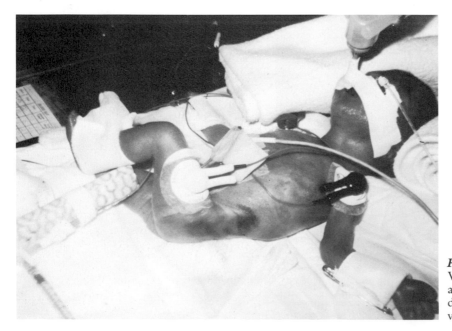

FIG. 24-16
Vascular compromise in the left buttock and loin owing to a complication of UAC displaced into the internal iliac artery. For vascular anatomy see Figure 24-4.

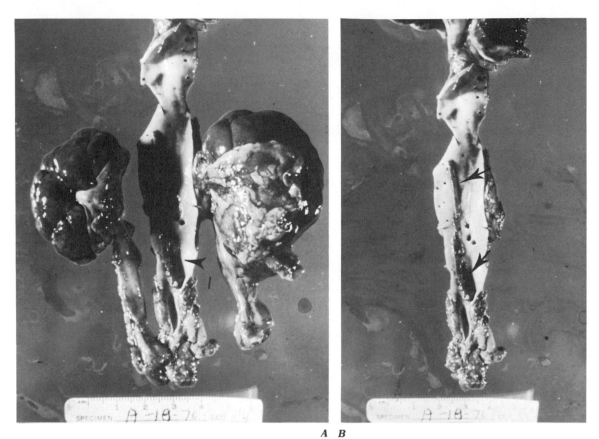

A **B**

FIG. 24-17
Arrows indicate mural thrombus in the abdominal aorta, which was associated with an umbilical arterial line. The left renal artery was found to be occluded by thrombus on further dissection of this autopsy specimen. The left kidney is showing a degree of atrophy. Both kidneys showed scattered infarction.

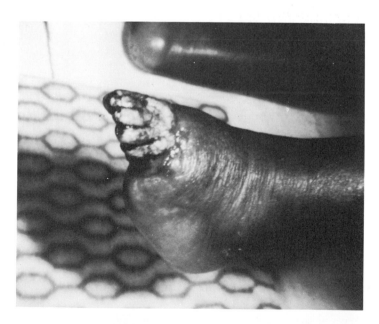

FIG. 24-18
Autoamputation of forefoot owing to vascular complication of UAC.

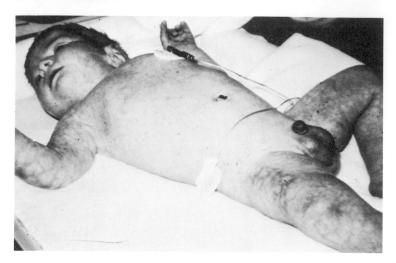

FIG. 24-19
Generalized mottling of skin in infant with severe hypertension secondary to UAC associated thrombus in renal artery.

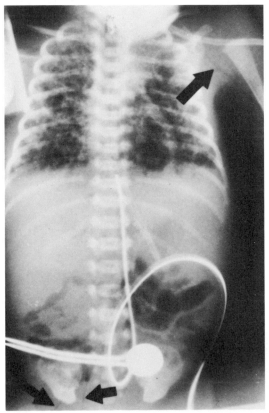

FIG. 24-20
AP roentgenogram demonstrating air embolism, from a UAC, in the left subclavian artery (upper arrow) and the femoral arteries (lower arrows).

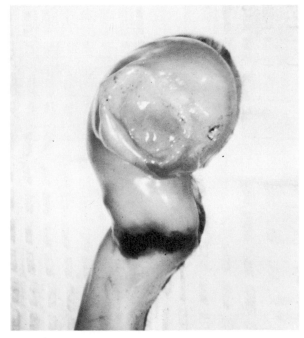

FIG. 24-21
Small omphalocele. This gut-containing hernia was transected during placement of a UAC.

c. Necrotizing enterocolitis[35,73]

d. Intestinal necrosis or perforation[102]
   (1) Vascular accident
   (2) Infusion of hypertonic solution[103]

e. Transection of omphalocele (Fig. 24-21)[104]

f. Herniation of appendix through umbilical ring[105]

g. Cotton-fiber embolus[106]

h. Wharton-jelly embolus[107]

i. Hypernatremia
   (1) True[6]
   (2) Factitious[108]

j. Factitious hyperkalemia[108]

k. Bladder injury (ascites)[109-111]

l. Curving back of the catheter on itself due to catching in the intima[112]

m. Pseudo coarctation of the aorta[113]

References

1. KANAREK SK, KUZNICKI MB, BLAIR RC: Infusion of total parenteral nutrition via the umbilical artery. J Parenter Enteral Nutr 15:71, 1991

2. CLAWSON CC, BOROS SJ: Surface morphology of polyvinyl chloride and silicone elastomere umbilical artery catheters by scanning electron microscopy. Pediatrics 62:702, 1978

3. HECKER JF: Thrombogenicity of tips of umbilical catheters. Pediatrics 67:467, 1981

4. BOROS SJ, THOMPSON TR, REYNOLDS JW, ET AL: Reduced thrombus formation with silicone elastomere (silastic) umbilical artery catheters. Pediatrics 56:981, 1975

5. JACKSON JC, TRUOG WE, WATCHKO JF, ET AL: Efficacy of thromboresistant umbilical artery catheters in reducing aortic thrombosis and related complications. J Pediatr 110:102, 1987

6. HAYDEN WR: Hypernatremia due to heparinized saline infusion through a radial artery catheter in a very low birth weight infant. J Pediatr 92:1025, 1978

7. RAJANI K, GOETZMAN BW, WENNBERG RP, ET AL: Effects of heparinization of fluids infused through an umbilical artery catheter on catheter patency and frequency of complications. Pediatrics 63:552, 1979

8. MERENSTEIN GB: Heparinized catheters and coagulation studies. J Pediatr 79:117, 1971

9. HORGAN MJ, BARTOLETTI A, POLANSKY S, ET AL: Effect of heparin infusates in umbilical arterial catheters on frequency of thrombotic complications. J Pediatr 111:774, 1987

10. BUTT W, SHANN F, MCDONNELL G, HUDSON I: Effect of heparin concentration and infusion rate on the patency of arterial catheters. Crit Care Med 15:230, 1987

11. BOSQUE E, WEAVER L: Continuous versus intermittent heparin infusion of umbilical artery catheters in the newborn infant. J Pediatr 108:141, 1986

12. HALL RT, RHODES PG, TURNER EA: Protamine sulphate titration for heparin activity in neonates with indwelling umbilical catheters. J Pediatr 88:467, 1976

13. WESTROM G, FINSTROM O, STENPORT G: Umbilical artery catheterization in newborns: Thrombosis in relation to catheter tip and position. Acta Paediatr Scand 68:575, 1979

14. OPPENHEIMER DA, CAROLL BA, GARTH KE, PARKER BR: Sonographic location of neonatal umbilical catheters. AJR 138:1025, 1982

15. POLLACI M, JACOBS HC, HOBBINS JC: Insertion of umbilical arterial catheters with guidance by ultrasound (Letter). N Engl J Med 320:805, 1989

16. BAKER DH, BERDON WE, JAMES LS: Proper localization of umbilical arterial and venous catheters by lateral roentgenograms. Pediatrics 43:34, 1969

17. WEBER AL, DELUCE S, SHANNON DL: Normal and abnormal position of umbilical artery and venous catheter on the roentgenogram and review of complications. AJR 20:361, 1974

18. MOKROHISKY ST, LEVINE RL, BLUMHAGEN JD, ET AL: Low positioning of umbilical artery catheters increases associated complications in newborn infants. N Engl J Med 229:561, 1978

19. LEDER ME, KLEIGMAN RE, FANAROFF AA: Severe symptomatic hypertension in the newborn (abstr). Pediatr Res 15:466, 1981

20. SHICK JB, BECK AL, DESILVA M: Umbilical artery catheter position and intraventricular hemorrhage. J Perinatol 9:382, 1989

21. GOETZMAN BW, STADALNICK RC, BOGEN HG, ET AL: Thrombotic complications of umbilical artery catheters: A clinical and radiographic study. Pediatrics 56:374, 1975

22. NEAL WA, REYNOLDS JW, JARVIS CW, WILLIAMS HJ: Umbilical artery catheterization: Demonstration of arterial thrombosis by aortography. Pediatrics 50:6, 1972

23. TOOLEY WH: What is the risk of an umbilical artery catheter? Pediatrics 50:1, 1972

24. AVERY ME, FLETCHER BD: The Lung and Its Disorders in the Newborn Infant. Philadelphia, WB Saunders, 1974

25. ADAM RD, EDWARDS LD, BECKER CC, SCHROM HM: Semi quantitative cultures and routine tip cultures on umbilical catheters. J Pediatr 100:123, 1982

26. DUNN P: Localization of the umbilical catheter by postmortem measurement. Arch Dis Child 41:69, 1966

27. ROSENFELD W, BIAGTAN J, SCHAEFFER H, ET AL: A new graph for insertion of umbilical artery catheters. J Pediatr 96:735, 1980

28. ROSENFELD W, ESTRADA R, JHAVERI R, ET AL: Evaluation of graphs for insertion of umbilical artery catheters below the diaphragm. J Pediatr 98:627, 1981

29. SHUKLA H, FERRARA A: Rapid estimation of insertional length of umbilical catheters in newborns. AJDC 140:786, 1986

30. WEAVER R, AHLGREN E: Umbilical artery catheterization in neonates. Am J Dis Child 122:499, 1971

31. RUBIN BK, McROBERT E, O'NEIL MB: An alternate technique to determine umbilical arterial catheter length. Clin Pediatr 25:407, 1986

32. BLOOM BT, NELSON RA, DIRKSEN HC: A new technique: Umbilical arterial catheter placement. J Perinatol 6:174, 1986

33. SQUIRE SJ, HORNUNG TL, KIRCHHOFF KT: Comparing two methods of umbilical artery catheter placement. Am J Perinatol 7:8, 1990

34. STEWART DL, WILKERSON S, FORTUNATE SJ: New technique for stabilizing umbilical artery catheters in very low birth weight infants. J Perinatol 9:458, 1989

35. LEHMILLER DJ, KANTO WP JR: Relationships of mesenteric thromboembolism, oral feeding and necrotizing enterocolitis. J Pediatr 92:96, 1978

36. BROWN R, FENTON LJ, TSANG RC: Blood sampling through umbilical catheters. Pediatrics 55:257, 1975

37. MILLER, D, KIRKPATRICK BV, KODROFF M, ET AL: Pelvic exsanguination following umbilical artery catheterization in neonates. J Pediatr Surg 14:264, 1979

38. RAO H, ELHASSANI S: *Primum non nocere:* Iatrogenic complications of procedures performed on newborn. Part I: Intravascular procedures. Perinatology-Neonatology 4:25, 1980

39. VIDYASAGER D, DOWNES JJ, BOGGS TR: Respiratory distress syndrome of newborn infants: Technique of catheterization of umbilical arteries and clinical results of treatment of 124 patients. Clin Pediatr 9:332, 1970

40. WESTROM G: Umbilical artery catheterization in newborns. V: A clinical follow-up study. Acta Paediatr Scand 69:371, 1980

41. MACDONALD MG, CHOU MM: Preventing complications from lines and tubes. Semin Perinatol 10:224, 1986

42. STRINGEL G, MERCER S, RICHLER M, McMURRAY B: Catheterization of the umbilical artery in neonates: Surgical implications. Can J Surg 28:143, 1985

43. SCHREIBER MD, PEREZ CA, KITTERMAN JA: A double-catheter technique for caudally misdirected umbilical arterial catheters. J Pediatr 104:768, 1984

44. CHIDI CC, KING DR, BATES E: An ultrastructural study of intimal injury induced by an indwelling umbilical artery catheter. J Pediatr Surg 18:109, 1983

45. CLARK JM, JUNG AL: Umbilical artery catheterization by a cut down procedure. Pediatrics [Neonatology Suppl] 59:1036, 1977

46. LEMONS JA, HONEYFIELD PR: Umbilical artery catheterization. Perinatal Care 2:17, 1978

47. HILLMAN LS, GOODWIN SL, SHERMAN WR: Identification of plasticizer in neonatal tissues after umbilical catheters and blood products. N Engl J Med 292:381, 1975

48. JAMES LS: Complications arising from catheterization of the umbilical vessels. In 59th Ross Conference on Pediatric Research, pp 36. Columbus, OH, Ross Laboratories, 1969

49. NAGEL JW, SIMS SJ, APLIN CE II, WESTMARK Er: Refractory hypoglycemia associated with a malpositioned umbilical artery catheter. Pediatrics 64:315, 1979

50. URBACH J, KAPLAN M, BLONDHEIM O, HIRSH HJ: Neonatal hypoglycemia related to umbilical artery catheter malposition. J Pediatr 106:825, 1985

51. CAREY BE, ZEILINGER TC: Hypoglycemia due to high positioning of umbilical artery catheters. J Perinatol 9:407, 1989

52. VAN LEEUWEN G, PATNEY M: Complications of umbilical artery catheterizations: Peritoneal perforation. Pediatrics 44:1028, 1969

53. MALLOY MH, NICHOLS MM: False abdominal aortic aneurism: An unusual complication of umbilical arterial catheterization for exchange transfusion. J Pediatr 90:285, 1977

54. WYNN ML, ROWEN M, RUCKER RW, ET AL: Pseudoaneurism of the thoracic aorta: A late complication of umbilical artery catheterization. Ann Thorac Surg 34:186, 1982

55. WIND ES, WISOFF G, BARON MG, ET AL: Mycotic aneurism in infancy: A complication of umbilical artery catheterization. J Pediatr Surg 17:324, 1982

56. DRUCKER DE, GREENFIELD LJ, SALZBERG AM: Aorto-iliac aneurisms following umbilical artery catheterization. J Pediatr Surg 21:725, 1986

57. LALLY KP, SHERMAN NJ: Iliac artery pseudoaneurism following umbilical artery catheterization. Surgery 101:636, 1987

58. KIRPEKAR M, AUGENSTEIN H, ABIRI M: Sequential development of multiple aortic aneurisms in a neonate post umbilical arterial catheter insertion. Pediatr Radiol 19:452, 1989

59. FOK TF, HA MH, LEUNG KW, WONG W: Sciatic nerve palsy complicating umbilical artery catheterization. Eur J Pediatr 145:308, 1986

60. LYNCH MC: Sciatic palsy after umbilical artery catheterization. Brief report. J Bone Joint Surg [Br] 70:151, 1988

61. HIMMEL PD, SUMNER DS, MONGKOLSMAI C, KHANNA N: Neonatal thrombosis associated with the umbilical arterial catheter: Successful management by transaortic thrombectomy. J Vasc Surg 4:119, 1986

62. MALIN SW, BAUMGART S, ROSENBERG HK, FOREMAN J: Nonsurgical management of obstructive aortic thrombosis complicated by renovascular hypertension in the neonate. J Pediatr 106:630, 1985

63. SEIBERT JJ, NORTHINGTON FJ, MIERS JF, TAYLOR BJ: Aortic thrombosis after umbilical artery catheterization in neonates: Prevalence of complications on long-term follow-up. Am J Roentgenol 156:567, 1991

64. MARTIN JE, MORAN JF, COOK LS, ET AL: Neonatal

aortic thrombosis complicating umbilical artery catheterization: Successful treatment with retroperitoneal aortic thrombectomy. Surgery 105:793, 1989

65. COCHRANE WD, DAVIS HT, SMITH CA: Advantages and complications of umbilical artery catheterization in the newborn. Pediatrics 42:769, 1968

66. EGAN EA, EITZMAN DV: Umbilical vessel catheterization. Am J Dis Child 121:213, 1971

67. RUDOLPH N, HSINN-HONG W, DRAGTSY D: Gangrene of the buttock: A complication of umbilical artery catheterization. Pediatrics 53:106, 1974

68. WIGGER HJ, BRANSILVER BR, BLANC WA: Thromboses due to catheterization in infants and children. J Pediatr 76:1, 1970

69. COLE ARF, ROLGIN SH: A technique for rapid catheterization of the umbilical artery. Anesthesiology 53:254, 1980

70. DORAND RD, COOK LN, ANDREW BF: Umbilical vessel catheterization. The low incidence of complications in a series of 200 newborn infants. Clin Pediatr 16:569, 1977

71. GUPTA JM, ROBERTON NRC, WIGGLESWORTH JS: Umbilical artery catheterization in the newborn. Arch Dis Child 43:382, 1968

72. KITTERMAN JA, PHIBBS RH, TOOLEY WH: Catheterization of umbilical vessels in newborn infants. Pediatr Clin North Am 17:895, 1970

73. LIVIDATIS A, WALLGREN G, FAXELIUS G: Necrotizing enterocolitis after catheterization of the umbilical vessels. Acta Paediatr Scand 63:277, 1974

74. BAUER SB, FELDMAN SM, GELLIS SS, RETIK AB: Neonatal hypertension: A complication of umbilical artery catheterization. N Engl J Med 293:1032, 1975

75. FORD KT, TEPLICK SK, CLARK RE: Renal artery embolism causing neonatal hypertension: A complication of umbilical artery catheterization. Radiology 113:169, 1974

76. PLUMER LB, KAPLAN GW, MENDOZA SA: Hypertension in infants: A complication of umbilical artery catheterization. J Pediatr 89:802, 1976

77. STEVENS PS, MANDELL J: Urologic complications of neonatal umbilical artery catheterization. J Urol 120:605, 1978

78. BUTT WW, GOW R, WHYTE H, ET AL: Complications resulting from use of arterial catheters: Retrograde flow and rapid elevation in blood pressure. Pediatrics 76:250, 1985

79. BROOKS WG, WEIBLING RE: Emergency department presentation of severe hypertension secondary to complications of umbilical artery catheterization. Pediatr Emerg Care 3:104, 1987

80. KREIGER TC, NEBLETT WW, O'NEILL, ET AL: Management of Aortic thrombosis secondary to umbilical artery catheters in neonates. J Pediatr Surg 20:328, 1985

81. AZIZ EM, ROBERTSON AF: Paraplegia: A complication of umbilical artery catheterization. J Pediatr 82:1051, 1973

82. LACKEY DA, TABER P: An unusual complication of umbilical artery catheterization. Pediatrics 49:281, 1972

83. HALDMAN S, FAWTER GW, ASHWAL S, SCHNEIDER S: Acute flaccid neonatal paraplegia: A case report. Neurology 33:93, 1983

84. BROWN MS, PHIBBS RH: Spinal cord injury in newborns from use of umbilical artery. J Perinatol 8:105, 1988

85. HENRY CG, GUTIERREZ F, JOSEPH I, ET AL: Aortic thrombosis presenting as congestive heart failure: An umbilical artery catheter complication. J Pediatr 98:820, 1981

86. KRISHNAMOORTHY KS, FERDNANDEZ, J, TODRES ID, DELONG GR: Paraplegia associated with umbilical artery catheterization in the newborn. Pediatrics 58:443, 1976

87. MARTIN GJ, IRELAND WR: Letter to the Editor: Broken umbilical catheters. Am J Dis Child 131:1405, 1977

88. WAGNER CW, VINOCUR CD, WEINTRAUB WH: Retrieval of an umbilical artery catheter: A potential for misadventure. South Med J 80:1434, 1987

89. COCHRANE WD: Umbilical artery catheterization. In Iatrogenic Problems in Neonatal Intensive Care. Report of the 69th Ross Conference of Pediatric Research, pp 28–32. Columbus, OH, Ross Laboratories, 1976

90. HILLIARD J, SCHREINER RL, PRIEST J: Hemoperitoneum associated with exchange transfusion through an umbilical arterial catheter. Am J Dis Child 133:216, 1979

91. SASIDHANAN P: Umbilical arterial rupture: A major complication of catheterization. Indiana Med 78:34, 1985

92. MONCINO MD, KURTZBERG J: Accidental heparinization in the newborn: A case report and brief review of the literature. J Perinatol 10:399, 1990

93. KNUDSEN FV, PETERSEN S: Neonatal septic osteoarthritis due to umbilical artery catheterization. Acta Paediatr Scand 66:225, 1977

94. KRAUSS AN, ALBERT RF, KANNAN MM: Contamination of umbilical catheters in the newborn infant. J Pediatr 77:965, 1970

95. LARROCHE JCL, BENNOUN M, KORN G: Umbilical catheterization: Its complications (anatomical study). Symposium on artificial ventilation. Biol Neonate 16:101, 1970

96. LIM MO, GRESHAM EL, FRANKEN EA: Osteomyelitis as a complication of umbilical artery catheterization. Am J Dis Child 131:142, 1977

97. POWERS WF, TOOLEY WH: Letter to the Editor: Contamination of umbilical vessel catheters. Encouraging information. Pediatrics 49:470, 1968

98. WHITE AA II, CRELINE ES, MCINTOSH S: Septic arthritis of the hip joint secondary to umbilical artery catheterization associated with transient femoral and sciatic neuropathy. Clin Orthop 100:190, 1974

99. RUDERMAN JW, MORGAN MA, KLEIN AH: Quantita-

tive blood cultures in the diagnosis of sepsis in infants with umbilical and Broviac catheters. J Pediatr 112:798, 1988

100. Pourcyrous M, Korones SB, Bada HS, et al: Indwelling umbilical arterial catheter: A preferred sampling site for blood culture. Pediatrics 81:821, 1988

101. Landers S, Moise AA, Fraley JK, et al: Factors associated with umbilical catheter related sepsis in neonates. Am J Dis Child 145:675, 1991

102. Castelman B, Scully RE, McNeely BV: Case records of the Massachusetts General Hospital. N Engl J Med 189:1027, 1973

103. Book LS, Herbst JJ: Intraarterial infusions and intestinal necrosis in the rabbit: Potential hazards of umbilical artery injections of ampicillin, glucose, and sodium bicarbonate. Pediatrics 65:114, 1980

104. Simpson JS: Misdiagnosis complicating umbilical vessel catheterization. Clin Pediatr 16:569, 1977

105. Biagtan J, Rosenfeld W, Salazard D, Velcek F: Herniation of the appendix through the umbilical ring following umbilical artery catheterization. J Pediatr Surg 15:672, 1980

106. Bavikatte K, Hillard J, Schreiner RL, et al: Systemic vascular cotton fiber emboli in the neonate. J Pediatr 95:61, 1979

107. Abramowsky CR, Chrenka B, Fanaroff A: Wharton jelly embolism: An unusual complication of umbilical catheterization. J Pediatr 96:739, 1980

108. Gaylord MS, Pittman PA, Bartness J: Release of benzalkonium chloride from a heparin-bonded umbilical catheter with resultant factitious hypernatremia and hyperkalemia. Pediatrics 87:631, 1991

109. Diamond DA, Ford C: Neonatal bladder rupture: Complication of umbilical artery catheterization. J Urol 142:1543, 1989

110. Mata JA, Livne PM, Gibbons MD: Urinary ascites: Complication of umbilical artery catheterization. Urology 30:375, 1987

111. Dmochowski RR, Crandell SS, Lowiere JN: Bladder injury and uroascites from umbilical artery catheterization. Pediatrics 77:421, 1986

112. McGravey VJ, Dabiri C, Bean MS: An unusual twist to umbilical artery catheterization. Clin Pediatr 22:587, 1983

113. Rodriquez M, Sosenko I: Catheter-induced aortic thrombosis masquerading as coarctation of the aorta. Clin Pediatr (Phila) 28:581, 1989

25 Umbilical Artery Cutdown

Mary Ann Fletcher

This method is most often successful even after failed insertion through the umbilical stump, as there is less tendency for false tracts. The most frequent reason for failed umbilical artery cutdown is mistaking the urachus for a vessel. Because of the time and risks associated with the cutdown procedure, standard insertion should be attempted first.

A. INDICATIONS

These are the same as for umbilical artery catheterization, described in Chapter 24.

B. CONTRAINDICATIONS

1. Bleeding diathesis
2. Omphalocele
3. Omphalitis
4. Peritonitis
5. Necrotizing enterocolitis
6. Extrophy of the bladder

C. EQUIPMENT

Sterile

1. Gown and gloves
2. Povidone iodine surgical scrub and swabs
3. Surgical drapes including aperture drape, preferably transparent
4. Towel clips
5. Surgical sponges (4 × 4 gauze pads)
6. 1% lidocaine HCl without epinephrine in 3-ml syringe with 25- to 27-gauge needle
7. No. 15 surgical blade and holder
8. Vessel probe or catheter introducer (optional)
9. Curved delicate dressing forceps, 2 pair (¼ or ½ curved)
10. Tissue forceps
11. Self-retaining retractor (such as eyelid retractor)
12. Absorbable suture, plain 4-0
13. Absorbable suture on small cutting needle 4-0
14. Nonabsorbable suture on a small, curved needle 5-0

15. Needle holder
16. Suture scissors
17. Skin closure tapes
18. Umbilical catheter
19. Stopcock
20. Flush solution in 3-ml syringe
21. Empty 3- to 5-ml syringe for blood withdrawal

Unsterile

1. Mask and cap
2. 0.5- to 1-inch porous adhesive tape
3. Surgical light source

D. PRECAUTIONS

1. See precautions for UAC (Chap. 24).
2. If possible, leave catheter from previously attempted standard procedure in place to aid in vessel identification.
3. Ensure that abdominal incision is on abdominal wall and not too close to umbilical stump.
4. Identify landmarks carefully to avoid cutting or catheterizing urachus.
5. Take care when incising mesenchymal sheath to avoid transecting vessel.
6. Secure the catheter with an internal ligature that is just tight enough to prevent accidental removal but loose enough for elective removal.

E. TECHNIQUE[1,2]

See Figure 25-1.

1. Insert an oral gastric tube to keep the bowel as decompressed as possible.
2. Prepare infant and drape as for UAC (see Chap. 24).
3. If catheter has been left in place after previous attempt, include vessel and catheter in the preparation, leaving the catheter accessible for removal.
4. Anesthetize area of skin immediately below um-

175

bilicus, at umbilical stump–abdominal wall junction, with 0.5 ml of lidocaine.

5. Prepare UAC as for standard procedure, leaving catheter filled with flush solution. Estimate length for insertion based on patient size. Subtract 1 to 2 cm from that recommended for standard insertion as cutdown catheter will enter vessel further along course.

6. Make a smile-shaped incision from 4 to 8 o'clock through the skin of the abdominal wall at junction with umbilical stump.

7. Place self-retaining retractor to maintain exposure.

8. Using blunt dissection through the subcutaneous tissue with mosquito forceps, identify the fascia overlying the urachus and umbilical vessels.

> The mesenchymal sheath is composed of three layers of fascia and is from 1 to 3 mm thick. While barely perceptible in extremely premature infants, in term infants it may be thick enough to require making an incision through the sheath prior to blunt dissection.

9. While elevating the fascia with two forceps, make a small incision between their tips. Enlarge incision with scissors to the same size as skin incision. In very immature infants, simple dissection should suffice.

10. With curved mosquito forceps dissect in the midline and identify the urachus (Fig. 25-1).

> The urachus is a white, glistening, cordlike struc-

ture in the midline. Its position may be confirmed by traction cephalad, pulling the dome of the bladder into view. The umbilical arteries lie posterolaterally on either side but not touching the urachus.

11. Identify the umbilical arteries lying to either side of the urachus.

> The vessels with their surrounding tissues appear larger than expected. When elevated, there will be no caudal bulge, distinguishing them from the urachus. If a previously attempted catheter was left "in place," palpation of the area allows more ready identification of the vessel. Previously unsuccessful attempts, with failure to pass more than a few centimeters, are usually associated with perivascular hematoma formation from unrecognized perforation and dissection through a false tract. Visualization of a hematoma helps distinguish the vessel from the urachus.

12. Try to avoid entering the peritoneum. In infants with very little subcutaneous tissue, it may be impossible to avoid penetrating the peritoneum. Should this occur, replace any bowel that may protrude and carefully close the peritoneum with absorbable suture, taking extreme care not to include any bowel within the suture.

13. Insert the tip of the mosquito forceps under the vessel and pull a doubled strand of plain absorbable suture under the vessel. Position sutures 1 cm apart.

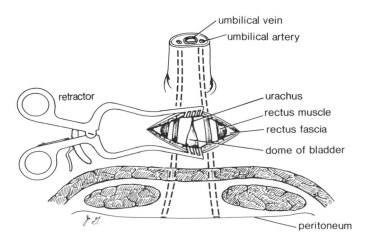

FIG. 25-1
Subumbilical cutdown. Anatomical view through incision. (Redrawn by permission from Sherman NJ: Umbilical artery cutdown. J Pediatr Surg 12:723, 1977)

14. While elevating the sutures and with suture scissors directed cephalad, make a V-shaped incision through ¾ of the diameter of the vessel. Take care not to transect the vessel but cut cleanly into the lumen.

    If the artery is accidentally transected and if the catheter insertion is unsuccessful, tie off the caudal end of the artery to prevent hemorrhage.

15. Use curved tissue forceps or a catheter introducer to dilate the artery.
16. Pass the catheter through the opening for the predetermined distance, checking for blood return after a few centimeters. The catheter should advance without resistance.
17. When the catheter is properly positioned, have an assistant check the perfusion in the lower extremities. If satisfactory, secure the catheter by tying the lower ligature firmly around the catheter.
18. Using absorbable suture, close the fascia and approximate the subcutaneous tissues.
19. Close the skin with nonabsorbable suture or with skin closure tape after cleaning the area.
20. The catheter may be further secured with a tape bridge (Fig. 36-16).
21. Verify the catheter position by radiograph.

F. REMOVAL OF CATHETER

1. Remove any tape.
2. Withdraw catheter until tip is approximately 2 cm from incision.
3. Observe catheter contents for cessation of pulsation.
4. When pulsation is absent, slowly withdraw remainder of catheter.

If the internal ligature around a catheter is too tight to allow removal with reasonable traction, it may be necessary to dissect and cut the ligature after sterile skin preparation.

5. Apply pressure for hemostasis.
6. Approximate wound edges with skin closure tape.

G. COMPLICATIONS (see also Chap. 24, Umbilical Artery Catheterization)

1. Catheterization of urachus[3]
2. Vesicoumbilical fistula[3]
3. Transection of urachus with urinary ascites[4]
4. Perforation of urinary bladder[5,6]
5. Transection of umbilical artery with hemorrhage
6. Incision of peritoneum (with possible evisceration)
7. Bleeding from incision

References

1. CLARK JM, JUNG AL: Umbilical artery catheterization by a cutdown procedure. Pediatrics 59:1036, 1977
2. SHERMAN NJ: Umbilical artery cutdown. J Pediatr Surg 12:723, 1977
3. WAFFARN F, DEVASKAR UP, HODGMAN JE: Vesico-umbilical fistula: A complication of umbilical artery cutdown. J Pediatr Surg 15:211, 1980
4. HEPWORTH RC, MILSTEIN JM: The transected urachus: An unusual cause of neonatal ascites. Pediatrics 73:397, 1984
5. DMOCHOWSKI RR, CRANDELL SS, CORRIERE JN JR: Bladder injury and uroascites from umbilical artery catheterization. Pediatrics 77:421, 1986
6. DIAMOND DA, FORD C: Neonatal bladder rupture: A complication of umbilical artery catheterization. J Urol 142:1543, 1989

26 Umbilical Vein Catheterization

Mhairi G. MacDonald

A. INDICATIONS

1. Primary
   a. Emergency vascular access for fluid and medication infusion and for blood drawing
   b. Central-venous-pressure monitoring (if catheter across ductus venosus)
   c. Exchange transfusion
2. Secondary
   a. Long-term central venous access in low birth weight infants
   b. Diagnosis of total anomalous pulmonary venous drainage below the diaphragm[1]

B. CONTRAINDICATIONS

   a. Omphalitis
   b. Omphalocele
   c. Necrotizing enterocolitis
   d. Peritonitis

C. EQUIPMENT

1. Catheter: Same as for umbilical artery catheterization, except
   a. 5 Fr catheter for infants weighing <3.5 kg
   b. 8 Fr catheter for infants weighing >3.5 kg
   c. Catheter used for exchange transfusion (removed after procedure) should have side holes.

   Reduces risk of sucking thin wall of inferior vena cava against catheter tip, with possible vascular perforation[2]

2. Other equipment as for UAC, but omit 2% lidocaine (see Chap. 24, C)

D. PRECAUTIONS

1. Keep catheter tip away from origin of hepatic vessels, portal vein, and foramen ovale. Catheter tip should lie in ductus venosus or inferior vena cava.[3]

Sometimes it will not be possible to advance the catheter through the ductus venosus. Vigorous attempts to advance are to be avoided. *In an emergency*, vital infusions (avoid very hypertonic solutions) may be given *slowly* after pulling catheter back into umbilical vein (approximately 2 cm) and checking blood return.

2. Check catheter position prior to exchange transfusion. Avoid performing exchange transfusion with catheter tip in portal system or intrahepatic venous branch (see E).
3. Once secured, do not advance catheter into vein.
4. Avoid infusion of hypertonic solutions when catheter tip is not in inferior vena cava.
5. Do not leave catheter open to atmosphere (danger of air embolus).
6. Avoid use of central-venous-pressure monitoring catheter for concomitant infusion of parenteral nutrition (risk of sepsis).
7. Be aware of potential inaccuracies of venous-pressure measurements in inferior vena cava (see Chap. 28).

E. TECHNIQUE

Anatomical Note: In the full term infant, the umbilical vein (UV) is 2 to 3 cm in length and 4 to 5 mm in diameter. From the umbilicus, it passes cephalad and a little to the right, where it joins the left branch of the portal vein after giving off several large intrahepatic branches that are distributed directly to the liver tissue. The ductus venosus becomes a continuation of the UV by arising from the left branch of the portal vein, directly opposite where the UV joins it. At birth it is 2 to 3 cm long and 4 to 5 mm in diameter, and it is located in a groove between the right and left lobes of the liver in the median sagittal plane of the body, at a level between the ninth and tenth thoracic vertebrae. It terminates in the inferior vena cava along with hepatic veins, as shown in Figure 26-1.

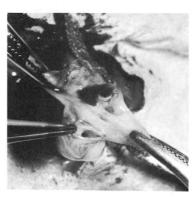

FIG. 26-2
The umbilical stump. Vein is indicated with nontoothed forceps.

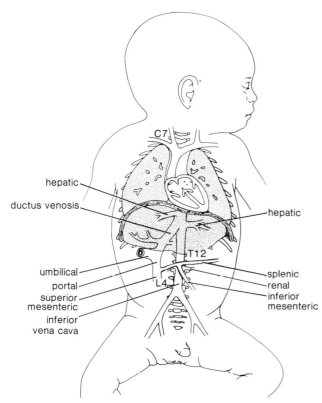

FIG. 26-1
Anatomy of the umbilical and associated veins, with reference to external landmarks.

1. Make necessary measurements to determine length of catheter to be inserted, adding length of umbilical stump (Figs. 24-1 and 24-3).[4]
2. Prepare for procedure as for UAC (see Chap. 24, E).
3. Identify thin-walled vein, close to periphery of umbilical stump (Fig. 26-2).
4. Grasp cord stump with toothed forceps.
5. Gently insert tips of iris forceps into lumen of vein and remove any clots.
6. Introduce fluid-filled catheter, *attached to the stopcock and syringe,* 2 to 3 cm into vein (measuring from anterior abdominal wall).
7. Apply gentle suction to syringe.
   a. If there is not easy blood return, catheter may have a clot in tip. Withdraw catheter, while maintaining gentle suction. Remove clot and reinsert catheter.
   b. If there is smooth blood flow, continue to insert catheter for full estimated distance.
8. If catheter meets any obstruction prior to measured distance
   a. It has most commonly
      (1) Entered portal system, or
      (2) Wedged in an intrahepatic branch of umbilical vein
   b. Withdraw catheter 2 to 3 cm, gently rotate and reinsert in an attempt to get tip through ductus venosus
9. Obtain x-ray-film verification of catheter position. A lateral x-ray film is often necessary for exact localization (Figs. 26-3A and 26-3B).[5,6] Desired location is D9-10, just above the right diaphragm.

   Position of catheter tip may be estimated clinically by measurement of venous pressure[2] and observation of waveform (Figs. 26-4 A-C and 26-5 A,B

   a. As soon as catheter has been advanced 2 to 3 cm into the vein have an assistant connect to pressure monitoring system (see Chap. 8).
   b. While continuing to advance catheter, measure venous pressure and note pressure changes with respiration (Fig. 26-4).

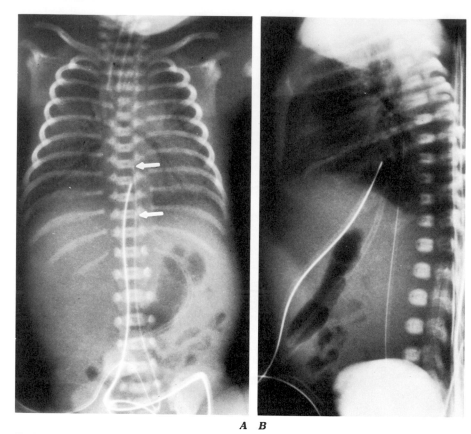

A B

FIG. 26-3
AP (*A*) and lateral (*B*) radiographs demonstrating the normal course of an umbilical venous catheter with an umbilical artery catheter (*arrows*) in position for comparison. Note how the venous catheter swings immediately superior from the umbilicus, slightly to the right as it traverses the ductus venosus into the inferior vena cava. The distal tip of this line is just superior to the right atrial/IVC junction, and it might optimally be pulled back slightly into the IVC. Note how the thinner umbilical artery catheter (*arrows*) heads inferiorly as it proceeds to the iliac artery, and then ascends posteriorly and to the left until it reaches the level of D7.

Ideal position is with catheter tip in inferior vena cava, near right atrium, although placement in ductus venosus is acceptable for purposes other than measurement of central venous pressure.

10. Secure catheter as for UAC (see Chap. 24, E).

There may be more bleeding from the umbilical vein than the artery because it is not a contractile vessel. Local pressure is usually sufficient to stop oozing.

For care of indwelling catheter sampling technique and removal of catheter, see Chapter 24.

F. COMPLICATIONS

1. Infections[5,7–16]
2. Thromboembolic[7,11,17,18]

Emboli from a venous catheter may be widely distributed. If catheter tip lies in the portal system and ductus venosus has closed, emboli will lodge in liver. If catheter has passed through ductus venosus, emboli will go to lungs, or, because of right-to-left shunting of blood through foramen ovale or ductus arteriosus in sick newborn

FIG. 26-4

Venous and arterial pressure tracings may be used to facilitate placement and detect misplacement. (*A*) The catheter has been pulled back through the ductus venosus and the tip lies in the portal system. The portal venous pressure is higher than central venous pressure, there are no venous pressure waves, and there is a small positive deflection during inspiration.

(*B*) Tip of catheter in the superior vena cava near the right atrium, shows a deflection of more than 4 mm Hg during spontaneous inspiration (I) and a large negative deflection of more than 15 mm Hg during a sigh (S). *Atrial tracing* shows an "ac" and a "v" wave. Ac wave occurs with atrial contraction and closure of atrioventricular valve after P wave of electrocardiogram. V wave occurs with ventricular contraction near T wave of electrocardiogram. (Based on data of Kitterman JA, Phibbs RH, Tooley WH: Catheterization of umbilical vessels in newborn infants. Pediatr Clin N Amer 17, No. 4:895, 1970.)

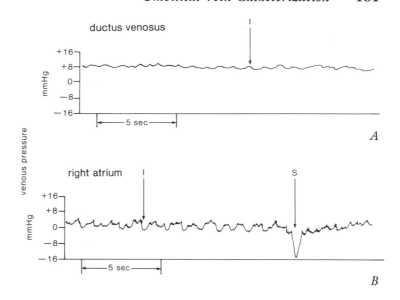

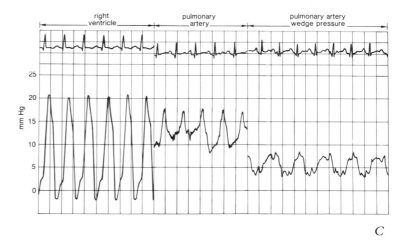

(*C*) Pressure tracing from Rt ventricle and pulmonary artery. *Right ventricular pressure tracing* shows a single large rise and fall, beginning just after onset of QRS complex. *Pulmonary-artery tracing* usually shows a dicrotic notch at end of T wave. Diastolic pressure is higher than that in right ventricle. *Pulmonary capillary wedge (PCW) tracing* should resemble atrial tracing, inasmuch as it reflects left atrial pressure transmitted to catheter tip when anterograde pulmonary arterial flow is occluded.

Note: The marked negative deflection in the right atrial (RA) tracing would be more typically seen in infants who are receiving mechanical ventilation and, thus, have a positive airway pressure which exceeds ventricular filling pressures during each inspiration. *In a spontaneously breathing neonate,* positive airway pressure occurs only during expiration, and never exceeds ventricular filling pressures. There are extremely small changes in cardiac pressures (i.e., on inspiration: RA mean pressure ↑ 1 mm Hg; Left atrial (LA) mean pressure ↓ 1 mm Hg. On expiration: RA pressure ↓ 1 mm Hg; LA pressure ↑ 1 mm Hg) during the respiratory cycle due to changes in venous filling or preload. RA and LA pressures remain approximately equal in both inspiration and expiration.[39]

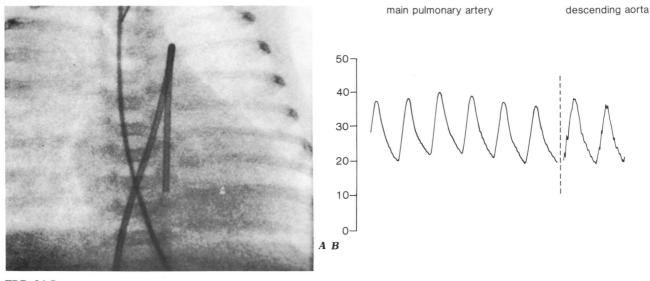

FIG. 26-5
(*A*) Radiograph showing venous catheter which has crossed the ductus arteriosus into the thoracic aorta. (*B*) In this situation the arterial pressure markings were not helpful because the presence of pulmonary hypertension in the patient rendered the tracings from the pulmonary artery and descending aorta virtually identical.

infants, emboli may be distributed throughout entire systemic circulation. These emboli may be infected and therefore may cause widespread abscesses.

3. Catheter malpositioned in heart and great vessels (Figs. 26-6 and 26-5 A,B)
   a. Pericardial effusion/cardiac tamponade (cardiac perforation)[3,19–21]
   b. Cardiac arrhythmias[22]
   c. Thrombotic endocarditis[23]
   d. Hemorrhagic infarction of lung[6]
   e. Hyrothorax (catheter lodged in or perforated pulmonary vein)[24]
4. Catheter malpositioned in portal system
   a. Necrotizing enterocolitis[25,26]
   b. Perforation of colon[27,28]

   c. Hepatic necrosis (thrombosis of hepatic veins or infusion of hypertonic or vasospastic solutions into liver tissues) (Fig. 26-7)[11,12,18,29,30]
   d. Hepatic cyst[31]
5. Other
   a. Perforation of peritoneum[32]
   b. Obstruction of pulmonary venous return (in infant with anomalous pulmonary venous drainage)[1]
   c. Plasticizer in tissues[33]
   d. Portal hypertension[17,23,34,35]
   e. Electrical hazard (see Chap. 24, I3c)[2]
   f. Fungal mass in right atrium[36]
   g. Pseudomass in left atrium[37]
   h. Digital ischemia[38]

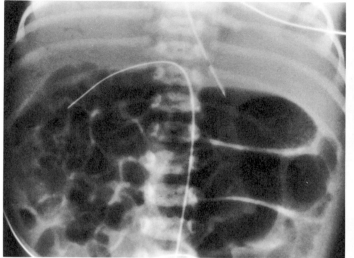

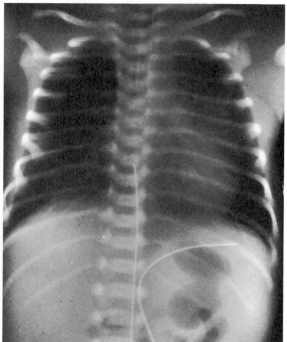

A B
C

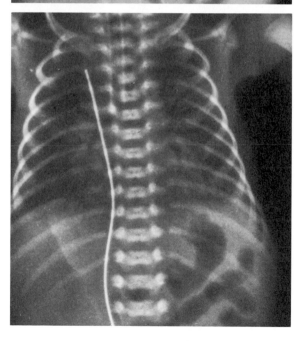

FIG. 26-6, A-C
Spectrum of malpositions of umbilical venous catheters
(UVC). (*A*) UVC in right portal vein with secondary
air embolization into portal venous system. (*B*) UVC in
splenic vein. UAC catheter in good position with its tip
at D7. (*C*) UVC extending through heart into the superior vena cava.

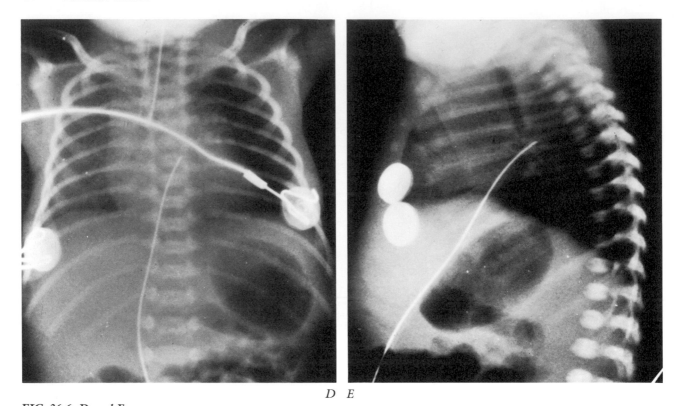

D E

FIG. 26-6, D and E

Spectrum of malpositions of umbilical venous catheters (UVC). The AP film (*D*) shows an indeterminate position of the UVC catheter. The right atrium, the right ventricle, and the left atrium are all possibilities. The lateral (*E*) shows its posterior position, confirming its presence in the left atrium. The lateral film is particularly important in making this distinction. Measurement of the PO_2 in blood from the catheter will be diagnostic of misplacement, unless the infant has severe persistent pulmonary hypertension or other cause of severe intracardiac shunting.

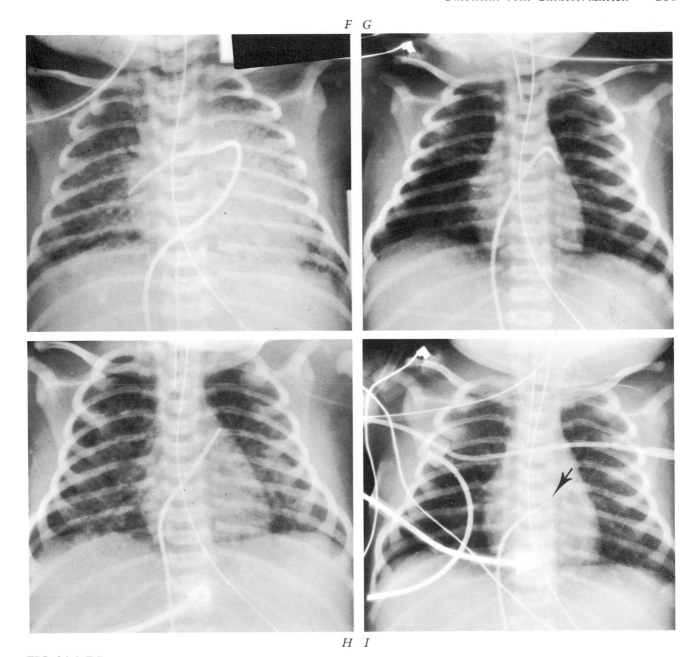

FIG. 26-6, F-I
Spectrum of malpositions of umbilical venous catheters (UVC). Series of radiographs demonstrating various malpositions of a venous catheter. (*F*) Right pulmonary artery. (*G*) Left main pulmonary artery. (*H*) Main pulmonary artery. (*I*) Right ventricle.

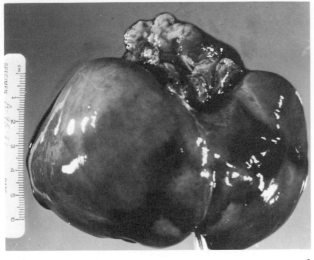 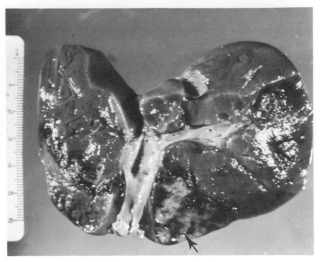

A B

FIG. 26-7

(*A*) Hepatic infarction (darkened areas on anterior aspect of liver) related to umbilical vein catheter. (*B*) Section through inferior aspect of liver to show internal appearance of infarcted areas (*arrow*).

References

1. Nickerson BG, Sahn DJ, Goldberg SJ, Allen HD: Hazards of inadvertent venous catheterization in a patient with anomalous pulmonary venous drainage: A case report. Pediatrics 63:929, 1979
2. Kitterman JA, Phibbs RH, Tooley WH: Catheterization of umbilical vessels in newborn infants. Pediatr Clin North Am 17:895, 1970
3. Johns AW, Kitchen WH, Leslie DW: Complications of umbilical vessel catheters. Med J Aust 2:810, 1972
4. Dunn P: Localization of the umbilical catheter by postmortem measurement. Arch Dis Child 41:69, 1966
5. Baker DH, Berdon WE, James LS: Proper localization of umbilical arterial and venous catheters by lateral roentgenograms. Pediatrics 43:34, 1969
6. Weber AL, Deluce S, Shannan DL: Normal and abnormal position of the umbilical artery and venous catheter on the roentgenogram and review of complications. Am J Roentgenol 20:361, 1974
7. Anagnostakis D, Kamba A, Petrochilou V, et al: Risk of infection associated with umbilical vein catheterization: A prospective study in 75 newborn infants. J Pediatr 86:759, 1975
8. Balagtas RC, Bell CE, Edward LD, Levine S: Risk of local and systemic infections associated with umbilical vein catheterization: A prospective study in 86 newborn patients. Pediatrics 48:359, 1971
9. Brans YW, Ceballos R, Cassady G: Umbilical catheters and hepatic abscesses. Pediatrics 53:264, 1974
10. Krauss AN, Albert RF, Kannan MM: Contamination of umbilical catheters in the newborn infant. J Pediatr 77:965, 1970
11. Larroche JCL, Bennoun M, Korn G: Umbilical catheterization: Its complications (anatomical study). Symposium on artificial ventilation. Biol Neonat 16:101, 1970
12. Scott JM: Iatrogenic lesions in babies following umbilical vein catheterization. Arch Dis Child 40:426, 1965
13. Tariq AA, Rudolph N, Levine EJ: Solitary hepatic abscess in a newborn infant: A sequel of umbilical vein catheterization and infusion of hypertonic glucose solutions. Clin Pediatr 16:577, 1977
14. Williams JW, Rittenberry A, Dillard R, Allen RG: Liver abscess in the newborn: Complication of umbilical vein catheterization. Am J Dis Child 125:111, 1973
15. Noel GJ, O'Loughlin JE, Edelson PJ: Neonatal staphylococcus epidermitis right sided endocarditis: Description of five catheterized infants. Pediatrics 82:234, 1988
16. Wilkins EG, Manning D, Roberts C, Davidson DC: Quantitative bacteriology of peripheral venous cannulae in neonates. J Hosp Infect 6:209, 1985
17. Oski FA, Allen DM, Diamond LK: Portal hypertension—a complication of umbilical vein catheterization. Pediatrics 31:297, 1963

18. Sarrut S, Alain J, Allison F: Early complications of umbilical vein perfusion in the premature infant. Arch Fr Pediatr 26:651, 1969

19. Purohit DM, Levkoff AH: Pericardial effusion complicating umbilical venous catheterizations. Arch Dis Child 52:520, 1977

20. Walker D, Pellet JR: Pericardial tamponade secondary to umbilical vein catheters. J Pediatr Surg 7:79, 1972

21. Savani RC, Valentini RP, Mimouni F (Vinstein AL, Section Editor): Pericardial effusion as a complication of umbilical venous catheterization. J Perinatol 10:443, 1990

22. Egan EA, Eitzman DV: Umbilical vessel catheterization. Am J Dis Child 121:213, 1971

23. Symchych PS, Krauss AN, Winchester P: Endocarditis following intracardiac placement of umbilical venous catheters in neonates. J Pediatr 90:287, 1977

24. Kulkarni PB, Dorand RD: Hydrothorax: A complication of intracardiac placement of umbilical venous catheters. J Pediatr 94:813, 1979

25. Livaditis A, Wallgren G, Faxelius G: Necrotizing enterocolitis after catheterization of the umbilical vessels. Acta Pediatr Scand 63:277, 1974

26. Shah KJ, Corkery JJ: Necrotizing enterocolitis following umbilical vein catheterization. Clin Radiol 29:295, 1978

27. Friedman A, Abellera R, Lidsky I, Lubert M: Perforation of the colon after exchange transfusion in the newborn. N Engl J Med 282:796, 1970

28. Lucey JF: Colonic perforation after exchange transfusion. N Engl J Med 280:724, 1969

29. Venkatavaman PS, Babcock DS, Tsang RC, Ballard JL: Hepatic injury: A possible complication of Dopamine infusion through an inappropriately placed umbilical vein catheter. Am J Perinatol 1:351, 1984

30. Richter E, Gl'obl H, Hoethusen W, Lassrich MA: Intrahepatic calcifications in infants following umbilical venous catheterization. Ann Radiol (Paris) 27:117, 1984

31. Levkoff AH, MacPherson RI: Intrahepatic encystment of umbilical vein catheter infusate. Pediatr Radiol 20:360, 1990

32. Kanto WP, Parrish RA: Perforation of the peritoneum and intraabdominal hemorrhage. Am J Dis Child 131:1102, 1977

33. Hillman LS, Goodwin SL, Sherwin WR: Identification and measurement of plasticizer in neonatal tissues after umbilical catheters and blood products. N Engl J Med 292:381, 1975

34. Erkan V, Blankenship W, Stahlman MT: The complications of chronic umbilical vessel catheterization (abstr). Pediatr Res 2:317, 1968

35. Lauridsen UB, Enk B, Gammeltoft A: Oesophageal varices as a late complication of neonatal umbilical vein catheterization. Acta Paediatr Scand 67:633, 1978

36. Johnson DE, Bass JL, Thomson TR, et al: Candida septicemia and right atrial mass secondary to umbilical vein catheterization. Am J Dis Child 135:275, 1981

37. Crie JS, Hajar R, Folger G: Umbilical catheter masquerading at echocardiography as a left atrial mass. Clin Cardiol 12:728, 1989

38. Welibé MA, Moore JH: Digital ischemia in the neonate following intravenous therapy. Pediatrics 76:99, 1985

39. Long WA: Pneumopericardium. In Long WA (ed): Fetal and Neonatal Cardiology. Philadelphia, WB Saunders, 1990, p 382

27 *Peripheral Arterial Cannulation*

Mhairi G. MacDonald
Martin Raymond Eichelberger

Cannulation of the Radial Artery

Cannulation of the axillary artery has also been reported in neonates.[1,2] However, although the axillary artery has better collateral supply than the brachial artery, which should be avoided, it is more difficult to cannulate than the radial artery. As a general rule, the most peripheral available artery should be used to reduce potential sequelae from any associated vascular compromise.

A. INDICATIONS

1. Frequent monitoring of blood gases
    a. When catheterization of umbilical artery is not possible for technical or clinical reasons.
    b. When preductal Po_2 measurement is required (e.g., persistent fetal circulation)
2. Direct monitoring of arterial blood pressure in presence of coarctation of aorta

B. CONTRAINDICATIONS

1. Bleeding disorder that cannot be corrected
2. Inadequate collateral flow from ulnar artery
3. Pre-existing evidence of circulatory insufficiency in upper limb
4. Local skin infection
5. Malformation of upper extremity

C. EQUIPMENT

Sterile

1. Gloves
2. Antiseptic solution (e.g., an iodophor)
3. 4 cm × 4 cm gauze squares
4. 0.24N–0.5N saline with heparin, 1 unit/ml

    Hypernatremia may occur in very small premature infants who receive excess sodium in flush solution.[3] In our experience 0.25N saline has been used without complications at infusion rates no greater than 1 ml/hr.

5. 5-ml syringe
6. 20-gauge venipuncture needle
7. 22-gauge × 1-inch (2.5 cm) tapered or nontapered cannula with stylet[4]
8. Antiseptic ointment (e.g., an iodophor)
9. Arterial pressure line or extension tubing (see Chap. 8)
10. 5-0 nylon suture with curved needle
11. Needle holder
12. Suture scissors
13. "T" connector primed with heparinized flush solution.
14. Transparent, semipermeable dressing.

Unsterile

1. Equipment for transillumination (see Chap. 11)

    Use of Doppler ultrasound for localization of the artery and assessment of the adequacy of the palmar circulation has also been described.[4-6]

2. 1/2-inch, water-resistant adhesive tape
3. Materials for forearm restraint (see Chap. 3)
4. A constant infusion pump capable of delivering flush solution at rate of 1 ml/hr against back pressure

ADDITIONAL EQUIPMENT REQUIRED FOR CUTDOWN PROCEDURE

All equipment is sterile, except mask.

1. Gown and mask
2. 0.5% lidocaine hydrochloride in labeled, 3-ml syringe
3. No. 11 scalpel and holder
4. Two curved mosquito hemostats
5. Nerve hook
6. 5-0 nylon suture

D. PRECAUTIONS

1. *Always* check ulnar collateral circulation prior to undertaking procedure using the Allen test (see Chap. 13) or Doppler ultrasound).[5,7-9]
2. Avoid excessive hyperextension of wrist, because this may result in occlusion of artery.
3. Leave *all* fingertips exposed so that circulatory status may be monitored. Examine limb frequently for changes in perfusion.
4. Never ligate artery.
5. Take care not to introduce air bubbles into cannula while assembling infusion system or taking blood samples.
6. Make sure that a continuous pressure waveform tracing is displayed on a monitor screen at all times.
7. Do not administer a rapid bolus injection of fluid via line, because there is a danger of retrograde embolization of clot or air.[10] Flush infusion after sampling should be:
   a. Minimal volume (0.3 ml-0.5 ml)
   b. Injected *slowly*

To reverse arteriospasm, see Chapter 15.

8. Use cannula for sampling only: no fluids other than heparinized saline flush solution should be administered via cannula.

9. Remove cannula at first indication of cloth formation or circulatory compromise, e.g., dampening of waveform on monitor. Do not flush to remove clots.
10. Remove cannula *as soon as* indications no longer exist.

E. TECHNIQUE

Standard Technique for Percutaneous Cannulation of the Radial Artery

Cutdown technique is better for the very small neonate, because trauma to the artery causes vasospasm, which makes percutaneous cannulation of a small vessel very difficult.

1. Perform Allen's test to check adequacy of ulnar collateral circulation (see Chap. 13).[11]

   In a small number of infants the ulnar artery may be more easily located than the radial artery. If Allen's test indicates that the collateral blood supply is adequate, the ulnar artery may be cannulated as described for the radial artery.[12] How the complication rate for cannulation of the ulnar artery compares with that of the radial artery has not yet been recorded in the literature.

2. Restrain infant's forearm and hand, with wrist in extension (Fig. 27-1).

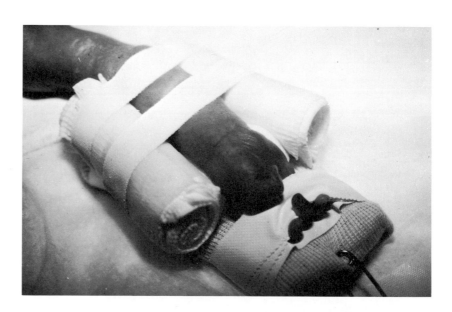

FIG. 27-1
Restraint for procedures on the radial artery.

3. Identify artery by
   a. Palpation at proximal wrist crease, just lateral to flexor carpi radialis (Fig. 27-2)
   b. Transillumination (see Color Fig. 11-1 at the beginning of this book; also see Chap. 11)[13,14]
   c. Doppler ultrasound[4,6,14]
4. Scrub and put on gloves.
5. Prepare skin over radial artery at wrist with antiseptic (e.g., an iodophor).
6. Make small skin puncture with venipuncture needle over radial artery, just proximal to proximal skin crease (to ease passage of cannula through skin and reduce changes of penetrating the posterial wall of the vessel).
7. Accomplish cannulation of artery (Fig. 27-3A).

Method A

a. Puncture artery directly at angle of 10 to 15 degrees to skin, with needle *bevel down*.
b. Advance slowly. There will be arterospasm when the vessel is touched and blood return may be delayed.
c. Withdraw needle stylet (blood should appear in the cannula) and advance cannula into artery as far as possible.

Method B

a. Pass needle stylet (*with bevel up*) and cannula *through* artery at 30-degree to 40-degree angle to skin.

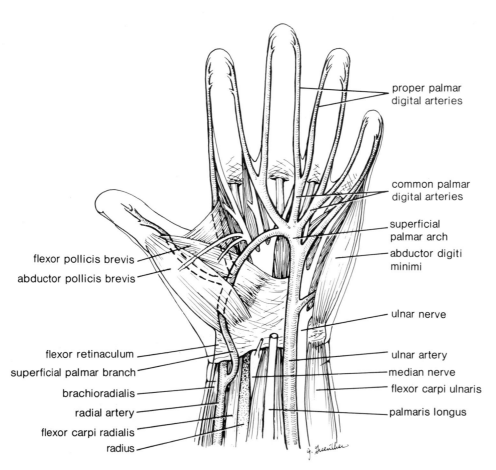

proper palmar digital arteries

common palmar digital arteries

superficial palmar arch

abductor digiti minimi

ulnar nerve

ulnar artery

median nerve

flexor carpi ulnaris

palmaris longus

flexor pollicis brevis

abductor pollicis brevis

flexor retinaculum

superficial palmar branch

brachioradialis

radial artery

flexor carpi radialis

radius

FIG. 27-2
Anatomical relations of the major arteries of the wrist and hand.

FIG. 27-3
(*A*) Cannulation of artery using method A (see text). (*B*) Cannulation of artery using method B (see text). (Redrawn from Filston HC, Johnson DG: Percutaneous venous cannulation in neonates and infants: A method for catheter insertion without "cutdown." Pediatrics 48:896, 1971. Copyright © American Academy of Pediatrics, 1971.

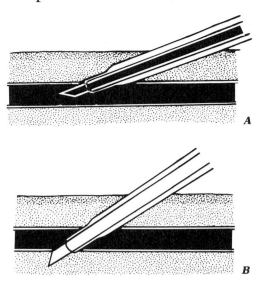

   b. Remove stylet and withdraw cannula slowly until arterial flow is established.
   c. Advance cannula into artery.

> Inability to insert the cannula into the lumen usually indicates failure to puncture the artery centrally. This often results in laceration of the lateral wall of the artery with formation of a hematoma, which can be seen on transillumination.

8. Suture cannula to skin with 5-0 nylon suture if desired.

> This step may be omitted as long as cannula is securely taped (see Fig. 23-3, page 146); use of sutures may produce a more unsightly scar.

9. Attach cannula firmly to "T" connector to permit infusion of 1 ml/hr of heparinized flush solution by constant infusion pump.
10. Apply iodophor ointment (optional) and pressure dressing (which should be checked every 5 minutes) for 30 minutes to puncture site.
11. Secure cannula, as shown in Figure 23-3. Transparent semipermeable dressing may be used in place of tape to allow continuous visualization of

skin entry site. Guarantee that all digits are visible for frequent inspection.
12. Maintain patency with heparinized saline solution.
13. Change IV tubing and flushing solution every 24 hours. Clean site of arterial entry, and apply topical iodophor ointment.

> Note that Ducharme et al reported that routine changing of infusion fluid, tubing, dressing, and insertion site did not alter the incidence of infection.[15]

Radial Artery Cutdown

Technique I: Cutdown at Wrist

The artery is initially exposed by cutdown and a catheter is inserted under direct vision.

1. Prepare as for percutaneous procedure E, 1–3.
2. Scrub and prepare as for major procedure (see Chap. 4).
3. Infiltrate site of incision (point of maximum pulsation just proximal to proximal wrist crease) with 0.5 to 1 ml lidocaine.
4. Wait 5 minutes for anesthesia.

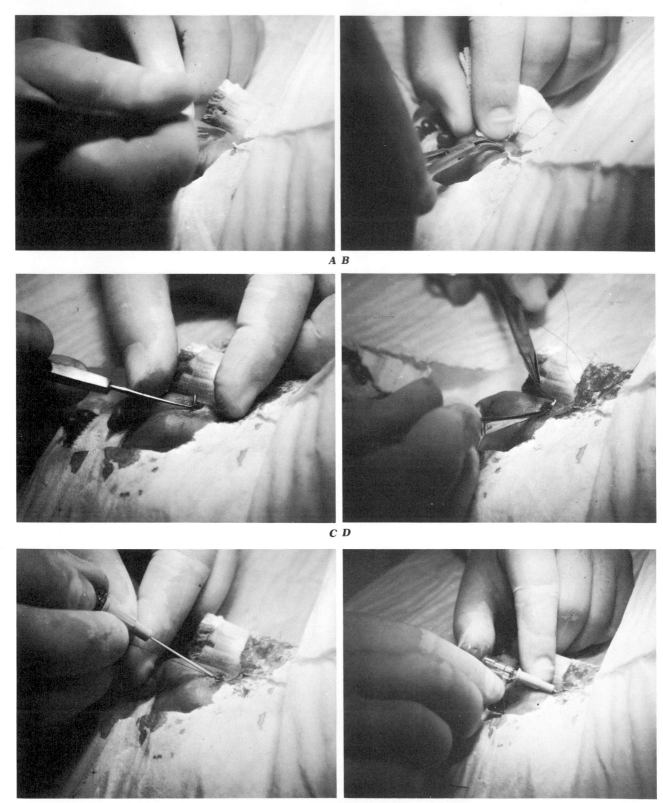

A B

C D

E F

FIG. 27-4
Radial-artery cannulation by cutdown. (*A*) Making transverse skin incision. (*B*) Blunt dissection with mosquito hemostat. (*C*) Elevating artery with artery hook. (*D*) Looping ligature around artery. (*E*) Introducing cannula into artery while gentle "back traction" is applied to suture. (*F*) Cannula advanced to hub.

5. Make a 0.5-cm transverse skin incision (Fig. 27-4A)
6. Deepen incision into subcutaneous tissue by blunt longitudinal dissection with curved mosquito hemostat (Fig. 27-4B).
7. Use curved mosquito hemostat to dissect artery free.

   Be gentle to avoid arteriospasm.

8. Elevate artery with hemostat or nerve hook (Fig. 27-4C).
9. Loop ligature (5-0 nylon) around artery for traction purposes (Fig. 27-4D). *Do not tie* ligature.
10. Advance cannula stylet into artery with bevel down, until cannula is clearly within vessel lumen (Fig. 27-4E).
11. Remove stylet and advance cannula to hub (Fig. 27-4F)
12. Remove ligature.
13. See percutaneous method, E, 8 to 13, for fixation and care of cannula.

The incision can usually be kept small enough so that the hub of the cannula fills it and no closing suture is needed.

Technique II: Cannulation at Anatomic Snuff-Box

1. Described by Amato and associates[16]
2. May be used in infants who have undergone previous arterial cutdown at wrist.
3. Should not be a primary approach to radial artery (particularly if cannulation is achieved by cutdown)
   a. Site is not easy to expose.
   b. Scar tends to be more disfiguring than at wrist.
4. The radial artery passes dorsally at wrist and traverses anatomical snuff-box, which is bounded medially by extensor pollicus longus and extensor pollicus brevis muscles (Fig. 27-5A).
5. Artery becomes superficial immediately after passing extensor pollicus longus and before passing beneath first dorsal interosseous muscle.

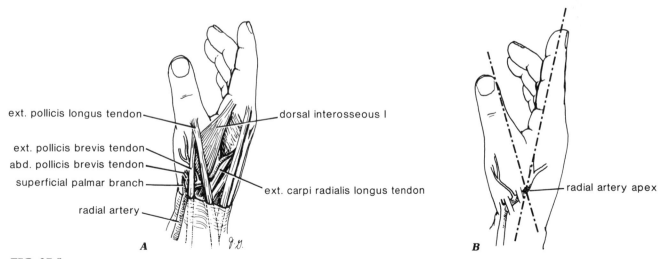

ext. pollicis longus tendon — dorsal interosseous I

ext. pollicis brevis tendon
abd. pollicis brevis tendon
superficial palmar branch — ext. carpi radialis longus tendon

radial artery

A

— radial artery apex

B

FIG. 27-5
(*A*) Anatomical relations of the radial artery on the volar aspect of the wrist. (*B*) Point for cannulation of the radial artery is indicated by the junction of the dotted lines. (Redrawn by permission from Amato JJ, Solod E, Cleveland RJ: A "second" radial artery for monitoring the perioperative pediatric cardiac patient. J Pediatr Surg 12:715, 1977).

6. Point for cannulation is located at junction of a line drawn along medial aspect of extended thumb and another line drawn along lateral aspect of extended index finger (Fig. 27-5).

Cannulation of the Temporal Artery[17,18]

We do not recommend this procedure because of the serious central nervous system sequelae that have been reported.[19-22] These sequelae are thought to be thromboembolic and result from clots dislodged from the cannula (which is in close proximity to the carotid bifurcation) into the internal carotid circulation during irrigation (Fig. 27-6).

Cannulation of the Posterior Tribial Artery

A. INDICATIONS

Blood-gas sampling or blood pressure monitoring.

B. CONTRAINDICATIONS

1. See Cannulation of the Radial Artery, B.
2. Pre-existing evidence of circulatory insufficiency in lower limb
3. Malformations of lower extremity

C. EQUIPMENT

See Cannulation of the Radial Artery, C.

D. PRECAUTIONS

1. See Radial Artery Cannulation, D 4 to 10
2. Document adequate perfusion of foot, via dorsalis pedis artery, prior to procedure.
 a. Adequate dorsalis pedis pulse should be present on palpation or Doppler ultrasound.
 b. Raise foot and perform Allen's test by occluding dorsalis pedis and posterior tibial artery. Tissue perfusion should return within 10 seconds of releasing pressure on dorsalis pedis artery (with posterior tibial artery remaining occluded).

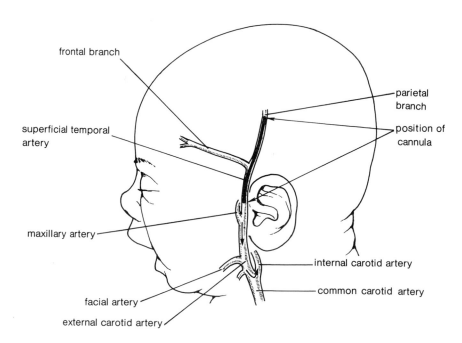

FIG. 27-6
Cannulation of the temporal artery showing the position of the tip of the cannula relative to the carotid bifurcation. Arrows indicate the route of emboli into the cerebral arterial system.

3. Always leave toes exposed to allow evaluation of distal circulation.
4. Be aware that the systolic blood pressure measured in the most peripheral arteries may be erroneously elevated.

E. TECHNIQUE

Percutaneous Cannulation

1. Document adequate perfusion of foot (see Precautions).
2. Restrain foot in equinovarus position (see Chap. 3).
3. Locate artery by
   a. Manual palpation
   b. Transillumination
      Place light source posterior to lateral malleolus. Pulsation can usually be seen posterior to medial malleolus (see Color Fig. 11-1 at the beginning of this book).[23]
   c. Doppler ultrasound.
4. Scrub and put on gloves.
5. Prepare skin over artery with antiseptic (e.g., an iodophor).
6. Cannulate, secure, and dress as for radial artery.
7. Leave all toes exposed.

Cannulation by a Cutdown Procedure

1. Prepare as for percutaneous method.
2. Put on mask.

3. Tape foot to footboard in equinovarus position (see Chap. 3).
4. Scrub and prepare as for major procedure (see Chap. 4).
5. Infiltrate incision site with 0.5 to 1 ml 0.5% lidocaine (Fig. 27-7).
6. Wait 5 minutes for anesthesia.
7. Make transverse incision (0.5 cm) posterior–inferior to medial malleolus (see Fig. 27-7).

   A vertical, rather than a transverse, incision is optional. The former has the advantage that it offers the opportunity to extend the incision cephalad, should the posterior wall of the vein be perforated on the initial attempt at cannulation. However, it has the disadvantage that it may be made too far lateral or medial to the artery.

8. Identify artery by longitudinal dissection with mosquito hemostat. The artery is usually found just anterior to Achilles tendon and adjacent to tibial nerve.
9. Place mosquito hemostat behind artery, and loop 5-0 nylon suture loosely around it.

   Be gentle to avoid arteriospasm.

10. Elevate artery in wound with suture. *Do not ligate artery.*
11. While stabilizing artery with suture, insert needle and cannula, with bevel down.

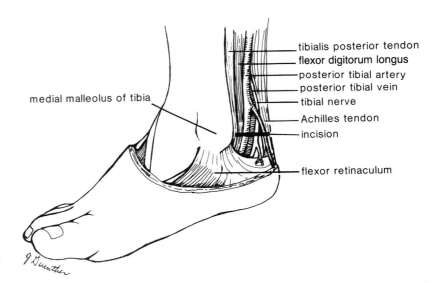

tibialis posterior tendon
flexor digitorum longus
posterior tibial artery
posterior tibial vein
tibial nerve
Achilles tendon
incision
flexor retinaculum

medial malleolus of tibia

FIG. 27-7
Anatomical relations of the posterior tibial artery, showing site of incision for cutdown.

12. Withdraw stylet, and advance cannula to hub.
13. Remove nylon suture.
14. Close wound with 5-0 nylon suture (usually requires only one suture).
15. Secure cannula as for radial artery.

F. CARE OF THE CANNULA

1. Change tubing and fluids every 24 hours.
2. Do not infuse fluid other than heparinized saline solution through the line.
3. Inspect cannula insertion site at least daily.
   a. If signs of cellulitis are present remove the cannula and send the cannula tip for culture. Also send a wound culture if there is inflammation at the cutdown site.
   b. Obtain a blood culture from a peripheral site if signs of sepsis are present.
   c. Inspect the area distal and proximal to the insertion site for blanching, redness, cyanosis, or changes in temperature or capillary refill time.

G. OBTAINING ARTERIAL SAMPLES

Equipment
1. Gloves
2. Alcohol swabs
3. Sterile 2 × 2 gauze squares
4. 25-gauge straight needle
5. Appropriate-sized syringe for sample
6. Rubber-tipped or disposable clamp
7. Syringe with 0.6 flushing solution (0.25–0.5 N saline with 1 unit heparin/ml)
8. Ice if necessary for sample preservation
9. Requisition slips and labels

Technique: 3 drop method
1. Wash hands and put on gloves.
2. Clean diaphragm of "T" connector with antiseptic solution and allow to dry.
3. Clamp "T" connector tubing, with attached clamp, close to the hub.
4. Place sterile gauze squares directly beneath hub on "T" connector.
5. Introduce 25-gauge needle through diaphragm and allow 3 to 4 drops of fluid and blood to drip out onto gauze squares.
6. Attach syringe to needle, and withdraw sample.

For blood gases use a heparinized tuberculine syringe and withdraw a 0.3- to 0.5-ml sample. Withdraw sample slowly and gently since the small syringe can produce a high suction pressure that could potentially damage very tiny arteries. Vented syringes are being developed to reduce the vacuum but are not yet commercially available.

7. Flush cannula slowly
   a. Unclamp "T" connector, and allow residual pump pressure in the line to flush catheter.[24]

Avoid increasing IV rate to flush lines.

   b. Or, flush over 30 to 60 seconds with no more than 0.3 to 0.5 ml of flush solution.

A study by Stanford and co-workers has suggested that the catheter remains functional longer when residual pump pressure is used to flush the line.[25]

H. REMOVAL OF THE CANNULA

Indications
1. Stabilization or resolution of the indications for cannulation of the artery
2. Cannula-related infection
3. Evidence of thrombosis or mechanical occlusion of the artery

Technique
1. Cut stitch securing cannula to skin.
2. Remove cannula gently.
3. Apply local pressure for 5 to 10 minutes.

I. COMPLICATIONS OF PERIPHERAL ARTERIAL CANNULIZATION[26-28]

1. Thromboembolism/vasospasm/thrombosis[26-35]
   a. Blanching of hand and partial loss of digits[36,37]
   b. Gangrene of fingertips and hemiplegia[38]
   c. Necrosis of forearm and hand (Fig. 27-8)[35,39,40]
   d. Skin ulcers[40,41]
   e. Ischemia/necrosis of toes (Fig. 27-9)[12,34]
   f. Cerebral emboli[19,22]
   g. Reversible occlusion of artery[31,42]
   h. Abnormal leg growth[43,44] (Femoral artery lines)

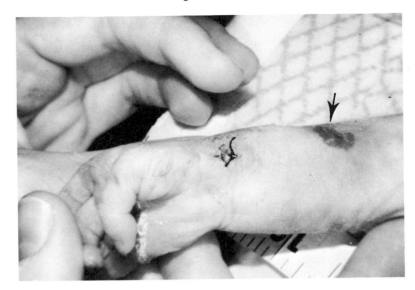

FIG. 27-8
Complication of cannulation of the radial artery. Arrow indicates necrotic area on forearm.

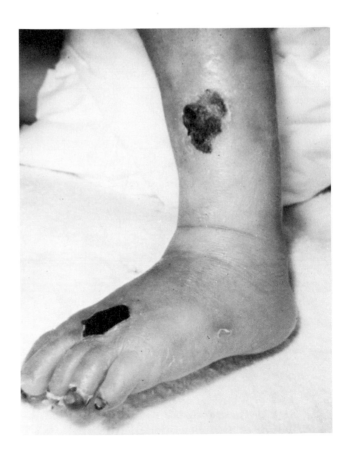

FIG. 27-9
Complication of cannulation of dorsalis pedis artery. Healing areas of sloughed skin are seen at site of skin puncture on dorsum of foot and also on anterior aspect of lower leg. Tips of toes 1, 3, 4, and 5 are necrotic.

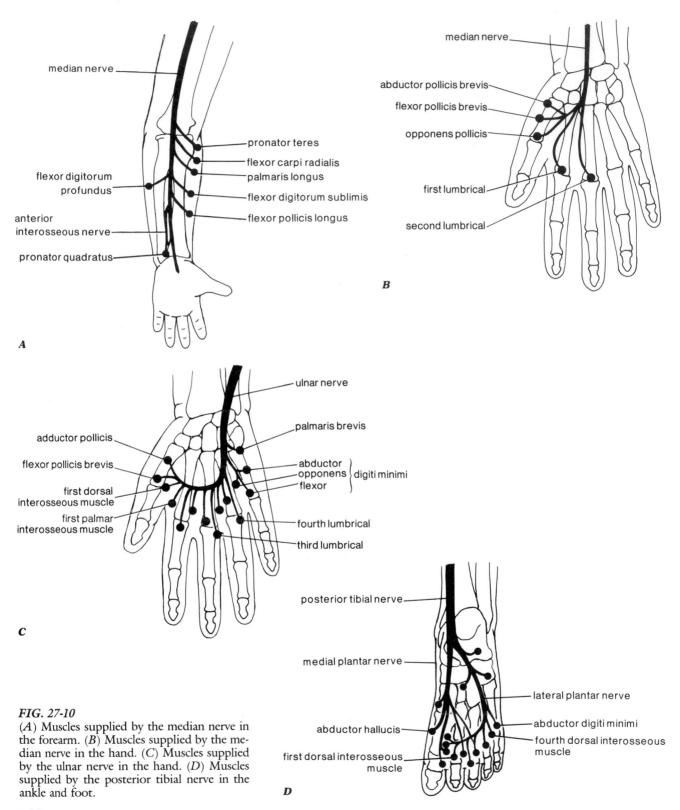

FIG. 27-10
(*A*) Muscles supplied by the median nerve in the forearm. (*B*) Muscles supplied by the median nerve in the hand. (*C*) Muscles supplied by the ulnar nerve in the hand. (*D*) Muscles supplied by the posterior tibial nerve in the ankle and foot.

198

2. Infiltration of infusate[34]
3. Infection[15,24,45-49]
4. Hematoma[29,50]
5. Damage to peripheral nerves, for example,
    a. Median nerve above medial epicondyle of humerus (Fig. 27-10A) may affect the following:
        (1) Pronation of forearm
        (2) Abduction of wrist
        (3) Flexion of wrist and distal phalanges of middle and index fingers
        (4) Opposition, abduction, and flexion of thumb (atrophy of thenar eminence)
        (5) Sensation—maximally over volar aspect index and middle fingers
        (6) Vasomotor control in limb
    b. Median nerve at wrist causes (Fig. 27-10B) carpal tunnel syndrome[51]
    c. Ulnar nerve at wrist causes (Fig. 27-10C)
        (1) Atrophy of small hand muscles
        (2) Sensory loss over dorsal and palmar surfaces of ring and little fingers and ulnar portion of hand and wrist
    d. Peripheral portion of deep peroneal nerve—anesthesia of the lateral aspect of the dorsum of the hand which results in no significant disability.
    e. Posterior tibial nerve at medial malleolus (Fig. 27-10D) may affect
        (1) Flexor hallucis brevis muscle
        (2) Flexor of proximal phalanx of big toe
        (3) Muscles of foot that spread and close toes and flex proximal phalanx of toes
        (4) Sensation on plantar surface of foot

Lesions of posterior tibial nerve may be difficult to detect on examination but may lead to significant discomfort in later life owing to loss of plantar arches on weight bearing.

6. False cortical thumbs[52]
7. Burns from transilluminator[23,53]
8. Hemorrhage (including accidental dislodgement of cannula)[31,34,54,55]
9. Hypernatremia caused by heparinized saline infusion through cannula[3]
10. Hypervolemia related to continuous flush device
11. Air embolism[53,57]
12. Pseudoaneurysm[47]
13. Acquired bone dysplasia[58]

References

1. GREENWALD BM, NOTTERMAN DA, DEBRUIN WJ, MC-CREADY M: Percutaneous axillary artery catheterization in critically ill infants and children. J Pediatr 117:442, 1990
2. LAWLESS S, ORR R: Axillary monitoring of pediatric patients. Pediatrics 84:273, 1989
3. HAYDEN WR: Hypernatremia due to heparinized saline infusion through a radial artery catheter in a very low birth weight infant. J Pediatr 92:1025, 1978
4. BUAKHAM C, KIM JM: Cannulation of a nonpalpable artery with the aid of a Doppler monitor. Anesth Analg (Cleve) 56:125, 1977
5. MOZERSKY DJ, BUCKLEY CJ, HAYWOOD CO JR, ET AL: Ultrasound evaluation of the palmar circulation: A useful adjunct to radial artery cannulation. Am J Surg 126:810, 1973
6. NAGABHUSHAN S, COLELLA JJ, WAGNER R: Use of Doppler ultrasound in performing percutaneous cannulation of the radial artery. Crit Care Med 4:327, 1976
7. MARCILLON M, MAESTRACCI P, GUILLOT F, ET AL: Control par la vélocimétrie Doppler de la fiabilité du test d'Allen pour le cathétérisime de l'arlère radiale. Ann Fr Anesth Réanim 1:403, 1982
8. FELDMAN BH: Letter to the Editor. J Pediatr 93:161, 1978
9. MORRAY JP, BRANDFORD HG, BARNES LF, ET AL: Doppler-assisted radial artery cannulation in infants and children. Anesth Analg 63:346, 1984
10. LOEWENSTEIN E, LITTLE JW, HING HC: Prevention of cerebral embolization from flushing radial artery cannulae. N Engl J Med 285:1414, 1971
11. ALLEN EV: Thromboangiitis obliterans: Methods of diagnosis of chronic occlusive arterial lesions distal to the wrist with illustrative cases. Am J Med Sci 178:237, 1929
12. BARR PA, SUMMERS J, WIRTSHAFTER D, ET AL: Percutaneous peripheral arterial cannulation in the neonate. Pediatrics [Neonatology Suppl] 59:1058, 1977
13. COLE FS, TODRES ID, SHANNON DC: Technique for percutaneous cannulation of the radial artery in the newborn infant. J Pediatr 92:105, 1978
14. WALL PM, KUHNS LR: Percutaneous arterial sampling using transillumination. Pediatrics 59:1032, 1977
15. DUCHARNE FM, GARTHIER M, LACROIX J, LAMENS L: Incidence of infection related to arterial catheterization in children: A prospective study. Crit Care Med 16:272, 1988

16. AMATO JJ, SOLOD E, CLEVELAND RJ: A "second" radial artery for monitoring the perioperative pediatric cardiac patient. J Pediatr Surg 12:715, 1977

17. AU-YEUNG JB, SUGG VM, KANTOR NM, ET AL: Percutaneous catheterization of scalp arteries in sick infants. J Pediatr 91:106, 1977

18. PRIAN G: A new technique for long-term arterial access in the high risk newborn (abstr). Pediatr Res 10:431, 1976

19. AU-YEUNG JB, SUGG VM, KANTOR NM ET AL: Letter to the Editor: Sequelae of temporal artery catheterization. J Pediatr 93:895, 1978

20. BULL MJ, SCHREINER RL, BHUWAN PG, ET AL: Neurologic complications following temporal artery catheterization. J Pediatr 96:1071, 1980

21. PRIAN GW, WRIGHT GB, RUMACK CM, O'MEARA OP: Apparent cerebral embolization after temporal artery catheterization. J Pediatr 93:115, 1978

22. SIMMONS MA, LEVINE RL, LUBCHENCO LO, GUGGENHEIM MA: Warning: Serious sequelae of temporal artery catheterization. J Pediatr 92:284, 1978

23. UY J, KUHNS LR, WALL PM, ET AL: Light filtration during transillumination. A method to reduce heat build-up in the skin. Pediatrics 60:308, 1977

24. TODRES ID, ROGERS MC, SHANNON DE, ET AL: Percutaneous catheterization of the radial artery in the critically ill neonate. J Pediatr 87:273, 1975

25. STANFORD VF, GARCIA-PRATS JA, ADAMS JM: Radial artery catheters (RAC) in newborns: Maintenance techniques and factors affecting duration (abstr 1338). Pediatr Res 16:310A, 1982

26. GOETZMAN BW: Arterial access in the newborn. Am J Dis Child 141:841, 1987

27. RANDEL SN, TSANG BHL, WUNG JT, ET AL: Experience with percutaneous indwelling percutaneous catheterization in neonates. Am J Dis Child 141:848, 1987

28. SELLDEN H, NISSEN K, LARSSON LE, EKSTROM-JUDAL B: Radial artery catheterization in children and neonates. Crit Care Med 15:1106, 1987

29. ADAMS JM, RUDOLPH AJ: The use of indwelling radial artery catheters in neonates. Pediatrics 55:261, 1975

30. BEDFORD RF: Removal of radial-artery thrombi following percutaneous cannulation for monitoring. Anesthesiology 46:430, 1977

31. MIYASAKA K, EDMONDS JF, CONN AW: Complications of radial artery lines in the pediatric patient. Can Anaesth Soc J 23:9, 1976

32. PUPPALA BL, BENAWRA R, MANGURTEN HH, ET AL: Doppler flow and radionuclide scan studies in the evaluation and management of peripheral artery thrombosis in the neonate. J Pediatr 99:791, 1981

33. RYAN JF, RAINES J, DALTON BC, MATHIEU A: Arterial dynamics of radial artery cannulation. Anesth Analg (Cleve) 52:1017, 1973

34. SPAHR RC, MacDONALD HM, HOLZMAN IR: Catheterization of the posterior tibial artery in the neonate. Am J Dis Child 133:945, 1979

35. HACK WW, VOS A, OKKEN A: Incidence of forearm and hand ischemia related to radial artery cannulation in newborn infants. Intensive Care Medicine 16:50, 1990

36. ADAMS JM: Iatrogenic Problems in Neonatal Intensive Care: Report of the 69th Ross Conference on Pediatric Research. Columbus, Ohio, Ross Laboratories, 1976, p 32.

37. CARTWRIGHT GW, SCHREINER RL: Major complications secondary to percutaneous radial artery catheterization in the neonate. Pediatrics 65:139, 1980

38. SAMMAAN HA: The hazards of radial artery pressure monitoring. J Cardiovasc Surg (Torino) 12:342, 1971

39. MAYER T, MATLAK ME, THOMSON JA: Necrosis of the forearm following radial artery catheterization in a patient with Reye's syndrome. Pediatrics 65:141, 1980

40. WYATT R, GLAVES I, COOPER DJ: Proximal skin necrosis after radial artery cannulation. Lancet I (II):1135, 1974

41. WARD RJ, GREEN HD: Arterial puncture as a safe diagnostic aid. Surgery 57:672, 1965

42. HACK WW, VOS A, VANDERLEI J, OKKEN A: Incidence and duration of total occlusion of the radial artery in newborn infants after catheter removal. Eur J Pediatr 149:275, 1990

43. MERTENSSON W: Effects of percutaneous femoral artery catheterization on leg growth in infants and children. Acta Pathologica Diagnosis 21:297, 1979

44. GUY RL, HOLLAND JP, SHAW DG, FIXSEN JA: Limb shortening secondary to complications of vascular cannulae in the neonatal period. Skeletal Radiol 19:423, 1990

45. ADAMS JM, SPEER ME, RUDOLPH AJ: Bacterial colonization of radial artery catheters. Pediatrics 65:94, 1980

46. BAND JD, MAKI DG: Infections caused by arterial catheters used for hemodynamic monitoring. Am J Med 67:735, 1979

47. COHEN A, REYES R, KIRK M, FOLKS RM: Oster's nodes, pseudoaneurysm formation and sepsis complicating percutaneous radial artery cannulation. Crit Care Med 12:1078, 1984

48. RICARD P, MARTIN R, MARCOUX A: Protection of indwelling vascular catheters: Incidence of bacterial contamination and catheter-related sepsis. Crit Care Med 13:541, 1985

49. GALVIS AG, DONAHOO JS, WHITE JJ: An improved technique for prolonged arterial catheterization in infants and children. Crit Care Med 4:166, 1976

50. BROWN AE, SWEENY DB, TUMLEY J: Percutaneous radial artery cannulation. Anesthesia 24:532, 1969

51. KOENIGSBERGER MR, MOESSINGER AC: Iatrongenic carpal tunnel syndrome in the newborn infant. J Pediatr 91:443, 1977

52. SKOGLUND RR, GILES EE: The false cortical thumb. Am J Dis Child 140:375, 1986

53. STEIN RT, KUHNS LR: Letter to the Editor. J Pediatr 93:162, 1978

54. BEDFORD RF, WOLLMAN H: Complications of percutaneous radial artery cannulation: An objective perspective in man. Anesthesiology 38:228, 1973

55. DOWNS JB, RACKSTEIN AD, KLEIN EF, HAWKINS IF: Hazards of radial artery catheterization. Anesthesiology 38:283, 1973

56. MORRAY J, TODD S: A hazard of continuous flush systems for vascular pressure monitoring in infants. Anesthesiology 38:187, 1983

57. CHANG C, DUGHI J, SHITBATA P, ET AL: Air embolism and the radial artery line. Crit Care Med 16:141, 1988

58. SEIBERT JT, McCARTHY RE, ALEXANDER JE, ET AL: Acquired bone dysplasia secondary to catheter related complications in the neonate. Pediatr Radiol 16:43, 1986

28 *General Principles of Central Venous Catheterization*

Mhairi G. MacDonald
Martin Raymond Eichelberger
Claire Bohince Pagano

Opinion varies regarding the optimal site and method of insertion of a central venous catheter in the neonate. Technical considerations are customized by each surgeon. Consequently, this chapter presents general principles and several methods that have proven to be relatively safe.

Optimal conditions for catheter placement are provided in the operating room, but not all patients are stable enough to be transported to the operating room and temperature maintenance may be a problem in the extremely low birth weight infant. With creation of a sterile "area" and strict attention to asepsis, central lines can be placed in the NICU without an associated increase in complications.[1]

A. INDICATIONS

1. To administer parenteral nutrition when osmolarity of solution is too high for peripheral vessels
2. To monitor central venous pressure
3. For long-term IV access for administration of medications

B. CONTRAINDICATIONS

1. Skin infection at insertion site
2. Uncorrected bleeding diathesis (except for distal peripheral venous sites)
3. When infant can be optimally treated using peripheral intravenous line

C. POSITION OF CATHETER TIP

1. Ideally, should be in superior vena cava (SVC), just proximal to right atrium
   a. Reduces complication rate

b. Increases accuracy of central venous pressure (CVP) measurement[2,3]
   c. Reduces incidence of cardiac arrhythmia
2. Vessels above diaphragm are preferable for access, thus reducing the incidence of
   a. Catheter contamination in the groin
   b. Thrombus formation[2] (because the flow through the vessels is greater)

   Silastic catheters may reduce this risk.[4]

   c. Inaccurate CVP measurement in the neonate[5] (Varying intra-abdominal pressure makes interpretation inconsistent [e.g., respiratory distress with abdominal breathing, abdominal distention].)

D. METHODS OF VASCULAR ACCESS

1. Venous cannulation may be percutaneous as by direct visualization ("cutdown").

Percutaneous Technique (Chap. 29)
   a. Advantages
      (1) Less likely to require general anesthesia
      (2) Vessel not ligated, therefore reusable
      (3) Decreases potential for wound infection
      (4) Simpler to perform and relatively rapid procedure
      (5) Smaller residual scar
   b. Disadvantages
      (a) Blind technique
      (b) Increases potential for damage to adjacent organs

Cutdown Technique (Chap. 30)

a. Advantages
  (1) Decreases trauma to vessel
  (2) Decreases risk of injury to adjacent structures
  (3) Facilitates insertion of silastic catheter
b. Disadvantages
  (1) More likely to require general anesthesia
  (2) Requires surgical incision
  (3) Increases potential for wound infection

E. GENERAL PRECAUTIONS

Central venous catheterization is a major and stressful procedure for the neonate. Cutdown procedures for central venous catheterization should be undertaken only by a surgeon experienced with the technique. They are described to promote better understanding of line care by pediatric staff and to prevent complications.

1. Sterile technique is *mandatory* regardless of technique, because sepsis is most common complication.[6]
2. Central venous catheter system must not be used for parenteral alimentation while in use to monitor CVP. Line may be used for hyperalimentation when CVP measurements are no longer necessary *only* after taking the following steps:
   a. Disconnect all monitoring devices from line.
   b. Culture blood obtained through catheter.
   c. Replace all IV tubing.
   d. Insert micropore filter in line.
   e. Infuse dextrose/electrolyte solution for 48 hours.
3. If catheter is used for parenteral feeding, avoid
   a. Use for any other purpose (e.g., infusing medications or blood products)
   b. Use of stopcock in line (increased potential for infection)
   c. The line should be cared for by specifically trained personnel.[7]
4. Always confirm the position of the catheter tip by x-ray after line placement.
5. Take care when placing sutures to secure silastic catheters because they are very easily occluded.
6. Avoid use of the internal jugular vein in infants with increased intracranial pressure.
7. Avoid use of adhesive tape on silastic catheters, because adhesive may react with the silastic and in-

crease the risk of catheter tears. Transparent semipermeable dressing can be used to adhere these lines to the skin.

F. SITES FOR CATHETER INSERTION

Only the most commonly used sites are listed. More peripheral veins can be used, such as the brachial and temporal veins, using the smallest diameter silastic catheters (O.D. approx. 0.6 mm).

1. External jugular vein
   Advantages
     Readily accessible
   Disadvantages
   a. May be excessively tortuous, especially on the left side
   b. Sharp angulation at junction with subclavian vein difficult to negotiate
   c. Movement of head and neck increases:
     (1) Risk of dislodgement and difficulty of nursing care
     (2) Risk of traumatic complications caused by mobility of catheter tip
2. Internal jugular vein
   Disadvantages
   a. Percutaneous technique places carotid artery at risk.
   b. Increased incidence of hydrocephalus or superior vena cava syndrome, especially if vessel is thrombosed bilaterally
   c. Mobility of catheter tip with head movement (see external jugular vein)
3. Facial vein
   Advantages
   a. Provides indirect route into internal jugular vein without ligation of this vessel
   b. Exposure is less difficult than for internal jugular vein.
   c. Can be accomplished at the bedside using local anesthesia
   Disadvantages
   May be too small for cannulation in very low birth weight infants
4. Cephalic or basilic vein
   Disadvantages
   a. Small-caliber vessel
   b. Long catheter required

5. Subclavian vein
   Disadvantages
   a. Expertise required
   b. Blind technique
   c. Relatively stiff (e.g. PVC) catheter required
   d. Risk of pneumothorax
6. Proximal saphenous vein
   Disadvantages
   a. Incision in groin
   b. Long tunnel required to exit catheter above level of umbilicus (to avoid contaminated area in groin)
   c. Catheter indwelling in inferior vena cava (IVC) passing adjacent to renal outflow tract
   d. Catheter cannot be reliably used to monitor central venous pressure in presence of increased intra-abdominal pressure.

G. CATHETERS

1. **Generic Characteristics** (For generic information on surgical tray and suture characteristics, see Appendix B)

   Bearing in mind that an "ideal" central venous catheter does not currently exist, the desirable characteristics include
   a. Rapidity and ease of placement
   b. Longevity
   c. Minimal tissue reactivity
   d. Low probability of septic and mechanical complications
   e. Size
      (1) Neck/subclavian *maximum* size 3 Fr (O.D. approx. 1 mm; 20 gauge) *minimum* length 10 cm.
      (2) Femoral *maximum* size 3 Fr; *minimum* length 30 cm.

   Bargy et al[8] measured the SVC in newborns weighing between 500 and 5000 grams, using radiologic and histologic measurements. They were able to show a good correlation between the body weight of the infant and the caliber of the SVC (r = 0.834).

   Using the criteria used by Burri et al[9] to minimize the risk of thrombosis (ratio between caliber of the catheter and vein 1/20 to 1/13), their recommendations for selecting catheter sizes

TABLE 28-1
Catheter Size Selection Relative to Body Weight*[8]

Weight	Catheter (O.D.)
<1.8 K	0.6 mm
1.9 to 2.6 Kg	1.0 mm (approx 3 Fr. 20 gauge)
2.7 to 4.5 Kg	1.3 mm
>4.8 Kg	1.8 mm

*For SVC.

(using commercially available catheters) are shown in Table 28-1.

2. **Types of Catheter**

   This is not intended to be an exhaustive list of catheter types, but merely an indication of some of the catheters that are commercially available and in fairly common use as this book goes to press.

   a. **Silastic (polymeric silicone)**[10–13]

   Possible generic advantages include
      (1) Reduced thrombogenicity
      (2) More pliable than PVC and polyurethane

   The advantages above are theoretical and based on the characteristics of the material and its behavior in vitro. However, clinically, there is no question that silastic catheters can cause thrombogenesis and can also perforate a vessel or viscus, particularly in very small premature infants (see K, Complications).

   Disadvantages

   May be more difficult to insert percutaneously than PVC or polyurethane catheters because of flexibility.
      (1) Nonprepared catheter tubing, 0.3 mm (0.012 inch) internal diameter × 0.64 mm (0.025 inch) outer diameter or 0.64 mm (0.025 inch) inner diameter × 1.19 (0.47 inch) outer diameter*
      Advantages
      (a) Readily available
      (b) Less expensive
      Disadvantages
      (a) Nonradiopaque
      (b) Supplied unsterilized

*For example, V. Mueller Company, Chicago, IL.

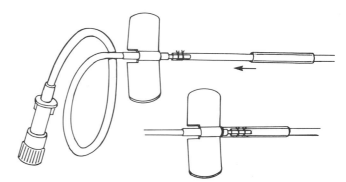

FIG. 28-1
Use of a blunt scalp-vein needle to form a hub for a silastic catheter. The plastic needle cover is used to stabilize the needle–catheter junction. A commercially available blunt-needle adapter may be inserted and fixed in a similar manner.

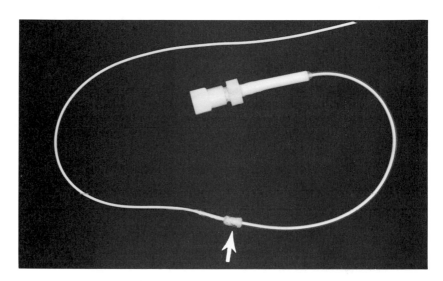

FIG. 28-2
An infant Broviac-type catheter. Dacron cuff is indicated by arrow.

Gas sterilization should not be used for catheters made of silastic materials. 2-chloroethanol or oxide residues may be associated with increased incidence of catheter-related thrombosis.[14]

    (c) Hub must be formed with blunt needle with increased risk of catheter shearing (Fig. 28-1).

    (d) Fixation of catheter to skin may be difficult (see Section F).

(2) Prepared catheter, 20 gauge × 22.9 cm (inches)*
  Advantages
  (a) Supplied sterile

(b) Has hub with plastic wings for suturing to skin

(c) Radiopaque

(3) Infant Cook (Broviac) catheter—small dacron (polyester fiber) cuff glued to catheter; plastic hub with cap (Fig. 28-2)† 3 Fr (20 gauge); length 8 cm. Minimum volume for heparin lock-0.1 ml. (Note: The smallest Broviac catheter‡ is 4.2 Fr)
  Advantages
  (a) Dacron cuff allows catheter fixation in subcutaneous tissues and may reduce incidence of infection.

*Vicra, Travenol Laboratories, Inc., Deerfield, IL 60015.

†Cook Inc., Bloomington, IN 47401.
‡Broviac Catheter, Medina, WA 98039.

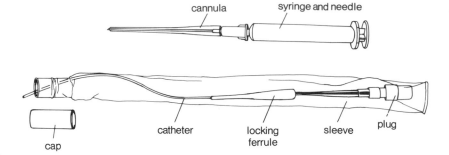

FIG. 28-3
Argyle Intramedicut cannula-stylet (*top*) and PVC catheter.

(b) Relatively easy to repair with repair kit available from manufacturer.

(c) Catheter fixed to skin only at site of exit from skin and is easily cleaned.

Disadvantages

Minimally radiopaque. Contrast should be used if there is question regarding catheter position or complication.

(4) Catheter placement kits, e.g., Geno, Vygon, and Ven-a-cath*

Advantages

(a) Designed for placement percutaneously and thus avoid cutdown

(b) Small size suitable for very low birth weight infant (23 gauge; 1–9 Fr; length 33.5 cm)

(c) Small size allows placement via peripheral veins.

Disadvantages

(a) Small size makes threading more difficult.

(b) Small size *may* increase risk of breakage with traction on withdrawal (see K, Complications).

b. **Polyvinylchloride (PVC) and Polyurethane (Fig. 28-3)**†

Advantages

(1) Catheters slightly more rigid than silastic, which facilitates percutaneous insertion

(2) More radiopaque

(3) More easily fixed to skin

Polyurethane catheters coated with hydromere may be less thrombogenic than silastic catheters, but this question is still being researched.

Disadvantages

(1) Increased incidence of thrombotic complications (PVC)

(2) PVC catheters have been associated with significant levels of plasticizer in neonatal tissues.[15]

(3) Greater rigidity than silastic *may* increase likelihood of mechanical complications (see K, Complications).

3. Some Methods of Fixation for Silastic Catheters

No method is entirely satisfactory.

a. Fixation of external catheter, tubing

(1) Suture plastic wings on hub to skin, using 5-0 silk suture.

If hub is not flanged, place a small piece of gauze behind hub to prevent pressure necrosis of skin. Place a small piece of adhesive tape across hub to hold in place. This tape should be removed when dressing is changed, so that hub area can be cleaned.

(2) Make external catheter adherent to skin with tincture of benzoin. Do not place adhesive tape on catheter or sutures over catheter.

(3) Cover skin entrance site and catheter, up to hub, with sterile, transparent semipermeable dressing.

*(Per-Q-cath) Gesco International Inc., San Antonio, TX 78217.

†For example, Argyle Intramedicut, Sherwood Medical Industries, St. Louis, MO 63103. Consists of a one-piece plastic cannula that tapers to a "hub" end; a smaller-caliber metal needle stylet, with attached syringe that is used for initial insertion; and a catheter made of very pliable PVC and engineered to pass through the plastic cannula.

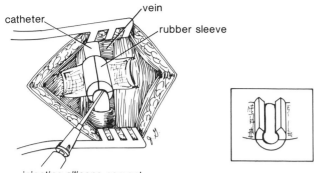

catheter

vein

rubber sleeve

injecting silicone cement
between sleeve and catheter

FIG. 28-4
Fixation of a silastic catheter using a silicone rubber sheath with dacron wings, which are sutured to the superficial muscle layer. (*Inset*) The sleeve is open to receive the catheter.

b. Use of silicon rubber/dacron sleeve (Fig. 28-4)*
Placement
  (1) Pass ready-made silicone rubber sleeve under catheter at its entry into the vein.
  (2) Suture dacron wings to superficial muscle layer with interrupted sutures of 5-0 nylon.
  (3) Inject silicone rubber cement between sleeve and catheter, as illustrated in Figure 28-4.
  (4) Close skin over sleeve.
Removal
  (1) Reopen wound after cleaning skin and infiltration with local anesthetic.
  (2) Dissect away dacron wings from tissues to which they have become fixed, using mosquito forceps.
  (3) Divide catheter above sleeve and withdraw distal catheter from its exit site.
  (4) Withdraw portion of catheter within vein from wound and reclose incision.
c. Silastic sheeting sandwich
  (1) Glue two sheets of silastic, approximately 1 × 1 cm, with silicone rubber cement to make a sandwich of the catheter, as shown in Figure 30-3A.

*Medical Devices, Inc., 1250 Mercer Street, Seattle, WA 98100. Part #13982. Silicon rubber catheter sleeve to which Dacron (polyester fiber) wings are bonded. The sleeves are supplied in 1-cm lengths with internal diameter of 0.19 cm (0.082 inch) and outside diameter of 0.43 cm (0.188 inch).

  (2) Suture four corners of sheeting to skin.
d. Use of silicone rubber cement (see Fig. 30-4)
e. Fixation of Per-Q-Cath (see Chap. 29) Broviac catheter (see Chap. 30)

H. STERILE DRESSING FOR CENTRAL VENOUS LINES

Indications
To protect the site from contamination and to prevent infection[16–19]

Levy et al reported a reduction of catheter contamination when iodophor-impregnated sterile film was placed on the skin prior to surgical insertion of lines.[20]

Some studies have shown a correlation between positive skin cultures and development of line sepsis,[21] while others have not.[22] More recent evidence suggests that the organisms present on the skin are less likely to give rise to sepsis than those contaminating hub connections.[23] This might explain why skin tunneling of catheters has a questionable effect upon the incidence of sepsis.[24] Application of antibiotic ointment, however, has been shown to reduce the incidence of catheter-related infection.[25] Maki et al reported that 2% aqueous chlorhexidine is more effective in preventing infection when repeatedly applied to the catheter entry site than 10% povidone-iodine or 70% alcohol, when used in adults.[26]

An attachable silver-impregnated cuff has been reported to reduce the incidence of catheter-related sepsis in adults.[27,28]

Equipment
Strict sterile technique is used for all central line dressings.
  1. Material for major skin preparation (see Chap. 4)
  2. Gown, mask, and hair cover
  3. Two pairs of gloves
  4. Scissors
  5. Cup with antiseptic solution
  6. Antiseptic ointment (e.g., an iodophor)
  7. Cotton-tipped applicators
  8. 4 × 4 gauze squares

9. Dressing of choice
   a. Semipermeable transparent*

   Note: These dressings have been associated with a significantly heavier growth of bacteria on the underlying skin when compared to gauze dressings, and result in a higher incidence of CVC contamination.[29]

   b. Sterile 2 × 2 cm gauze squares or presplit 2 × 2 cm gauze dressing†

10. Normal saline
11. Culture materials
12. Hydrogen peroxide
13. Adhesive tape (if sterile tape not available, use unused roll)
14. Tincture of benzoin (optional)

Precautions

1. Procedure should be undertaken by personnel specially trained in the technique.[16,30]
2. Ensure that all personnel wear masks if within 6-foot radius of sterile area.
3. Use strict aseptic technique.
4. Remove dressing with care, to avoid cutting or dislodging catheter.
5. Always use a clamp with padded blades (e.g., with rubber tubing) if necessary to clamp catheter.
6. Never place a clamp on plastic hub of catheter.
7. Never advance a dislodged catheter into the patient.
8. Do not include IV tubing connector in dressing.
9. Do not cut dressing and tape until immediately prior to the procedure.
10. Do not use aerosolized preparation of benzoin (see Complications, in this section).
11. Do not place adhesive tape on silastic tubing, because this may occlude or damage catheter.

Technique

When subcutaneous tunnel is used, occlusive dressing should be applied to both cutdown site and catheter exit site.

---

*For example, Op-Site, J.J. Smith and Nephew, Ltd., Hull, England. (Distributed by Acme United Company, Bridgeport, CT) or Tegaderm—3M Company, St. Paul, MN.

†For example, Soft Wick, Johnson and Johnson Products, Inc., New Brunswick, NJ 08903.

1. Restrain patient appropriately.
2. Put on head cover and mask.
3. Scrub as for major procedure (see Chap. 4).
4. Put on gown and gloves.
5. Prepare sterile work area, using "no-touch" technique.
6. Remove old dressing and discard.
7. Inspect catheter site carefully (Table 28-2).
8. Culture site if there is drainage or it appears inflamed.
9. If area around catheter is contaminated with dried blood or drainage, clean with hydrogen peroxide.
10. Change gloves.
11. Cleanse area with antiseptic solution, starting at catheter site and working outward in circular motion for 2 to 4 cm. Repeat twice.
12. Apply small amount of topical antibiotic (e.g., polymixin in combination with neomycin and bacitracin) ointment to catheter entrance site with cotton-tipped applicator.

    Topical antiobiotics have been shown to decrease the total risk of catheter-associated infection, although at the expense of a higher risk of acquiring fungal (candidal) infection.[25]

13. Allow area to dry, and apply dressing of choice.
    a. Clear, adhesive, hypoallergenic, polyurethane dressing, such as Op-Site or Tegoderm

    Allows continuous inspection of catheter insertion site. Water vapor may pass through the film but not bacteria. Film is thin, yet strong, and conforms to the contours of the body. Skin irritation is reduced.[30,31] However, may increase risk of infection compared with gauze dressings.[32]

    (1) Pat off excess antiseptic with sterile gauze and allow to dry.
    (2) Cut dressing to desired size.
    (3) Free small area of adhesive back.
    (4) Anchor dressing to skin above catheter skin entry site, so that the point of skin entry will be in the center of the dressing.
    (5) Remove remainder of adhesive backing, while applying dressing smoothly over site.
    b. Standard occlusive gauze dressing
    (1) Cut gauze halfway across. Place around catheter, as shown in Fig. 28-5.

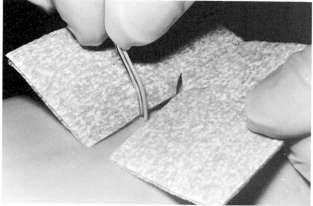

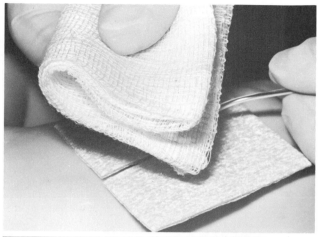

A B
C

FIG. 28-5
Occlusive dressing for a central venous line using pre-split gauze. (*A*) Placing split gauze over the skin entry site. (*B*) Covering split gauze and the catheter with sterile gauze. (*C*) Entire dressing is covered with adhesive tape.

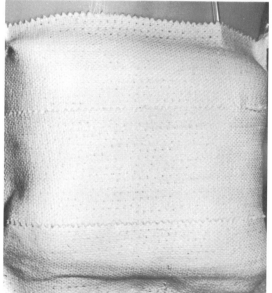

(2) Cover remainder of external catheter length (not hub) with sterile gauze (Fig. 28-5).

(3) Apply tincture of benzoin to skin area 1 to 2 cm around gauze for better adhesion (optional).

(4) If sterile tape not available, discard outer layer of tape on roll.

(5) Cover gauze with tape (Fig. 28-5C).

(6) Label dressing with initials and date.

14. Secure IV tubing with tape to prevent tension on the catheter.

15. Change gauze dressing Monday, Wednesday, and Friday and whenever dressing is loose or wet. The frequency of changing semipermeable dressings is not resolved, although there is general agreement that they may remain in place for longer than gauze dressings.

16. Confirm position of line by chest x-ray study at least once a week. Chest x-ray films obtained for any reason should be scrutinized for catheter position and complications (e.g., accumulation of fluid in hemithorax).

If extravascular position is suspected or catheter is nonradiopaque, inject 1 ml of 30% Renografin through catheter immediately prior to x-ray study.

1. Dilute 1 ml of Renografin-60 with 1 ml of saline. Inject rapidly, using palm to push syringe plunger as soon as x-ray technician is ready.

2. Have technician make exposure on agreed signal ("shout," etc.) as the last 0.5 ml is being injected.

TABLE 28-2

Examination of the Catheter Site

Problem	Comment
Erythema	Accept mild erythema. Document extent in patient record. Ensure more reliable monitoring by keeping consistent caregiver.
Drainage from incision	Obtain culture: 1. Clean area with sterile normal saline, to remove antiseptic ointment. 2. Swab drainage and place in culture tubes for bacterial and fungal studies. 3. Remove catheter if drainage purulent. Culture tip of catheter.
Catheter dislodgement	Mark catheter at exit site. Consider displacement if 1. Edema of site or subcutaneous tunnel 2. Oozing of solution from cutdown site—obtain x-ray film for catheter position. Restrain infant and remove or fix catheter as appropriate.
Dislodged anchoring sutures	Replace sutures.
Catheter kinking	Reposition catheter. Wear sterile gloves if it is necessary to manipulate sterile sections of catheter.
Catheter leakage	Clamp catheter between patient and point of leak, to avoid air embolus or infection. Ideally, catheter should be removed and replaced. However, risk–benefit considerations may indicate repair by insertion of sterile, blunt-end adapter after trimming the catheter beyond site of leak. Some catheters may be repaired using kit supplied by manufacturer.
Loss of skin integrity	Consider skin sensitivity to tape if blistering. Avoid covering sensitive areas with tape.
Catheter removed from body	Cover site with occlusive dressing until healed. 1. Prevents possible infection. 2. Prevents formation of a vein–skin sinus.

Complications
1. Infection[23,25–30,32]
2. Catheter dislodgement/leakage
3. Skin breakdown
4. Loose dressing
5. Catheter kinking
6. Respiratory distress precipitated by acetone defatting solution or aerosolized benzoin.[33–35]

I. CARE OF THE CATHETER WHEN NOT IN USE FOR CONTINUOUS INFUSION

Indications
To irrigate and maintain patency of the catheter using aseptic technique to minimize risk of infection and prevent clotting of the catheter

Equipment
1. 5 ml heparin saline solution: 10 U/ml
2. Antiseptic solution
3. Catheter clamps (must have no teeth or be padded)
4. Clean gloves
5. IV catheter plug

Technique
1. Converting to a heparin lock
   a. Prepare as for major procedure (see Chap. 4).
   b. Prepare sterile work area.
   c. Using sterile technique, clean hub–IV tubing connection with six successive applications of antiseptic.
      (1) Use sterile cotton pads.
      (2) Begin at catheter–IV tubing junction and work outwards in both directions.
   d. Clamp catheter with padded hemostat.
   e. Holding hub with alcohol swab, disconnect catheter hub from IV tubing.
   f. Release clamp and flush line with 3 ml heparinized saline.
   g. Reclamp catheter while plunger of heparin syringe is depressed.
   h. Prime sterile cap or injection plug with flush solution to remove air.

i. Screw cap (or plug) into hub of catheter and tape junction to prevent loosening.
j. Remove clamp.
k. Coil catheter and tape to chest or abdomen.
l. Flush catheter every 12 hours.

2. Flushing catheters
(Equipment is same as for heparin lock.)
   a. Put on gloves and prepare sterile work area.
   b. Prepare IV catheter plug (injection cap) with antiseptic solution.
   c. Insert needle into IV catheter plug. Always use a 1-inch needle. A longer needle can puncture the catheter.
   d. Slowly inject 2 ml heparin solution. While continuing to inject another 0.5 to 1 ml, withdraw needle from cap. By injecting while withdrawing, constant pressure will prevent blood from backflowing into catheter.

3. Changing IV catheter plug (injection cap)
(Equipment is same as for heparin lock.)
   a. Clamp catheter with special clamp.
   b. Clean around old cap with antiseptic solution.
   c. Remove old cap and discard.
   d. Flush IV catheter plug with heparin flush.
   e. Attach new catheter plug into catheter hub.
   f. Unclamp.
   g. Heparin-flush catheter following above procedure.

J. CATHETER REMOVAL

Indications

1. Patient's condition no longer necessitates use
2. Clotted catheter
3. Local infection/phlebitis
4. Sepsis and/or positive blood cultures obtained through the catheter (catheter colonization)

> There are clinical circumstances when a line is left in place and antibiotic or antifungal therapy is administered via the central line.

Technique

1. Remove dressing.
2. Pull catheter from vessel slowly over 2 to 3 minutes.

> Avoid excessive traction if catheter is fettered because the catheter may snap. Gladman et al[36] have reported four cases of tethering of silastic percutaneous microcatheters, apparently associated with formation of septic thromboses. Two

of the catheters snapped on firm traction. Two catheters were successfully removed after prolonged gentle traction using a splint.

3. Apply continuous pressure to the catheter insertion site for 5 to 10 minutes, until no bleeding is noted.
4. Inspect catheter (without contaminating tip) to ensure that entire length has been removed.

> The cuff on the Cook/Broviac catheter may not exit with the catheter. If retained the cuffs rarely cause more than a persistent small subcutaneous lump, although they can occasionally extrude through the skin. If desired, the cuff may be removed, after application of local anesthesia, by making a small incision over the cuff. The wound is closed with a single suture.

5. Send tip of catheter for culture.
6. If desired, antibiotic ointment may be placed over site.
7. Dress with small, self-adhesive bandage or gauze pad and inspect daily until healing occurs.

K. COMPLICATIONS OF CENTRAL VENOUS LINES[37–41]

Whether there is any significant difference in the rate of complications associated with percutaneously versus surgically introduced lines is unclear from the available literature. The incidence of infection and thrombotic complications is higher in preterm than in term infants.[42–44]

1. Infection (most common complication) (Fig. 28-6)[42–53]
2. Vascular accident–thrombosis, embolism[42–44,54–56]
   For example:
   a. Pulmonary embolism (Fig. 28-7)[57–60]
   b. Air embolism (Fig. 28-7)[61]
   c. Superior vena cava (SVC) syndrome[62–64]

> There is no standard treatment for SVC syndrome. There have been reports of success in dissolving catheter-related thrombosis using heparin and urokinase/streptokinase infusion,[64–67] but there is also a high rate of failure with these treatments. Because there is also a significant rate of spontaneous resolution it is difficult to interpret some reports of successful treatment. Newer therapeutic agents, such as tissue plasminogen activator,[68] require clinical trials. Surgical embolectomy has been advocated in life-threatening events, but repair of the SVC is technically difficult and is often associated with poor outcome.

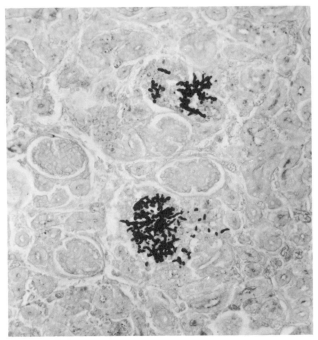

FIG. 28-6
Light micrograph of renal tissue from a premature infant with an infected central venous line. Deposits of *Candida albicans* have formed pseudomycelia (hyphae).

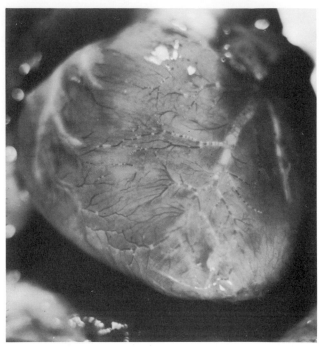

FIG. 28-7
Air in coronary vessels. The patient suffered massive air embolus via a central venous line placed in the superior vena cava. The infant had multiple anomalies, including a left superior vena cava that drained into the coronary sinus.

A   **B**

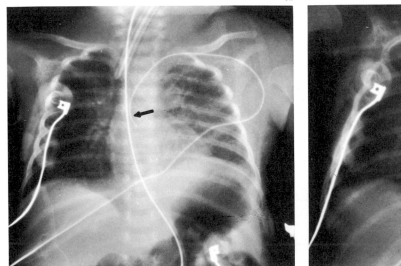
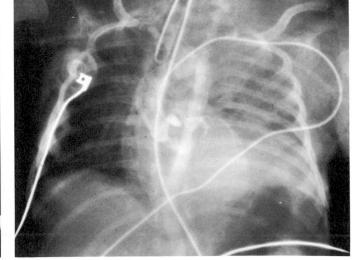

FIG. 28-8
In the initial radiograph (*A*), the presumed subclavian venous catheter had an unusual medial curve in its distal tip (*arrow*). An injection of contrast material (*B*) showed that this was an inadvertent subclavian *arterial* catheter with tip in the root of the aorta.

d. Renal vein thrombosis
e. Intracardiac thrombus[69]
f. Infected thrombus[36,53,66,70]
3. Damage to other vessels and organs
   a. Pneumothorax[46,47]
   b. Puncture of subclavian artery (Fig. 28-8)[39,46,47]
   c. Perforation of first intercostal vessel[2]
   d. Myocardial perforation (see also J4)[71,72]

e. Pneumomediastinum[47]
f. Damage to brachial plexus[46]
4. Extravascular collection of fluid
   For example:
   a. Pleural effusion (Fig. 28-9)[6,14]
   b. Pericardial effusion[14,42,44,73,74]
   c. Mediastinal extravasation (Fig. 28-10)[46,75]
   d. Hemothorax[39,46,76]

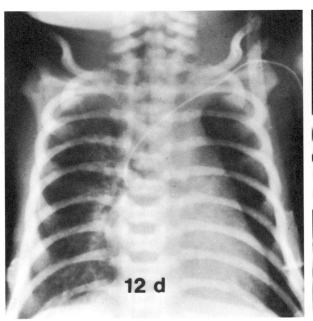
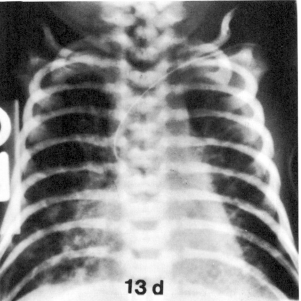
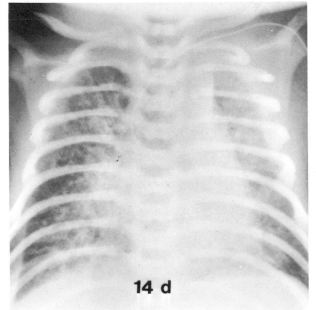

A B
C

FIG. 28-9
Sequential radiographs showing the development of a slightly asymmetric pulmonary venous obstructive pattern and pleural effusions (more obvious on right). Removal of the central line was followed by the rapid resolution of the abnormalities.

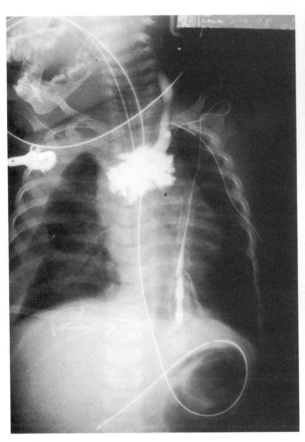 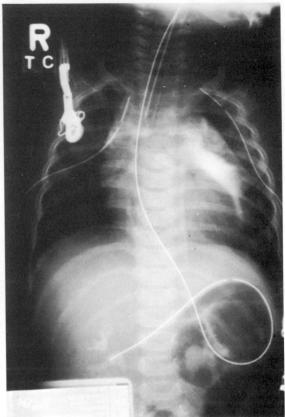

A B

FIG. 28-10
Left extrapleural effusion due to perforation of a central venous catheter through the vessel wall at the junction of the innominate vein with the superior vena cava. (*A*) Contrast material is passing from the catheter tip into the mediastinal tissues. (*B*) Follow-up film at 48 hours showing residual contrast material in the mediastinum.

e. Hydrothorax[13,42–44,75,77–79]

f. Chylothorax[80,81]

g. Ascites[5,13]

h. Effusion in subarachnoid space[83,84]

i. Retroperitoneal, extrapleural effusion[3,38,82]

Caused by:

(1) Vessel perforation/misplaced catheter or[74,75,85–87]

(2) Myocardial necrosis/perforation[72,74]

(3) Thrombophlebitis of lymphatic duct or vein leading to obstruction of vessel or compromise of vessel wall integrity (Fig. 28-11), or

(4) Hyperosmolar parenteral nutrition fluid, causing compromise of vessel wall integrity and fluid shifts

There is no evidence that silastic catheters that are misplaced into the right atrium are any less likely to perforate the heart than are catheters made of more rigid materials. In addition, because they are so flexible, the catheter tip can be directed into the foramen ovale, thus increasing the risk of systemic embolism.[88]

5. Hemorrhage/hematoma[41,46,47,76]

6. Catheter

a. Misplacement,[3,47] including intracardiac (Fig. 28-12)[72,89]

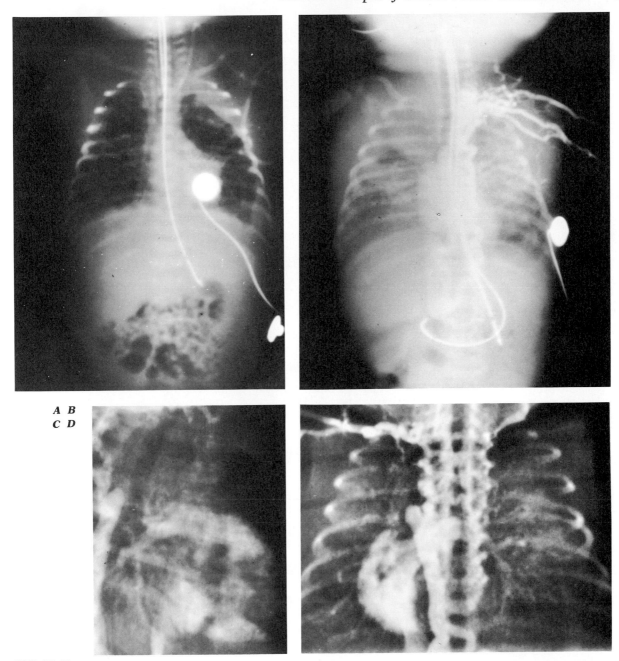

A B
C D

FIG. 28-11
(*A*) AP chest film demonstrating a left pleural effusion in an infant, with the catheter tip in the left innominate vein. (*B*) Venogram with injection in the left arm showing obstruction of the superior vena cava with collateral flow via the hemiazygous system to the lumbar collaterals and the inferior vena cava. (*C* and *D*) Left neck and right subclavian venous injection showing obstruction of the superior vena cava with major collateral pathways via the azygous system to the inferior vena cava. Such obstructions of the brachycephalic venous systems have been associated with blockage of the thoracic duct and consequent pleural effusions.

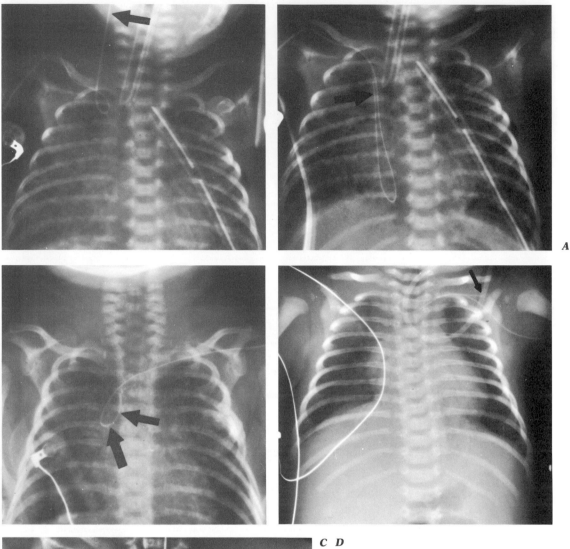

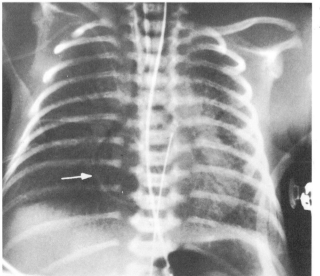

A B

C D

E

FIG. 28-12
Various venous malpositions of subclavian
venous catheters. (*A*) Jugular. (*B*) Looped
in the right atrium with the tip in the superior vena cava. (*C*) Looped in the superior
vena cava. (*D*) Looped in the innominate
vein with the tip overlying the left scapula.
(*E*) Knotted in the left atrium.

b. Migration[3,90]
c. Occlusion[38,57,91]
d. Breaks[92]
e. Dislodgement[38,57,93]
f. Transection/embolism[39,46]
g. Occlusion (other than by thrombus)
   (1) Fungus[70]
   (2) Mineral deposits[94,95,96]
      (avoidance and clearance[94,95])
h. Tethered in vein[36]
i. Knot (see Fig. 28-12E)
7. Hydrocephalus[96]/Dural venous thrombosis[97]
8. Cardiac arrhythmia[6]
9. Polyvinyl catheters—plasticizers in tissues[15]
10. Glomerulonephritis—similar to "shunt nephritis" related to infected ventriculoatrial shunts[98]
11. Paralysis of the diaphragm due to phrenic nerve injury[99,100]
12. Acquired bone dysplasia[101]

References

1. LALLY P, HARDIN WD, BOETTCHER M, ET AL: Broviac catheter insertion: Operating room or neonatal intensive care unit? J Pediatr Surg 22:823, 1987
2. BAUSMER G, KEITH BA, TESLUK H: Complications following use of indwelling catheter of inferior vena cava. JAMA 167:1606, 1958
3. EFFMAN L, ABLOW RC, TOULOUKIAN RJ, SEASHORE JH: Radiographic aspects of total parenteral nutrition. Radiology 127:195, 1978
4. KIELY EM: Placement of central feeding catheters. Br Med J (Pract Obstet) II:1123, 1978
5. TALBERT JL, HALLER JA: Technic of central venous pressure monitoring in infants. Am Surg 32:767, 1966
6. EICHELBERGER MR, ROUS PG, HOELZER DJ, ET AL: Percutaneous subclavian venous catheters in neonates and children. J Pediatr Surg 16:547, 1981
7. PUNTIS JWL, HOLDEN CE, SMALLMAN S, ET AL: Staff training: A key factor in reducing intravascular catheter sepsis. Arch Dis Child 65:335, 1990
8. BARGY F, BARBET P, HOUETT A: Diameter of the superior vena cava in the newborn: Clinical applications in parenteral nutrition. Surg Radiol Anat 9:293, 1987
9. BURRI C, AHNEFELD FW: The Caval Catheter. New York, Springer-Verlag, 1982
10. BRALEY S: The silicones as subdermal engineering materials. Ann NY Acad Sci 146:148, 1968
11. COCKINGTON RA: Silicone elastomer for nasojejunal intubation and central venous cannulation in neonates. Anaesth Intensive Care 7:248, 1979
12. IRVING IM, CASTILLA P, HALL EG, RICKHAM PP: Tissue reaction to pure and impregnated silastic. J Pediatr Surg 6:24, 1971
13. SPRIGGS DW, BRANTLEY RC: Thoracic and abdominal extravasation: A complication of hyperalimentation in infants. AJR 128:419, 1977
14. DHANDE VG, KATTWINKEL J, ARFORD BA: Recurrent bilateral pleural effusions secondary to superior vena caval obstruction as a complication of central venous catheter (abstr). Pediatr Res 16:285A, 1982
15. HILLMAN LS, GOODWIN SL, SHERWIN WR: Identification and measurement of plasticizer in neonatal tissues after umbilical catheters and blood products. N Engl J Med 292:381, 1975
16. GODFREY D: The dressing care of hyperalimentation catheters. American Journal of IV Therapy and Clinical Nutrition 6:53, 1979
17. IVEY M: The status of parenteral nutrition. Nurs Clin North Am 14:285, 1979
18. KAMINSKY M: Prolonged uncomplicated intravascular catheterization. American Journal of IV Therapy 3:19, 1976
19. NITA Hyperalimentation Standards of Practice of the National Intravenous Therapy Association (NITA) 3:234, 1980
20. LEVY JH, NAGLE DM, CURLING PE, ET AL: Contamination reduction during central venous catheterization. Crit Care Med 16:165, 1988
21. GORBEA HF, MAJKA JA, PERRY LK: Predictive value of surveillance skin culture in total parenteral nutrition-related infection. Lancet 2:1385, 1982
22. JARRARD M, ORSON C, FREEMAN J: Daily dressing change: Effects on skin flora beneath subclavian catheter dressing during TPN. Journal of Parenteral and Enteral Nutrition 4:391, 1980
23. LINARES J, SITGES-SENA A, CSARAN J, ET AL: Pathogenesis of catheter sepsis: A prospective study with quantitative and semiquantitative cultures of catheter hub and segments. J Clin Microbiol 21:357, 1985
24. GARDEN OJ, SIM AJW: A comparison of tunnelled and non-tunnelled subclavian vein catheters: A prospective study of complications during parenteral feeding. Clin Nutr 2:51, 1983
25. MAKI DG, BAND JD: A comparative study of polyantibiotic and iodophar ointment in prevention of vascular catheter-related infection. Am J Med 70:739, 1981
26. MAKI DG, RINGER M, ALVARADO CJ: Prospective randomized trial of povidone-iodine, alcohol and chlorhexidine for prevention of infection associated with central venous and arterial catheters. Lancet 1:338, 1991
27. MAKI DG, COBB L, GARMAN JK, ET AL: An attachable silver-impregnated cuff for prevention of infection with central venous catheters: A prospective randomized trial. Am J Med 85:307, 1988

28. FLOWERS RH, SCHWENZER KJ, KOPEL RF, ET AL: Efficacy of an attachable subcutaneous cuff for the prevention of intravascular catheter-related infection. JAMA 261:878, 1989

29. HOFFMAN KK, WEBER DJ, SAMSA GP, RUTALA WA: Transparent polyurethane film as an intravenous catheter dressing: a meta-analysis of the infection risks. JAMA 267:2072, 1992

30. GOLDMAN D, MAKI D: Infection control—total parenteral nutrition. JAMA 223:1360, 1973

31. KELLMAN B, FRAZE DE, KANAREK KS: Central line dressing material and neonatal skin integrity. Nutrition in Clinical Practice 302:65, 1988

32. RAAD II, BODEY GP: Infectious complications of indwelling vascular catheters. Clin Infections Dis 15:197, 1992

33. GOLDFRANK LR, KIRSTEIN R, BRESNITZ EA: Hydrocarbons (mind boggling solutions). In Goldfrank LR (ed): Toxicologic Emergencies, 2nd Ed. New York, Appleton-Century-Crofts, 1982, p 337

34. LAHAM S, POTVIN M, SCHRADER K, ET AL: Studies on inhalation toxicity of 2-propranolol. Drug Chem Toxicol 3:343, 1980

35. WIGAEORS E, HOLM S, ASTRAND I: Human exposure to acetone vapor. 2nd Annual International Congress on Toxicology, Brussels, Belgium. Toxicol Lett (Special Issue) 1:45, 1980

36. GLADMAN G, SINHA S, SIMS DG, CHISWICK ML: Staphylococcus epidermitis and retention of neonatal percutaneous central venous catheters. Arch Dis Child 65:234, 1990

37. ALTMAN RP, RANDOLPH JG: Application and hazards of total parenteral nutrition in infants. Ann Surg 174:85, 1971

38. GROFF DB: Complications of intravenous hyperalimentation in newborns and infants. J Pediatr Surg 4:460, 1969

39. McGOON MD, BENEDETTO PW, GREEN BM: Complications of percutaneous central venous catheterization: A report of two cases and a review of the literature. Johns Hopkins Med J 145:1, 1979

40. RIELLA MC, SCUBAER BH: Five years' experience with a right atrial catheter for prolonged parenteral nutrition at home. Surg Gynecol Obstet 143:205, 1976

41. Voegele LD: Subclavian venipuncture for vascular access. South Med J 73:1288, 1980

42. GOUTAIL-FLAUD MF, SFEZ M, BERG A, ET AL: Central venous catheter-related complications in newborns and infants: A 587 case study. J Pediatr Surg 26:645, 1991

43. SADIQ HF, DEVASKAR S, KEENAN WJ, WEBSTER TR: Broviac catheterization in low birth weight infants: Incidence and treatment of associated complications. Crit Care Med 15:47, 1987

44. ARUSZKEWYCS V, HOLTROP PC, BATTON DG, ET AL: Complications associated with central venous catheters inserted in the critically ill neonates. Infect Control Hosp Admin 12:544, 1991

45. BOECKMAN CR, KRILL CE JR: Bacterial and fungal infections complicating parenteral alimentation in infants and children. J Pediatr 5:117, 1970

46. DEFALQUE RJ: The subclavian route—a critical review of the World literature up to 1970. Der Anaesthesist 21:325, 1972

47. FILSTON HC, GRANT JP: A safer system for percutaneous subclavian venous catheterization in newborn infants. J Pediatr Surg 14:564, 1979

48. Moran JM, Atwood RP, Rowe MI: A clinical and bacteriologic study of infections associated with venous cutdowns. N Engl J Med 272:554, 1965

49. KING DR, KOMER M, HOFFMAN J, ET AL: Broviac catheter sepsis: The natural history of an iatrogenic infection. J Pediatr Surg 20:728, 1985

50. FREEMAN J, GOLDMANN DA, SMITH NE, ET AL: Association of intravenous lipid emulsion and coagulase negative staphylococcus bacteremia in neonatal intensive care units. N Engl J Med 323:301, 1990

51. DATO VM, DAJAM AS: Candidemia in children with central venous catheters: Role of catheter removal and amphoteracin B Therapy. Pediatr Infect Dis J 9:309, 1990

52. POWELL DA, AUNGST J, SNEDDEN S, ET AL: Broviac catheter-related Malassezia furfur sepsis in five infants receiving intravenous fat emulsions. J Pediatr 105:987, 1987

53. RUPAR DG, HERZOG KD, FISCHER MC, LONG SS: Prolonged bacteremia with catheter-related central venous thrombosis. Am J Dis Child 144:879, 1990

54. FLEIGEL CP, SIGNER E, STAHL M: Thrombotic complications of long-term intravenous alimentation in infants. Ann Radiol 19:21, 1976

55. HOSHAL VL, AUSE RG, HOSKINS PA: Fibrin sheath formation on indwelling subclavian central venous catheters. Arch Surg 102:353, 1971

56. ROSS P, EHRENKRANZ R, KLEINMAN S, SEASHORE JH: Thombus associated with central venous catheters in infants and children. J Pediatr Surg 24:253, 1989

57. DIMMICK JE, ELLIS DR, HARDWICK DF: Complications of intravenous alimentation in seriously ill infants. Can J Surg 17:186, 1974

58. FIROV HV: Pulmonary embolization complicating total intravenous alimentation. J Pediatr Surg 7:81, 1972

59. WESLEY JR, KEENS TG, MILLER SW, PLATZKER ACG: Pulmonary embolism in the neonate: Occurrence during the course of total parenteral nutrition. J Pediatr 93:113, 1978

60. ROCKOFF MA, GANG DL, VANCANTI JP: Fatal pulmonary embolism following removal of a central venous catheter. J Pediatr Surg 19:307, 1984

61. PETERS JL, ARMSTRONG R: Air embolism occurring as a complication of central venous catheterization. Ann Surg 187:375, 1978

62. MULVIHILL SJ, FONKALSRUD EW: Complications of infant vena cava occlusion in infants receiving total parenteral nutrition. J Pediatr Surg 19:752, 1984

63. RASZKA WV, SMITH RF, PRATT SR: Superior vena cava syndrome in infants. Clin Pediatr 28:196, 1989

64. CAGLAR MK, TOLBOOM J: Successful treatment of superior vena cava syndrome with urokinase in an infant with a central venous catheter. Helv Pediatr Acta 43:483, 1989

65. WACHS T: Urokinase administration in pediatric patients with occluded central venous catheters. J Intravenous Nursing 13:100, 1990

66. LACEY SR, ZARITSKY AL, AZIZKHAN RG: Successful treatment of *candida*-infected caval thrombosis in critically ill infants by low-dose streptokinase infusion. J Pediatr Surg 23:1204, 1988

67. SUAREZ CR, OW EP, LAMBERT GH, ET AL: Urokinase therapy for a central venous catheter thrombus. Am J Hematol 31:269, 1989

68. ATKINSON JB, BAGNALL HA, GOMPERTS E: Investigational use of tissue plasminogen activator (T-PA) for occluded central venous catheters. JPEN 14:310, 1990

69. MAHONY L, SNIDER AR, SILVERMAN NH: Echocardiographic diagnosis of intracardiac thrombosis complicating total parenteral nutrition. J Pediatr 98:469, 1981

70. AZIMI PH, LEVERNIER K, LEFRAK LM, ET AL: *Malassezia* furfur: A cause of occlusion of percutaneous central venous catheters in infants in the intensive care nursery. Pediatr Infect Dis J 7:100, 1988

71. FISCHER GW, SCHERTZ RD: Neck vein catheters and pericardial tamponade. Pediatrics 52:868, 1973

72. FRANCIOSI RA, ELLEFSON RD, UDEN D, DRAKE RM: Sudden unexpected death during central hyperalimentation. Pediatrics 69:305, 1982

73. SEIBERT JJ, WEINSTEIN MM, ERENBERG A: Catheter-related complications of total parenteral nutrition in infants. Pediatr Radiol 4:233, 1976

74. OPITZ JC, TOYAMA W: Cardiac tamponade from central venous catheterization: Two cases in premature infants with survival. Pediatrics 70:139, 1982

75. DAVIS WS, AKERS DR: Catheterization of the subclavian vein. An unusual complication. Rocky Mountain Med J 64:72, 1967

76. BORJA AR: Current status of infraclavicular subclavian vein catheterization. Ann Thorac Surg 13:615, 1972

77. KNIGHT L, TOBIN J JR, L'HEUREUX P: Hydrothorax: A complication of hyperalimentation with radiologic manifestations. Radiology 111:693, 1974

78. RAFFENSPERGER JG, RAMENOFSKY ML: A fatal complication of hyperalimentation: A case report. Surgery 68:393, 1970

79. SHAW JCL: Parenteral nutrition in the management of sick low birth weight infants. Pediatr Clin North Am 20:333, 1973

80. HEIMBACH DM, IVEY TD: Technique for placement of a permanent home hyperalimentation catheter. Surg Gynecol Obstet 143:634, 1976

81. PIRO J, SAINTY JM, DEVEZE JL, FOGLIANI J: A propos de deux ca de chylothorax consecutifs a des Catheterismes des gros troncs veineux Gauches. Ann Anesthesiol Fr 16:1, 1975

82. WHITE LE, MONTES JE, CHAVEZ-CABALLO E, ET AL: Radiological case of the mouth. Am J Dis Child 141:903, 1987

83. GLASIER CM, HASSELL DR: Spinal canal extension of hyperalimentation catheter without neurological sequelae. Pediatr Radiol 19:206, 1989

84. JOHNSON DG: Total intravenous nutrition in newborn surgical patients: A three year perspective. J Pediatr Surg 5:601, 1970

85. BAR-JOSEPH G, GALVIS AG: Perforation of the heart by central venous catheter in infants: Guidelines to diagnosis and management. J Pediatr Surg 18:284, 1983

86. AGARWAL KC, ALI KHAN MA, FALLA A, AMATO JJ: Cardiac perforation from central venous catheters: Survival after cardiac tamponade in an infant. Pediatrics 73:333, 1984

87. ROGERS BB, BERNS SD, MAYNARD EC, HANSEN TWR: Pericardial tamponade secondary to central venous catheterization and hyperalimentation in a very low birth weight infant. Pediatr Pathol 10:819, 1990

88. HAUSDORF G, BITZAN M, COMMENTZ J, ET AL: Intra-atrial malpositions of silastic catheters in newborns. Crit Care Med 15:308, 1987

89. GEORGE RJ, LYONS J, TINKER J: Right atrial thrombi associated with silastic central venous catheters (abstr). Crit Care Med 9:203, 1981

90. MORGAN WW JR, HARKINS GA: Percutaneous introduction of longterm indwelling venous catheters in infants. J Pediatr Surg 7:538, 1972 (In discussion by GB Groff at end of paper)

91. WARNER BW, GORGONE P, SCHILLING S, ET AL: Multiple purpose central venous access in infants less than 1000 grams. J Pediatr Surg 22:820, 1987

92. FILLER RM, CORAN AG: Total parenteral nutrition in infants and children: Central and peripheral approaches. Surg Clin North Am 56:395, 1976

93. ALFIERIS GM, WING CW, HOY GR: Securing Broviac catheters in children. J Pediatr Surg 22:825, 1987

94. BREAUX CW, DUKE D, GEORGESON KE, MESTRE JR: Calcium phosphate crystal occlusion of central venous catheters used for total parenteral nutrition in infants and children. J Pediatr Surg 22:829, 1987

95. DUFFY LF, KERZNER B, GEBUS V, DICE J: Treatment of central venous catheter occlusions with hydrochloric acid. J Pediatr 114:1002, 1989

96. STEWART RD, JOHNSON DG, MYERS GG: Hydrocephalus as a complication of jugular catheterization during total parenteral nutrition. J Pediatr Surg 10:771, 1975

97. HURST RW, KERNS SR, MCILHENNY J, ET AL: Neonatal dural venous sinus thrombosis associated with central venous catheterization: CT and MR studies. J Computer Assisted Tomography 13:504, 1989

98. WYATT RJ, WALSH JW, HOLLAND NH: Shunt nephri-

tis: Role of the complement system in its pathogenesis and management. J Neurosurg 55:99, 1981

99. LAM DS, RAMOS AD, PLATZKER ACG, ET AL: Paralysis of the diaphragm complicating central venous alimentation. Am J Dis Child 135:382, 1981

100. PLEASURE JR, SHASHIKUMAS VL: Phrenic nerve damage in the tiny infant during vein cannulation for parenteral nutrition. Am J Perinatol 7:136, 1990

101. SEIBERT JJ, McCARTHY RE, ALEXANDER JE, ET AL: Acquired bone dysplasia secondary to catheter-related complications in the neonate. Pediatr Radiol 16:43, 1986

29 Percutaneous Central Venous Catheterization

Gail R. Knight
Martin Raymond Eichelberger
Mhairi G. MacDonald

A. BACKGROUND

The indications, contraindications, advantages, and disadvantages of percutaneous insertion of central venous lines are listed in Chapter 28, Sections A, B, and D.

There are three basic techniques used for percutaneous placement:

1. Through-the-needle Technique

a. Venous cannulation with a needle or cannula large enough to accommodate a catheter
b. Catheter is advanced through the needle or cannula.
c. Introducer needle or cannula is removed.

This method is illustrated by silastic microcatheter placement technique in Section B.

2. Seldinger Technique

a. Vessel is located using a small-gauge needle of adequate size to allow smooth passage of the guide wire, with syringe attached.
b. Syringe is removed from needle upon blood return.
c. Guide wire is passed through needle in vessel, advancing $1/3$ to $1/4$ of wire.
d. Needle is removed, leaving guide wire in place.
e. Catheter is inserted over wire to desired position, using a twisting motion and making sure that wire is visible at proximal end of catheter before advancing catheter.
f. Guide wire is removed gently.

3. Combined Technique (Fig. 29-1)

a. Vascular access is achieved, using guide wire as above.
b. Peel-away sheath is introduced over the wire into the vessel.
c. Guide wire is removed gently.
d. Catheter of smaller diameter than peel-away sheath is introduced into the vessel through the sheath and positioned as desired.
e. Sheath is pulled back and peeled off catheter.

In this chapter we will illustrate in detail only the through-the-needle technique. In our experience, this is the method most commonly used for percutaneous placement of central venous lines in neonates.

B. THROUGH-THE-NEEDLE TECHNIQUES

PLACEMENT OF MICROGAUGE SILASTIC CATHETER VIA PERIPHERAL VEINS[1,2]

1. Equipment*

Sterile
a. Gown and gloves
b. Antiseptic solution (see Chap. 4)
c. Alcohol prep

*Available as accessory insertion trays:
1. Gesco, P.O. Box 690188, San Antonio, TX 78269
2. VYGON, 1 Madison St., East Rutherford, NJ 07073
3. Ven-A-Cath, American IV Products, Inc., 7466 New Ridge Road, Bldg 21, Hanover, MD 21076

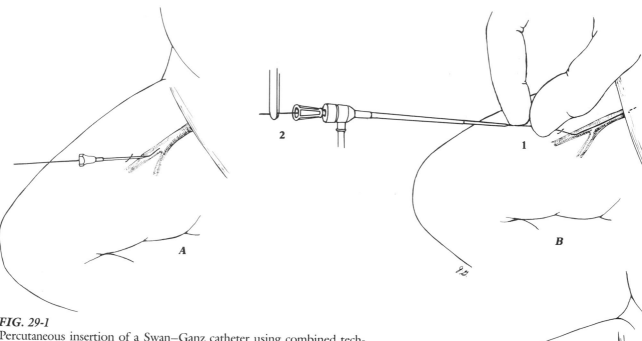

FIG. 29-1
Percutaneous insertion of a Swan–Ganz catheter using combined technique (see text). (*A*) A No. 18 wire has been passed into the femoral vein through a No. 21 AMC needle. (*B*) The needle has been withdrawn and a No. 5 sheath assembly is being passed over the wire, maintaining the position of the wire first (*1*) at the skin surface until the distal end appears beyond the sheath obturator, and second (*2*) beyond the obturator with a hemostat as the sheath is passed into the vein using the wire as a guide. (*C*) The obturator has been withdrawn, leaving the sheath ready for catheter insertion.

d. Heparinized saline solution (1 U/ml)
e. Fenestrated drape with tape
f. Surgical drapes
g. Nontoothed (half-curved) 4-inch forceps

> Stainless steel instruments preferred over plastic because of easier handling.

h. Fine-point scissors
i. 5- or 6-ml syringe with 18-gauge needle
j. *For infants weighing less than 2500 gm* or for smaller-caliber veins 23-gauge (approx. 2.0 F; 0.64 mm O.D.) silicone radiopaque catheter, approx. length, 30 cm, with introducer
   Select one:
   (1) 20- or 19-gauge Breakaway Introducer Needle
   (2) 20-gauge IV catheter placement unit

> Test to make sure silicone catheter fits easily through venous catheter lumen.

   (3) 19-gauge winged infusion needle†

> Refer to instructions enclosed with Vygon catheter and introducer.

k. *For infants weighing more than 2500 gm* (optional)

> The smaller gauge silicone catheter and introducer may be used for all infants.

†Vygon catheter

20-gauge (2.8 Fr) silicone radiopaque catheter, approximate length 30 cm, with introducer
Select one:
  (1) 18-gauge Breakaway Introducer Needle
  (2) 18-gauge IV catheter placement unit
l. 2 × 2 gauze squares
m. Skin closure tapes (e.g., Steri-strips)
n. Sterile, transparent, adhesive, semipermeable dressing

Unsterile

  a. Mask and head cover
  b. Materials for restraint
  c. Tape measure
  d. X-ray cassette and drape
  e. Tourniquet

2. Precautions

  a. Use strict sterile technique.
  b. Carefully restrain patient.
  c. Provide continuous direct patient observation during procedure.
  d. Recognize that apparent position of catheter tip may change when insertion site is in extremity and extremity is flexed or extended at shoulder or hip.
  e. Avoid leaving catheter in the lower right atrium, as migration of catheter or direct infusion of hypertonic solution can lead to myocardial tissue damage.[3]
  f. When securing the catheter prevent kinking or occlusion.
  g. Do not clamp the catheter directly.
  h. Do not place suture over catheter. The catheter is easily occluded or lacerated.
  i. Avoid withdrawing blood through the catheter. If it is necessary, flush the catheter with heparinized saline immediately after blood draw.
  j. Avoid flushing with a 1-ml syringe. Small syringes create sufficiently high pressures within the catheter to lead to rupture or thromboembolism.
  k. When removing the catheter, do not stretch it if there is resistance, as excessive tension may cause rupture. If resistance prevents removal, apply gentle intermittent tension every 2 to 4 hours until catheter is free.[4]

3. Placement of Catheter using Breakaway Introducer Needle

  a. Identify appropriate vein for insertion (See Fig. 12-1), for example:
  Basilic
  Easily accessible
  Relatively easy to thread to a central location
  Less risk of complications during insertion
  May enter in either the forearm or antecubital region
  Cephalic
  Same as for basilic site except that it can be difficult to thread catheter to a central position because of narrowing of vessel prior to entering the subclavian vein.

  With arm insertions, turn the infant's head toward the insertion site, to prevent the catheter from travelling cephalad through the ipsilateral jugular vein.

  Axillary
  Locate vein just medially and anterior to the axillary artery.
  Do not attempt procedure until the vein location is well defined.
  If arterial spasm occurs secondary to inadvertent puncture, see Chap. 15, Management of Arterial Spasm.
  Increased potential for pneumothorax
  Posterior auricular or superficial temporal
  Saphenous
  Can be more difficult to thread to central location secondary to valves and distance
  Popliteal
  Same as for saphenous
  External jugular
  Vein location should be carefully defined prior to attempting procedure.
  Can be more difficult to access
  Higher risk of pneumothorax
  b. Position radiograph cassette prior to skin preparation so the entire length of catheter will be visible on film when in place.
  c. Measure distance from proposed site of skin entry to right atrium.
  d. Prepare as for major procedure (see Chap. 4)

Rinse gloves in sterile saline to remove glove powder, which may adhere to catheter.

e. Attach syringe to catheter and flush with heparinized saline solution.

f. If using extremity, apply tourniquet to distend selected vessel.

g. Using Breakaway Introducer Needle, enter skin 1 cm distal to proposed site of entry into the vein.

h. Puncture vein.

i. With the forceps, grasp catheter 1 cm from the end and advance it through the introducer (Fig. 29-2A).

j. Advance catheter, grasping a few millimeters at a time for better control. After approximately 5 cm, remove the tourniquet. Catheter should advance easily if intraluminal. Stop at predetermined length.

To avoid shearing off the catheter, do not withdraw catheter while the introducer needle is in place.

k. Aspirate blood through catheter to confirm intravascular position and then flush with 1 ml of heparinized saline solution.

l. Secure the catheter during removal of the intro-

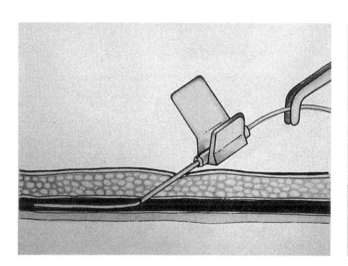

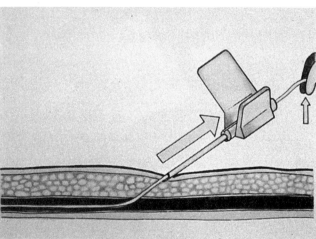

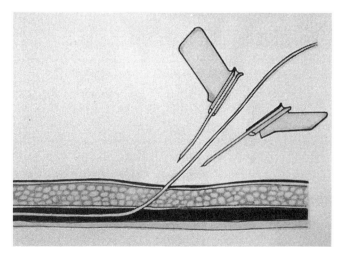

A B
C

FIG. 29-2
(*A*) Make venipuncture, thread catheter through introducer needle, and place catheter into position. (*B*) Hold catheter in place with forceps and withdraw introducer needle. (*C*) Pinch wings of needle together and strip needle cannula from catheter. *A–C*, with permission from Gesco International, San Antonio, TX.

ducer needle, by holding catheter with forceps during withdrawal (Fig. 29-2B).

m. Slowly withdraw the introducer needle until completely outside the skin.

n. Release introducer by either pinching or splitting wings and carefully peel the introducer needle apart, stripping it away from the catheter (Fig. 29-2C).

o. Verify correct catheter insertion length and adjust with forceps.

p. With a gauze pad, apply gentle pressure to insertion site, until hemostasis is achieved.

q. Secure the catheter and attached syringe temporarily with skin closure tapes and cover with sterile gauze until radiograph confirmation of position.*

4. Placement of Catheter Using an Introducer Cannula

a. Prepare as above, steps a to f.

b. Using Cathlon IV cannula with needle stylet, introduce needle through skin, 1 cm distal to point of entry into vein.

c. Puncture vein.

Do not advance further after receiving a flashback of blood, because the back wall of vessel may be pierced by the stylet.

d. Advance cannula into the vein 2 to 4 mm. If possible, leave at least 2 cm of cannula extending from the skin surface.

e. Remove needle stylet.

f. Cut off hub of introducer cannula.

g. With the forceps grasp the insertion end of the silastic catheter and advance it through introducer cannula. Advance catheter, grasping a few millimeters at a time for better control. After approximately 5 cm, remove the tourniquet.

h. The catheter should advance easily if intraluminal.

i. Advance catheter at least 1 cm further than premeasured length.

To accommodate for the length of the introducer

j. Aspirate blood through catheter to confirm intravascular placement and flush with 1 ml of heparinized saline solution.

k. Carefully remove the introducer cannula by pulling it straight out. The introducer will remain on the silastic catheter near the hub.

l. Verify the length of catheter inserted and adjust as necessary.

m. With a gauze pad, apply gentle pressure to insertion site until achieving hemostasis.

n. Secure catheter and attached syringe temporarily with skin closure tapes and cover with sterile gauze until radiographic confirmation of catheter tip position.

5. Dressing and Securing the Catheter

The catheters are small and fragile. They can easily migrate and break if not properly secured. (For other methods of securing silastic catheters, see Chapter 28, G3.)

a. Use sterile technique (see Chap. 28, H).

b. Clean area with alcohol and allow to dry.

c. Cut skin closure tapes (e.g., Steri-strips) to lengths of approximately 2 cm. Starting a few millimeters distal to insertion site, apply 4 to 5 slightly overlapping skin closure tapes, securing catheter to skin (Fig. 29-3A).

d. Apply a small dot of antibiotic ointment over insertion site (optional).

e. Cut a square of transparent semipermeable dressing to fit over insertion site and skin closure tapes.

Do not allow the transparent dressing or skin closure tapes to extend around the extremity. As the patient grows or with the occasional development of even mild venous congestion, the dressing will form a tourniquet.

f. Secure entire length of catheter to the patient (Fig. 29-3B).

  (1) Loosely coil the catheter or track it down the extremity to a comfortable position for securing the hub.

  (2) Adhere the catheter to the skin with narrow strips of transparent semipermeable dressing. Start by slightly overlapping with the first dressing applied near the insertion site and end at the hub of the catheter.

---

*If the catheter tip location is not visible on radiograph, instill 0.3 ml of water-soluble contrast medium (e.g., Renografin-60, diluted 1:1 with water).

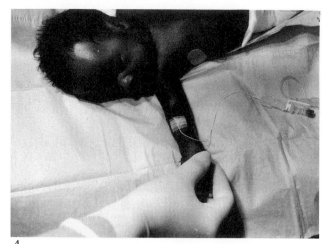

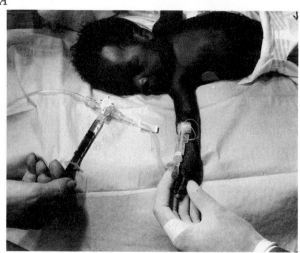

FIG. 29-3

(*A*) Shows five overlapping skin closure tapes just distal to skin entry site covered with one square of transparent semipermeable dressing. (*B*) Entire length of external catheter has been covered with sterile transparent semipermeable dressing.

    g. Criss-cross a single piece of tape under the hub and over the wings, to stabilize the connection between catheter and hub (Fig. 29-4A, B, C).

    h. Place a 2 × 2 gauze sponge or eyepad dressing under the hub. Tape over the hub and around the arm. This tape should be inspected weekly and changed if becoming too tight or loose.

    i. Make sure the catheter or connection of hub is not kinked.

6. Complications

See Chapter 28, K.

INTRACLAVICULAR PERCUTANEOUS CATHETERIZATION OF THE SUBCLAVIAN VEIN

A supraclavicular approach has also been described.[2]

1. Indications and Contraindications[5–14]

See Chapter 28, A.

2. Equipment

Sterile

    a. Gloves and gown

    b. Cup with antiseptic solution

    c. Gauze squares

    d. Roll of 4 × 4 gauze

    e. Transparent aperture drape

    f. 0.5% lidocaine-HCL in labeled 3-ml syringe with 25-gauge needle

    g. 18-gauge venipuncture needle

    h. 0.25N saline flush solution—heparinized 1 U/ml in labeled 5-ml syringe

    i. No. 20 Argyle Intramedicut (see Chap. 28, G2). Alternatively, a silastic catheter (e.g., Cook catheter) may be placed by this route, using the Seldinger technique (see A2).

    j. Needle holder

    k. 5-0 nylon suture with small, curved needle

    l. Suture scissors

    m. "T" connector

    n. Appropriate materials for occlusive dressing of choice (see Chap. 28, H)

Unsterile

    a. Appropriate heat source (see Chap. 2)

    b. X-ray cassette

    c. Materials for restraint (Fig. 29-5)

    d. Mask and head cover

3. Precautions

    a. Consider as a major operative procedure: approach accordingly, including performance by a surgeon experienced with procedure.

FIG. 29-4

(A–C) Securing the catheter hub. The Catheter hub should be properly secured to prevent development of tension at the catheter's entry point into the hub. **A.** The tape has been placed under hub of catheter. **B.** The tape is criss-crossed over hub to prevent tension at junction of catheter and hub. A–C, with permission from Gesco International, San Antonio, TX. **C.** Catheter is completely secured.

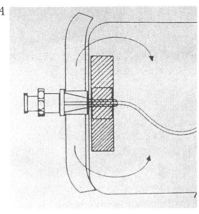

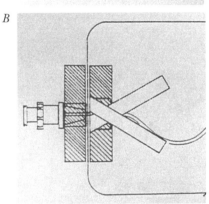

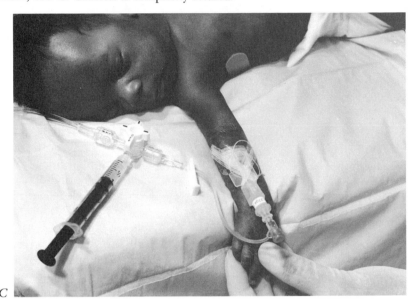

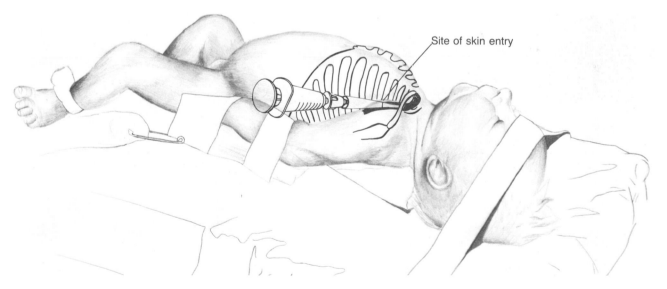

Site of skin entry

FIG. 29-5

Infant restrained for catheterization of the subclavian vein. (Eichelberger MR, Rous PG, Hoelzer DJ, Garcia VF, Koop CE: Percutaneous subclavian venous catheters in neonates and children. J Pediatr Surg 16, No. 4:547–553, 1981. Reprinted by permission)

b. Use strict sterile technique.

c. Perform only in an operating room or intensive care unit.

d. Recognize that adequate restraint of patient is mandatory.

e. Provide continuous direct patient observation during procedure.

f. Note anatomical differences between neonates and older children (Figs. 29-6, 29-7).

The subclavian vein runs more cephalad in neonates than in older patients. The apex of the pleura extends into the base of the neck.

g. Place neonate in head-down position only when prepared to insert catheter. Intraventricular hemorrhage may be associated with this positioning.[9]

h. Catheterize side of greatest compromise if there is asymmetric pulmonary defect, to ensure maximal preservation of lung function.

i. Confirm catheter position radiographically, and reconfirm weekly.

4. Technique

a. Use general anesthesia if child is difficult to immobilize or is undergoing concomitant surgical procedure.

b. Place patient supine and restrain extremities, with arms at sides pulled caudally (see Fig. 29-5).

With the arms pulled gently downward along the patient's side, the subclavian vein runs more parallel with the deltopectoral groove.

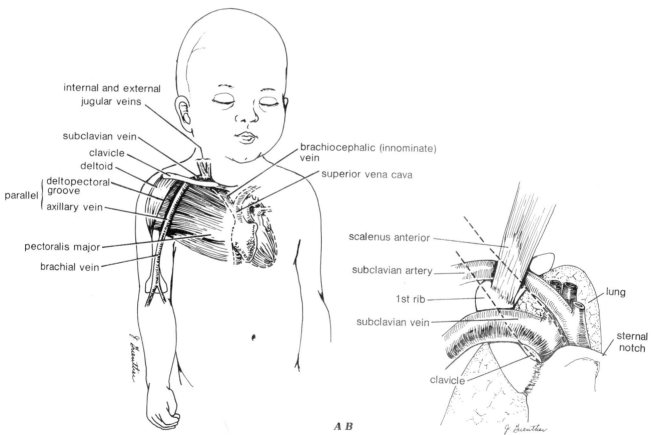

A B

FIG. 29-6
Anatomical relations of the subclavian vein in the neonate.

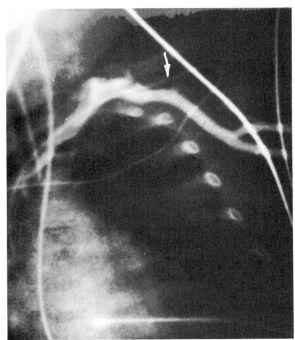

FIG. 29-7
Brachial venogram demonstrating the anatomical relationship of the subclavian vein to the first rib. Central venous line is in situ *(arrow)*.

c. Maintain head in midline position, with tape across forehead.

With the head in this position, the catheter is less likely to enter the jugular vein.

d. Prepare as for major procedure (see Chap. 4).
e. Prepare infraclavicular region with antiseptic, such as an iodophor.
f. Quarantine area with aperture drape.
g. Use 18-gauge venipuncture needle to puncture skin in deltopectoral groove, 2-cm from clavicle.
h. Palpate groove formed at point where clavicle and first rib cross. Subclavian vein consistently passes beneath clavicle and above first rib (Figs. 29-6, 29-7).
i. Place infant in Trendelenburg position.
    (1) Produces venous distention and improves access
    (2) Reduces risk of air embolus
j. Place needle/cannula through skin puncture previously made with venipuncture needle, with bevel down. Advance to inferior edge of clavicle in previously located groove
    (1) Subclavian vein is located immediately beneath clavicle.
    (2) Deep insertion is unnecessary in small patients.
k. Pass needle/cannula beneath clavicle and direct midway between sternal notch and chin, or to a point 1 cm above sternal notch.[8] Limit manipulation with the needle stylet in place to straight line insertion, without change in direction. If direction change is required, withdraw system completely, then reinsert.
l. Apply gentle, continuous aspiration to prevent inadvertent passage of needle through vein.

Cessation of blood return after needle has been advanced an adequate distance indicates penetration of back wall of vein. If this occurs, remove needle stylet and back plastic cannula out slowly. Once satisfactory blood flow is obtained from the cannula, insert catheter and advance it through cannula.

m. As soon as blood is noted in syringe, reinject blood (to distend vein at needle tip) and simultaneously advance cannula approximately 3 mm.
n. Remove needle, leaving cannula in situ (keep thumb over end of cannula until catheter is inserted *or* if using a Cook (Broviac-type) catheter, proceed using the Seldinger technique (see A2).
o. Remove catheter from plastic container. We also recommend removal of the locking ferrule because we have found that it interferes with fixation (see Fig. 28-3).
p. Place "T" connector in hub of catheter and flush connector/catheter with heparinized saline.
q. Clamp tubing of "T" connector.
r. Insert catheter into cannula (Fig. 29-8).
s. Continue insertion of catheter until 1 to 2 cm are intravascular
t. Use plastic cover from catheter to estimate length of catheter to be inserted.
    (1) Plastic cover is same length as catheter.
    (2) Measure combined length as follows:
        From midway between nipple and midpoint of clavicle to suprasternal notch
        From suprasternal notch to point of skin entry

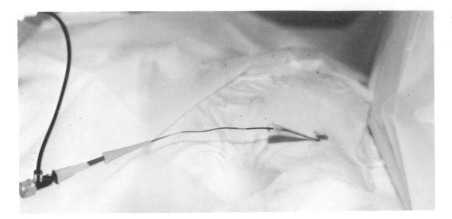

FIG. 29-8
Inserting an Argyle Intramedicut catheter into the subclavian vein via a cannula.

u. Insert catheter for estimated length.

Occasionally, manipulation under fluoroscope may be necessary. Catheter placement under electrocardiographic guidance has been described.[15,16]

Catheter should be inserted easily if cannula is intraluminal. If resistance to catheter is encountered
(1) Withdraw catheter into cannula
(2) Withdraw cannula slightly (1 to 2 mm)
(3) Reinsert catheter
(4) Repeat this maneuver until catheter is inserted or cannula is removed from beneath clavicle

v. Confirm intraluminal position by aspirating through catheter and noting free flow of blood.

w. Obtain x-ray film for catheter position.

x. Pull back plastic cannula out of skin, while holding catheter with opposite hand. Take care to avoid inadvertent displacement of catheter. Pull back cannula until it engages with hub of catheter (or locking ferrule).

y. Place a 5-0 nylon suture deep into skin, just distal to skin-entry site of catheter, and tie around catheter with half-hitch knot. (For alternative methods of securing silastic catheters, see Chap. 28, G3.)

z. Aspirate blood via "T" connector through catheter to confirm intravascular position, arrange external catheter across infant's chest, and place second nylon suture through skin; tie around

catheter 1 cm from first suture. For sterile dressing, see Chapter 28, H.

5. Complications

See Chapter 28, K.

References

1. MASOORLI S, ANGELES T: PICC lines: The latest home care challenge. RN Magazine, January 1990.
2. CHATHAS MK, PATON KB, FISHER DE: Percutaneous central venous catheterization. Am J Dis Child 11:144, 1990
3. KHILNANI P, TOCE S, REDDY R: Mechanical complications from very small percutaneous central venous Silastic catheters. Crit Care Med 18:12, 1990
4. GLADMAN G, SINHA S, SIMS DG, CHISWICK ML: Staphlococcus epidermitis and retention of neonatal percutaneous central venous catheters. Arch Dis Child 65:234, 1990
5. ALTMAN RP, RANDOLPH JG: Application and hazards of total parenteral nutrition in infants. Ann Surg 174:85, 1971
6. BORJA AR: Current status of infraclavicular subclavian vein catheterization. Ann Thorac Surg 13:165, 1972
7. COCKINGTON RA: Silicone Elastomer for nasojejunal intubation and central venous cannulation in neonates. Anaesth Intensive Care 7:248, 1979
8. DEFALQUE RJ: The subclavian route—a critical review of the World literature up to 1970. Der Anaesthesist 21:325, 1972
9. EICHELBERGER MR, ROUS PG, HOELZER DJ, ET AL:

Percutaneous subclavian venous catheters in neonates and children. J Pediatr Surg 16:547, 1981

10. FILSTON HC, GRANT JP: A safer system for percutaneous subclavian venous catheterization in newborn infants. J Pediatr Surg 14:564, 1979

11. FIROV HV: Pulmonary embolization complicating total intravenous alimentation. J Pediatr Surg 7:81, 1972

12. KLEIN MD, RUDD M: Successful central venous catheter placement from peripheral subcutaneous veins in children. Anesthesiology 52:447, 1980

13. SEIBERT JJ, WEINSTEIN MM, ERENBERG A: Catheter-related complications of total parenteral nutrition in infants. Pediatr Radiol 4:233, 1976

14. SHAW JCL: Parenteral nutrition in the management of sick low birth weight infants. Pediatr Clin North Am 20:333, 1973

15. MARTIN JT: Neuroanesthetic adjuncts for patients in the sitting position. III: Intravascular electrocardiography. Anesth Analg (Cleve) 49:793, 1970

16. RICHARDO CC, FREEMAN A: Intra-atrial catheter placement under electrocardiographic guidance. Anesthesiology 25:388, 1964

30 Placement of a Central Venous Line by Surgical Cutdown

Martin Raymond Eichelberger
Mhairi G. MacDonald

In this chapter no attempt has been made to provide a comprehensive review of all the possible techniques and sites of placement and available types of catheter.[1,2] The preference of the individual surgeon, catheter availability and the size and medical condition of the infant will play a significant role in determining the method, site, and catheter used. We hope, however, that the sites and methods that we have described are illustrative of important general principles.

A. INDICATIONS

See Chapter 28.

B. CONTRAINDICATIONS

1. See Chapter 28.
2. If using internal jugular vein
   a. Previous catheterization of contralateral jugular vein
   b. Thrombosis of jugular venous system on contralateral side
3. Infant with ventriculo-atrial shunt in place

C. EQUIPMENT

Sterile
1. Items necessary for major skin preparation (see Chap. 4)
2. Gown and gloves
3. Cup with antiseptic solution
4. Transparent aperture drape (e.g., Steridrape)*
5. 4 × 4 gauze squares

*3M Company, 3M Center, St. Paul, MN 55101

6. 0.5% lidocaine-HCL in labeled 3-ml syringe with 25-gauge venipuncture needle (optional)

   General anesthesia is preferred.

7. Catheter of choice (see Chap. 28)
8. Blunt-needle adapter, 21-gauge (only necessary if nonprepared catheter tubing used)
9. Heparinized 0.25N saline flush solution (1 unit/ml) in 5-ml syringe
10. 3-0 silk suture and 5-0 silk suture on a cutting needle (see Appendix B)
11. "T" connector
12. No. 11 scalpel blade and holder
13. Two small tissue retractors or self-retaining retractor
14. Tissue forceps
15. Fine vascular forceps
16. Two small, curved mosquito hemostats
17. Dissecting scissors
18. No. 15 Vim–Silverman needle with obturator
19. 5-0 silk suture on small, curved needle
20. Needle holder
21. Suture scissors
22. 30% Renografin (60% diluted, 1:1) in labeled 3-ml syringe (if using nonradiopaque catheter)
23. Appropriate materials for occlusive dressing of choice (see Chap. 28)

Unsterile
1. Cap and mask
2. Roll of 4 × 4 gauze
3. Safety razor

4. Tape measure
5. 1-inch adhesive tape
6. X-ray cassette

> Hoffman et al have described placement of central venous catheters using ECG guidance.[3]

D. PRECAUTIONS

1. See Chapter 28.

E. TECHNIQUES

1. Catheter Placement via Jugular veins, using Vim–Silverman Needle

a. Direct Approach

(1) Immobilize infant in position similar to that for percutaneous insertion of subclavian venous catheter (see Chap. 29, Subclavian Vein).

(2) If right side is to be catheterized, turn head to left and extend neck.

(3) Estimate length of catheter to be inserted by measuring from point midway between nipple and midpoint of the clavicle to point over sternocleidomastoid muscle at junction of middle and lower third of neck (Fig. 30-1).

(4) Have assistant shave area of head posterior to ear if this is intended position for subcutaneous tunnel.

(5) Put on cap and mask.

(6) Scrub as for major procedure, and put on gown and gloves (see Chap. 4).

(7) Prepare neck and scalp area or right chest wall with antiseptic solution, such as an Iodophor, and drape with transparent aperture drape.

(8) Make small, transverse incision (1 to 2 cm) through skin and platysma muscle.

(9) Free external jugular vein by blunt dissection with curved mosquito hemostat. If internal jugular vein is used, sternocleidomastoid muscle must be split to locate vein.

FIG. 30-1
The jugular veins in relation to major anatomical landmarks.

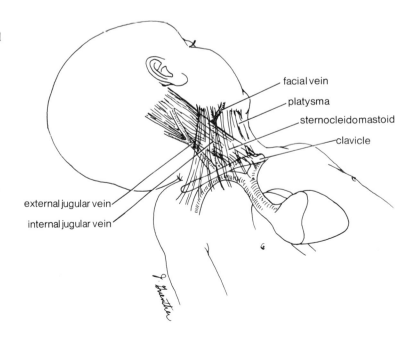

facial vein
platysma
sternocleidomastoid
clavicle
external jugular vein
internal jugular vein

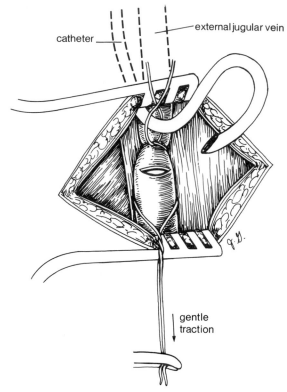

FIG. 30-2
Catheterization of the external jugular vein; venotomy has been performed prior to inserting the catheter.

(10) Pass curved mosquito hemostat behind vein, and place proximal and distal ligatures of 5-0 nylon loosely around vein (Fig. 30-2).

(11) Using Vim–Silverman needle with obturator in situ, tunnel a subcutaneous tract approximately 5 to 10 cm from neck to exit on
  (a) Anterior chest wall, a short distance medial to right nipple (Fig. 30-3A)
  (b) Scalp (Fig. 30-3B)

(12) Remove obturator, and pass catheter through needle.

(13) Remove needle, leaving catheter in subcutaneous tract.

(14) Place blunt-needle adapter on external end of catheter if nonprepared catheter tubing is used (see Fig. 28-1).
  (a) Remove plastic needle guard from 21-gauge scalp-vein needle.
  (b) Thread needle guard onto external end of catheter tubing.
  (c) Thread blunt-needle adapter onto end of catheter.
  (d) Use two 3-0 silk ties to hold catheter tubing onto adapter.
  (e) Slip plastic needle guard over junction

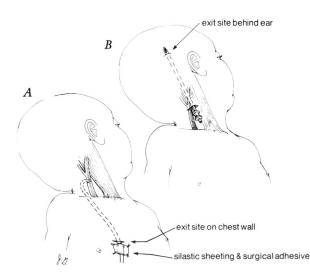

FIG. 30-3
Formation of a subcutaneous tunnel with a Vim–Silverman needle. (*A*) Tunnel on the anterior chest wall. The catheter is in situ and has been fixed using a "sandwich" of silastic sheeting. (*B*) Alternative route under the scalp.

between needle and adapter to prevent catheter shearing at this point.

(15) Attach "T" connector to hub of catheter.

(16) Fill catheter system with heparinized flush solution.

(17) Perform transverse venotomy (see Fig. 30-2)

For external jugular vein

(a) Tie cephalad venous ligature, and exert traction on both ligatures in opposite directions with aid of appropriately prepared assistant.

(b) Make short, transverse incision in anterior wall of vein, and enlarge gently by inserting and spreading tips of fine vascular forceps.

For internal jugular vein

(a) Use purse-string suture of 6-0 nylon, placed in vessel wall around point of catheter entrance, to avoid ligation of vessel.

(b) Make incision in vessel as for external jugular vein.

(18) Bevel intravascular end of catheter (optional).

(19) Grasp catheter gently with blunt non-toothed tissue forceps, introduce catheter tip and insert for premeasured distance.

(20) Leave loop of catheter in neck wound to dampen effect of head movement (see Fig. 30-4, *inset*)

(21) Close wound with subcuticular 5-0 absorbable suture, taking care not to penetrate the catheter.

(22) Use selected method for fixation and dressing (see Chap. 28).

b. Indirect Approach via the Common Facial vein[4–8]

Use of the common facial vein (CFV) to enter the jugular venous system offers the following advantages:

Ligation of internal jugular vein is avoided.
Procedure may be carried out bilaterally.
Internal jugular vein is potentially reusable for catheterization.

FIG. 30-4
Insertion of a catheter into the common facial vein. Incision is below the angle of the mandible at the level of the hyoid bone. The facial vein is ligated at the junction of the anterior and posterior tributaries. (*Inset*) The catheter is looped in the neck wound to "dampen" the effect of head movement. (Reproduced with permission from Zumbro GL, Mullin MJ, Nelson TG: Catheter placement in infants needing total parenteral nutrition utilizing common facial vein. Arch Surg 102:71, 1971. Copyright © 1971, American Medical Association) Alternatively, a subcutaneous tunnel may be made with a catheter exit site on the anterior chest wall.

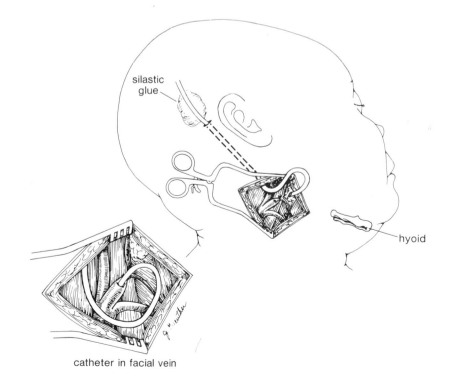

silastic glue

hyoid

catheter in facial vein

(1) Prepare for procedure as for direct cutdown on jugular veins.

    (a) Estimate length of catheter to be inserted ($\simeq$ 5 cm in term infants) by measuring from anterior border of sternocleidomastoid muscle, at level of hyoid bone, to point midway between nipple and clavicle.

    (b) Subcutaneous tunnel may be prepared either on scalp or anterior chest wall, as for jugular veins (Fig. 30-3).

(2) Make a 1- to 2-cm transverse incision over anterior border of sternocleidomastoid muscle at level of hyoid bone (Fig. 30-4).

(3) Deepen incision beneath muscle border by blunt dissection, using mosquito hemostat.

(4) Retract wound edges.

(5) Locate CFV just beyond its formation from anterior and posterior facial-vein tributaries (see Fig. 30-4, *inset*).

(6) Pass curved mosquito hemostat beneath vein.

(7) Pass two 5-0 nylon sutures around vein. Position one cephalad, at junction of anterior and posterior facial-vein tributaries. Position one caudad, at junction of CFV with internal jugular vein.

(8) Using ligatures to elevate vein in wound, make transverse incision in CFV, 1 cm from its junction with internal jugular vein.

If the lumen of the CFV is very narrow, the incision may be made immediately prior to the junction of the CFV with the internal jugular vein, where the lumen widens. Sufficient length of the CFV for distal ligation may be produced in the junctional area by "tenting up" the vein wall around the catheter.

(9) Introduce catheter for predetermined distance.

(10) Tie caudad ligature, taking care not to occlude catheter lumen.

(11) Complete procedure as for direct approach.

2. Proximal Saphenous Vein Cutdown Using Cook/Broviac Catheter[9-15]

Additional Equipment Required

  a. Infant Cook catheter (see Chap. 28, G2)

  b. Blunt vascular dilator

  c. 5-0 absorbable suture on curved cutting needle (e.g., vicryl, See Appendix B2).*

  d. Long tonsil hemostat to create subcutaneous tunnel

  e. Heparinized saline ($1-10\mu$/ml)†

Technique

The proximal saphenous vein is a useful site, because the vessel is of adequate size to take a Broviac catheter, even in extremely low birth weight premature infants. Potential disadvantages of this site are reduced by using a silastic catheter (may reduce thrombotic complications), and creating a subcutaneous tunnel to bring the point of exit above the umbilicus. The technique described is also applicable to the jugular veins.

  a. Scrub, and prepare as for major procedure (see Chap. 4).

  b. Prepare as for cutdown on jugular vein.

    (1) Choose right or left groin area for insertion.

    (2) Prepare groin/abdomen and chest on same side.

  c. Make incision 1 cm long: 1 cm caudad, and 1 cm lateral to pubic tubercule (Fig. 30-5).

  d. Spread incision into subcutaneous tissues, using curved mosquito hemostat.

    (1) Incise superficial fascia.

    (2) Identify saphenous vein lying medial and inferior to its junction with femoral vein at foramen ovale (see Fig. 30-5).

  e. Move 0.5 cm to 1 cm distally before

    (1) Passing curved mosquito hemostat behind vein. Avoids inadvertent damage to femoral vein.

    (2) Placing two 5-0 nylon sutures loosely around vein.

  f. Create tunnel, using tonsil hemostat, in subcutaneous plane laterally onto anterior thorax or abdomen, just above umbilicus (Fig. 30-6).

  g. Flush catheter with heparinized saline and replace cap.

  h. Pull catheter through tunnel into groin wound so that dacron cuff is just within abdominal/thoracic skin incision. Estimate length of catheter to be inserted so that tip will be in inferior vena cava at junction with right atrium.

---

*Vicryl sutures are made by Davis and Geck, Division of American Cyanamide, 1 Casper Street, Danbury, CT 06810

†Concentration depends on whether the line will be capped or immediately used for infusion.

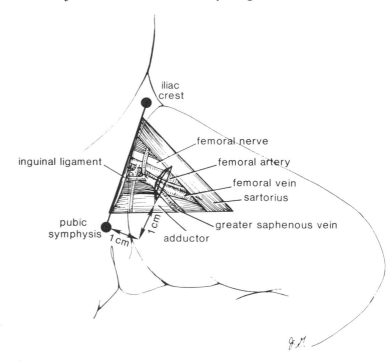

FIG. 30-5
Anatomical view of the site of incision for proximal saphenous vein cutdown with underlying femoral triangle.

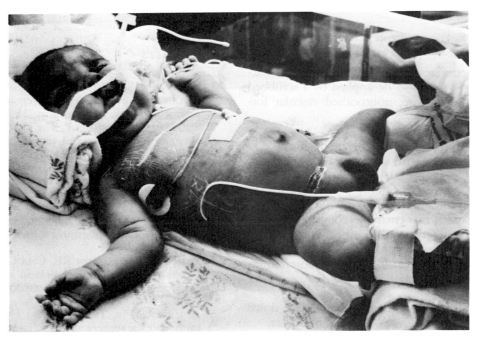

FIG. 30-6
Infant with two Broviac catheters in place. The catheter exiting from the subcutaneous tunnel from the chest wall enters the left common facial vein. The catheter exiting from the tunnel on the upper abdomen enters the proximal saphenous vein.

31 ECMO Cannulation and Decannulation

Billie Lou Short
Kathryn D. Anderson

Venoarterial Extracorporeal Membrane Oxygenation (ECMO) —Cannulation

A. INDICATIONS

Placement of carotid arterial and internal jugular venous catheters for use in venoarterial extracorporeal membrane oxygenation (ECMO). ECMO is used to treat term or near-term infants with reversible respiratory failure who do not respond to maximal oxygen and ventilator support.[1-3]

B. CONTRAINDICATIONS FOR ECMO IN THE NEONATAL PERIOD[1,2]

1. Gestational age < 34 weeks
2. Birth weight < 2000 gm
3. Severe coagulopathy or bleeding disorder
4. Congenital heart disease without lung disease
5. Irreversible lung pathology
6. Intracranial hemorrhage greater than grade I
7. Major congenital anomaly
8. Age greater than 10 to 14 days
9. Significant positive response to ventilator management

C. PRECAUTIONS

1. Ensure that the patient is paralyzed before placement of the venous catheter, to prevent air embolus.
2. Recognize that
   a. Internal jugular lines placed for IV access prior o ECMO may cause clot formation, resulting in the need for embolectomy prior to the placement of the venous ECMO catheter.
   b. Excessive manipulation of the internal jugular vein may cause spasm and inability to place a catheter of appropriate gauge.

   c. A lacerated vessel may result in the need for a sternotomy for vessel retrieval.

   Appropriate instruments should be on the beside tray or cart. A backup unit of blood should be available in the blood bank.

   d. Blood loss sufficient to produce hypotension can occur during a difficult cannulation.

   Blood should be available at the bedside (10–20 ml/kg).

   e. The vagus nerve is located next to the neck vessels.

   Manipulation can cause bradycardia or other arrhythmias.

   f. Vital signs and pulse oximetry values must be monitored at all times, because clinical observation of the infant is prevented by the surgical drapes.

D. PERSONNEL, EQUIPMENT (see Fig. 31-1), AND MEDICATIONS[4]

Personnel
1. Surgical team
   a. A senior surgeon (pediatric, cardiovascular, or thoracic) with assistant
   b. A surgical scrub nurse, and circulating nurse
2. Medical team
   a. A physician trained in management of ECMO patients and cannulation techniques, who will administer anesthetic agents and medically manage the infant during the procedure
   b. A bedside intensive care (NICU or PICU) nurse who will monitor vital signs, record events, and draw up medications as needed by the ECMO physician

VENOARTERIAL ECMO CIRCUIT

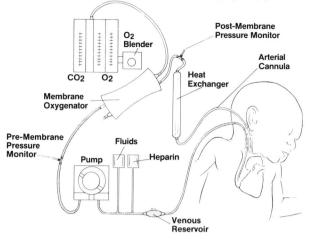

FIG. 31-1
Schematic diagram of venoarterial ECMO circuit showing the drainage from the right atrium into the bladder of the circuit, with flow through the membrane lung, heat exchanger, and return flow to the arch of the aorta via the carotid artery catheter. (With permission, Fetal and Neonatal Physiology, Volume 1, RA Polina and WC Rox, eds. Philadelphia, Sanders, 1992, p. 933.)

   c. A respiratory therapist who will change ventilator settings as necessary

3. Circuit specialists
   a. Cardiovascular perfusionist or an RN or RT specially trained in this procedure who will prime the pump
   b. A bedside ECMO Specialist (RN, RT, or CV perfusionist with special training in ECMO management) who will manage the ECMO system after the patient is on ECMO

Equipment—Sterile
  1. Arterial and venous catheters[5]
   a. Arterial
     (1) Determines the resistance of the ECMO circuit, because it is the part of the ECMO circuit with the smallest internal diameter, and thus the highest resistance
     (2) This catheter should be as short as possible, with a thin wall and a large internal diameter (resistance is directly related to

the length of the catheter and indirectly related to the diameter), e.g., BioMedicus Extracorporeal Circulation Cannula, 8 to 10 Fr (Biomedicus, Minneapolis, MN) and Elecath 8 to 10 Fr (Electro-Catheter Corp, Rahway, NJ).
   b. Venous
     (1) Should have as large an internal diameter as possible to allow maximal blood flow (blood flow rate is directly related to oxygenation of the patient)
     (2) Should be thin walled with a large internal diameter, e.g., Biomedicus Extracorporeal Circulation Cannula, 8 to 14 Fr; Elecath 8 to 14 Fr

2. Surgical instruments required are listed in Tables 31-1 and 31-2.
3. Sterile gowns and gloves
4. Sterile saline for injection
5. Syringes (1–20 ml) and needles (19–26 gauge)
6. Povidone iodine solution
7. Povidone iodine ointment
8. Semipermeable transparent membrane type dressing
9. Absorbable gelatin sponge, e.g., Gelfoam, Upjohn, Kalamazoo, MI
10. Surgical lubricant, bacteriostatic

Equipment—Nonsterile
1. Surgical head covers and mask
2. Pulse oximeter
3. Surgical head light
4. Electrocautery
5. Wall suction
6. Shoulder roll, e.g., small blanket to place under infant's shoulders
7. Tubing clamps

Medications
1. A long-acting paralysing agent, e.g., pancuronium bromide (0.1 mg/kg)
2. Fentanyl citrate (10–20 μg/kg)
3. Sodium heparin (100–150 U/kg)
4. Topical thrombin
5. Xylocaine, 0.25% with epinephrine
6. Xylocaine, 1% plain
7. Cryoprecipitate—thawed (optional)

TABLE 31-1

Surgical Instruments for ECMO Cannulation

(Place in a 12 × 18 mayo tray with a Huck towel on the bottom of the tray.)

Number	Item
Place on the tray	
2	Custard cup (place one inside of the other with a 3 × 4 sponge)
1	Medicine cup (place inside of the custard cup with a 3 × 4 sponge)
2	Straight bulldog clamps
1	Sauer eye retractor
1	Alm retractor
1	Mastoid Jansen retractor
2	Vein retractors
2	Octagonal forceps
2	7″ Gerald forceps
2	6″ Debakey forceps
1	Adson forcep, plain
2	Adson forcep with teeth
2	#3 knife handles
1	Castroviejo needleholder
2	Right angle retractors
2	Chops retractors
1	Set of Garrett dilators, 9 pcs (sizes 1.0, 1.5, 2.0, 2.5, 3.0, 3.5, 4.0, 4.5, 5.0)

String the following instruments left to right on two 9-inch sponge sticks or instrument stringer; then, place on top of a rolled Huck towel.

Number	Item
4	9″ sponge stick
1	Tonsil clamp (bleeder)
1	6½″ crile
1	5¾″ crile
1	Baby right angle clamp
4	Straight mosquitoes
6	Curved mosquitoes
3	Fine curved mosquitoes
2	Tubing clamp with guard
1	Ryder needleholder
1	Webster needleholder
1	Straight mayo scissor
1	5¾″ Metzenbaum scissor
1	Curved Steven scissor
1	Straight Iris scissor
4	Small towel clips (nonpenetrating)
1	Baby Satinsky clamp
1	Curved bulldog clamp
1	Straight bulldog clamp
1	Disposable ECMO tray (Table 31-2)

For information on suture material, see Appendix B2 at the end of this book.

TABLE 31-2

Contents of Disposable ECMO Tray

Number	Item
2	1-ml syringes
1	20-ml syringe
1	6-ml syringe
1	3-ml syringe
1	Needle adapter
3	Single cavity tray
2	Gauze packages
1	Betadine ointment
1	Surgical blade no. 15 carbon
2	Semipermeable transparent dressings
1	Handle, suction frazier, 8 Fr
1	Xylocaine insert
1	Mini yellow vessel loops
1	Hand control cautery
1	Suture, 4-0 vicryl
1	Suture 2-0 silk
1	Suture 6-0 prolene
4	Forceps, sponge
1	25-gauge needle
1	NaCL 5 ml amp.
1	3-gm foil package of surgilube
1	Surgical blade no. 11 carbon
2	Steridrapes
2	Connectors straight ¼ × ¼
1	Xylocaine 1%
1	Suction tubing ³⁄₁₆″ × 10′
1	Package sterile towels (12)

E. TECHNIQUE—PREPARATION FOR CANNULATION

1. Place infant with head to "foot" of warmer.
2. Hyperextend the patient's neck with a shoulder roll and turn the head to the left (Fig. 31-2).
3. Paralyze the patient with pancuronium.
4. Anesthetize the patient with fentanyl (10–20 µg/kg).

   Watch for hypotension.

5. Monitor vital signs and give additional fentanyl as needed (see Analgesia Chap. 5).
6. Clean a wide area of the right neck, chest, and ear with iodophor iodine solution.
7. Drape the infant and entire bed with sterile towels.

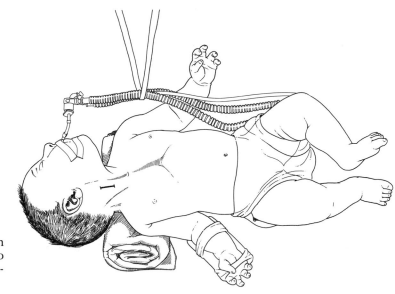

FIG. 31-2
Infant positioned for cannulation with shoulder-roll present and head extended to the left. Position of neck incision is indicated.

8. Use steri-drapes to secure the towels to the skin.
9. At the point of incision infiltrate the skin with xylocaine (0.25% with epinephrine) (see Fig. 31-2).
10. Wait at least 3 minutes for anesthesia.
11. Make a 1- to 2-cm vertical incision over the right sternocleidomastoid muscle, starting approximately 1 cm above the right clavicular head, using the electrocautery set on cutting current (Fig. 31-3).
12. Continue to use the electrocautery to cut through the subcutaneous tissue.
13. Coagulate all visible bleeding sites.

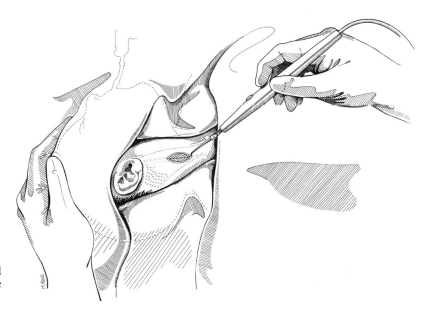

FIG. 31-3
Landmarks over the sternocleidomastoid muscle for making the incision with the electrocautery.

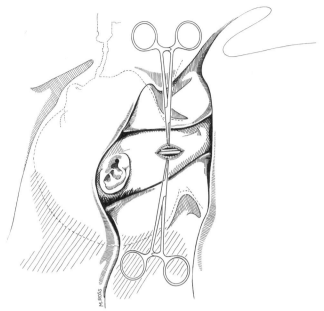

FIG. 31-4
Split sternocleidomastoid and open carotid sheath.

14. Spread the fibers of the sternocleidomastoid muscle apart with a hemostat and retract using hemostats clamped onto the muscle (Fig. 31-4).
15. Open the carotid sheath, taking care to avoid the vagus nerve.
16. Irrigate both common carotid artery and internal jugular vein with 1% plain xylocaine, to vasodilate the vessels.

17. Encircle the artery with proximal and distal 2-0 silk ties, held with clamps but not tied—avoid "sawing" the ties on the artery.
18. *Avoid contact with the internal jugular vein*—isolate after cannulation of carotid artery, to avoid spasm.
19. Estimate the length of the cannula to be inserted
    a. Identify the sternal notch and the xiphoid process.
    b. The arterial catheter is inserted approximately ⅓ of the distance between the sternal notch and the xiphoid process.
    c. The venous catheter is inserted approximately ½ the distance between the sternal notch and the xiphoid process.
    d. Mark these distances on the catheters with a 2-0 tie.
20. Heparinize the patient with a bolus of 100 to 150 U/kg of heparin, depending on the estimated risk of bleeding, and wait 60 to 90 seconds before proceeding.

Arterial Cannulation

1. Tie the distal ligature on the carotid artery and place a bulldog clamp on the proximal portion of the artery.

   Allow blood to dilate the artery before placing the bulldog clamp.

2. Make an arteriotomy using an no. 11 scalpel blade, and place two traction sutures of 6-0 proline on the proximal side of the arteriotomy (Fig. 31-5AB).

FIG. 31-5
(*A*) Carotid artery isolated with vessel clamp in place and with arteriotomy site showing the placement of the 6-0 proline traction sutures. (*B*) *Inset*, showing magnified view of Fig. 31-5A.

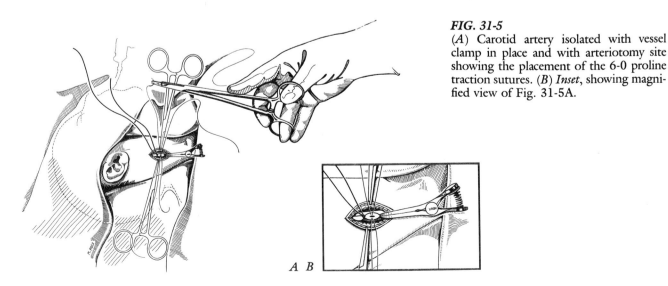

A   B

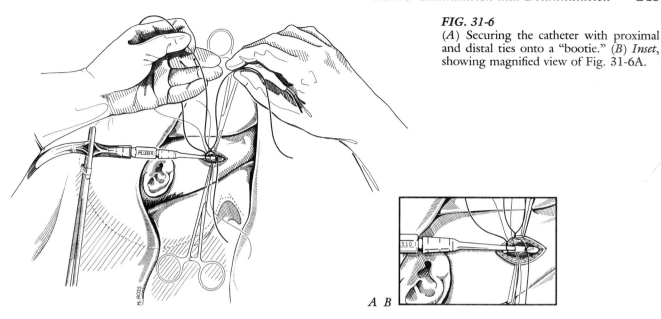

A B

Always use traction sutures to prevent intimal tears.

3. Lubricate Garrett dilators with sterile surgical lubricant and dilate the artery to the approximate size of the catheter.
4. Place a sterile tubing clamp on the catheter. Lubricate the catheter and insert the catheter into the vessel as the bulldog clamp is removed.
5. Secure the catheter with a 2-0 silk ligature tied over a 0.5- to 1-cm vessel loop ("bootie") (Fig. 31-6A,B)
6. Place a second 2-0 silk ligature. Tie the distal tie around the catheter, and then tie the distal and proximal ties together.
7. Allow blood to backup into the catheter to remove air.

Venous Cannulation

1. Dissect the vein and isolate with two 2-0 silk ties.

   Do not apply traction to the vein with the ties, to avoid spasm.

2. Place a bulldog clamp on the proximal end of the vein, allowing blood to distend the vein, then tie the distal end with the 2-0 silk ligature.

3. Make a venotomy with a no. 11 scalpel blade and place two stay sutures of 6-0 proline as traction sutures, as for arterial cannulation.
4. Lubricate the venous catheter, place a sterile tubing clamp on the catheter, and dilate the venotomy.
5. Insert the catheter as an assistant places traction on the proximal tie, and apply pressure over the liver to increase the back flow of blood out of the catheter (to decrease the risk of an air embolus).

   There will be a slight impedance to catheter advancement at the thoracic inlet—pushing against resistance will tear the vein. Use gentle downward and backward pressure.

6. Secure, as for the artery, and back blood into the catheter by pressing gently on the liver.
7. Pack the wound with absorbable gelatin sponge soaked in topical thrombin, to assist in hemostasis.

   Cryoprecipitate and topical thrombin can be used to form a fibrin clot if dropped onto the field from separate syringes in a 1:1 concentration. (If mixed together in one syringe, they will form a solid clot in the syringe.)

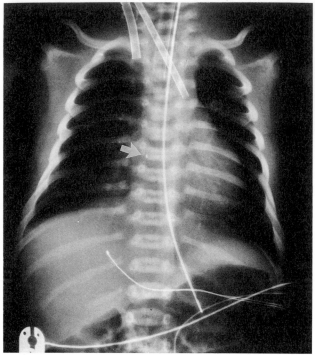

FIG. 31-7
X-ray at cannulation showing proper placement of the arterial and venous catheters. Note the radiopaque dot indicating the end of the Biomedicus venous ECMO catheter (arrow).

8. Confirm catheter placement by x-ray if the patient is stable (Fig. 31-7). If unstable, the patient can be placed on ECMO and the x-ray taken when adequate oxygenation is achieved, but prior to closing the surgical wound.

Placing the Patient on the ECMO Circuit
The circuit has been previously primed with packed cells/albumin. Priming of the circuit is beyond the scope of this chapter.

1. Fill catheters with sterile saline. Connect them to the ECMO circuit by inserting the $1/4 \times 1/4$-inch connectors into the tubing as the assistant drips sterile saline into the ends of the circuit tubing and the catheter to ensure that all residual air is eliminated prior to connection.
   a. Do not squeeze the tubing while attaching; air will enter when the tubing is released.
   b. If air is seen in the tubing, the catheters must be disconnected from the circuit. Prior to reconnection, air is removed, and the catheters are reconnected as described above.

2. Remove all sterile tubing clamps from the catheters and have a nonsterile assistant hold the catheters.

   Nonsterile tubing clamps remain in place on the arterial and venous sides of the circuit at this juncture.

3. Place the patient on ECMO by removing the arterial clamp, placing a clamp on the bridge, and removing the venous clamp.

   This will remove all nonsterile clamps from the circuit.

4. Increase ECMO flow in 50-ml increments over 20 minutes, until adequate oxygenation is achieved (usually at 120 ml/kg/min).

   Transfusion may be needed for hypotension.

5. Decrease the ventilator settings and oxygen concentration gradually as the ECMO flows are increased.

   Typical resting ventilator settings are: A rate of 10 to 15 breaths/min, a peak pressure limit of 15 cm H_2O, and $FIO_2 = 0.21$.

Closure of the Neck Wound
1. Ensure x-ray confirmation of appropriate catheter position and the achievement of an adequate flow rate through the ECMO circuit, prior to closure of the neck wound.
2. Cut and remove traction sutures.
3. Approximate the skin with a running 4-0 vicryl suture on an *atraumatic* needle.
4. Tie the vicryl suture, and use the tails of the suture to secure each catheter.
5. Tie catheters together with another silk tie.
6. Anesthetize the area behind the ear with 0.25% xylocaine with epinephrine.
7. Use 2-0 silk suture on a GI needle to place a stitch behind the ear and tie around the catheter to secure in place. Place a separate stitch for each catheter.
8. Tie catheters together, dress the incision with povidine iodine ointment, and cover the area with semipermeable membrane dressing.

9. Tape the circuit tubing securely to the bedside, to reduce traction on the catheters.

F. COMPLICATIONS

1. Torn vessels; more commonly the vein
   a. This risk is decreased if the 6-0 proline stay sutures are always used.
   b. Do not attempt to use too large a catheter.
2. Blood loss, particularly during the venous cannulation, when side-holes in the catheter are outside the vein
3. Venous spasm, resulting in inability to place large enough catheter

   > The rate of blood flow is impeded by the small gauge of the catheter, requiring that a second venus catheter be placed in the femoral vein. The two catheters must be "Y" connected together into the ECMO circuit.

4. Arrhythmias and/or bradycardia can occur, due to stimulation of the vagus nerve.
5. Hypotension, due to an increase in the intravascular space when the patient is connected to the ECMO circuit

Extracorporeal Membrane Oxygenation—Decannulation

A. INDICATIONS

1. Removal from ECMO after lung recovery
2. Removal from ECMO because of a complication such as uncontrolled bleeding or failure of lung recovery

B. CONTRAINDICATIONS

All intensive support is being withdrawn, and permission for autopsy is obtained; it is optimal to remove the catheters during the autopsy.

C. PRECAUTIONS

1. The patient must be paralyzed during the removal of the venous catheter, to avoid an air embolus.
2. The vessels are fragile and may tear. A backup unit of blood should be at the bedside.

3. Delay removing catheter for 24 hours in cases in which there is a high risk for reoccurrence of pulmonary hypertension, e.g., severe congenital diaphragmatic hernia.

D. PERSONNEL, EQUIPMENT, AND MEDICATIONS

Personnel

Same as for cannulation, with the exception of the primer who is not required

Equipment—Sterile

1. Surgical tray with towels and suture as for cannulation
2. Semipermeable transparent dressing
3. Povidine iodine ointment
4. Syringes (1–20 ml) and needles (18–26 gauge)
5. Unit of blood
6. Absorbable gelatin sponge

Nonsterile

Same as for cannulation

Medications

1. Fentanyl (10–15 μg/kg)
2. Vecuronium bromide (0.1 mg/kg $\times$ 2)

   > A short-acting paralyzing agent is used because of the relatively short duration of the procedure. Allowing the infant to breath spontaneously as soon as possible after decannulation will facilitate rapid weaning from ventilator support.

3. Xylocaine 0.25% with epinephrine
4. Topical thrombin
5. Protamine sulfate (1 mg only)

E. TECHNIQUE

Vessel reconstruction is beyond the scope of this chapter.

1. Place the neck in an extended position, using the shoulder roll.
2. Give fentanyl for relaxation, prior to giving vecuronium.

   > Because of the risk of air embolism during the removal of the venous catheter, the infant must not be allowed to breath during decannulation. If

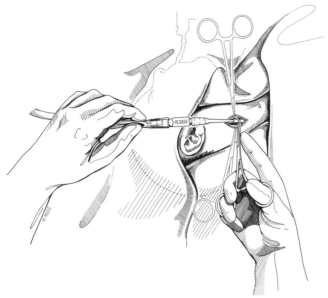

FIG. 31-8
Placement of Satinsky vessel clamp prior to removal of ECMO catheter.

two doses of vecuronium do not produce paralysis, give pancuronium.

3. Clean the neck, and drape as for cannulation.
4. Anesthetize with 0.25% xylocaine with epinephrine.
5. Cut and remove the vicryl suture.
6. Remove absorbable gelatin sponge packing, exposing the catheters and vessels.

   The venous catheter is usually removed first because it is most readily accessible.

7. Separate the catheter from surrounding tissue by blunt dissection.
8. Encircle the vein with a 2-0 silk tie, which is used for traction and hemostatic control.
9. Place a Satinsky clamp around the vein to stabilize the catheter (Fig. 31-8).
10. Place a 2-0 silk tie proximal to the clamp.
11. Cut the silk ties securing the catheter in the vein with a no. 11 scalpel blade.

    The two proximal ties should be cut where they cross the "bootie."

12. Ask the circuit specialists to remove the patient from the ECMO circuit.

13. Monitor vital signs and oxygen saturation as an indication that ventilator settings are appropriate.

    Settings may have to be increased when the patient is removed from the circuit.

14. Supply an inspiratory "hold" on the ventilator while the surgeon places pressure on the liver and removes the catheter.

    Failure to do this can result in air embolus.

15. Replace any significant blood loss.
16. Cut the 2-0 silk traction suture and tie the suture proximal to the Satinsky clamp. Remove the Satinsky clamp.
17. Isolate the arterial catheter, dissect free and remove.

    The procedure is the same as for the venous catheter, with the exception that an inspiratory hold is not required.

18. Give protamine after removal of both catheters.

    Administration of protamine is not mandatory if there is no significant bleeding.

19. Irrigate the wound with sterile saline and cauterize any bleeding sites.
20. Pack the wound with thrombin-soaked absorbable gelatin sponge and close the neck incision using subcuticular horizontal sutures of 4-0 vicryl.
21. Remove the sutures holding the cannula behind the right ear.
22. Place povidine iodine ointment over the incision and cover with semipermeable transparent dressing.

F. COMPLICATIONS

1. Vessel laceration, which may require a sternotomy for correction
2. Blood loss
3. Air embolus

References

1. STOLAR CJH, SNEDECOR SM, BARTLETT RH: Extracorporeal membrane oxygenation and neonatal respiratory failure: Experience from the extracorporeal life support organization. J Pediatr Surg 26:563, 1991

2. Beck R, Anderson KD, Pearson GD, et al: Criteria for extracorporeal membrane oxygenation in a population of infants with persistent pulmonary hypertension of the newborn. J Pediatr Surg 21:297, 1986

3. O'Rourke PP, Crone RK, Vacanti JP, et al: Extracorporeal membrane oxygenation and conventional medical therapy in neonates with persistent pulmonary hypertension of the newborn: A prospective randomized study. Pediatrics 84:957, 1989

4. Allison PL, Kurusz M, Graves DF, Zwischenberger JB: Devices and monitoring during neonatal ECMO: Survey results. Perfusion 5:193, 1990

5. VanMeurs KP, Mikesell GT, Seale WR, et al: Maximum blood flow rates for arterial cannulae used in neonatal ECMO. ASAIO Trans 36:M679, 1990

Part 6
Respiratory Care

32 Tracheal Intubation

Mary Ann Fletcher

Oral and Nasal Routes

A. INDICATIONS

1. Provide airway for mechanical respiratory support.
2. Relieve critical upper-airway obstruction (see Color Fig. 32-1).
3. Provide route for selective bronchial ventilation.
4. Provide route for direct tracheal suctioning.
5. Assist in bronchial hygiene when secretions cannot be cleared otherwise.

B. CONTRAINDICATIONS

None absolute

> In older patients the presence of cervical injuries is a contraindication to intubation with a laryngoscope, but because the occurrence of cervical injuries is infrequent in neonates and the performance of an emergency tracheotomy is particularly treacherous, we would consider intubation the less risky procedure.

C. EQUIPMENT

1. Humidified oxygen/air source, blender, and analyzer
2. Bag and mask for ventilation
3. Suction apparatus
4. Cardiorespiratory monitor
5. Oxygenation monitor: transcutaneous oxygen or oxygen saturation
6. Stethoscope
7. Gloves
8. Scissors
9. Endotracheal (ET) tube
   a. Magill tube (single end-hole), or
   b. Murphy tube (side-hole contralateral to direction of bevel)
   c. Flexible, soft tube
   d. Nonirritating material

   e. Nontapered shape without shoulder[1]
   f. Radiopaque marking for radiographic localization
   g. Diameter selected for infant size (Table 32-1)
   h. Length selected for infant's size[2-4]: normal tracheal length is 2.5 to 5 cm in infants from 0.6 to 5 kg.[5]

Because of short tracheas in neonates, there is little leeway between a tube that is too short (increased risk for extubation) or too long (increased risk for mainstem intubation or airway trauma). The appropriate length for an ET tube depends on a number of factors, including an infant's size and airway anatomy as well as whatever fixation devices are used. To resist putting an orotracheal tube in too far, a "rule of 1,2,3/7,8,9" for lip-to-lip distance is helpful.[4] For babies weighing 1 kg, the distance from lip to a safe location for the tip of ET tube is approximately 7 cm; 2 kg, 8 cm; more than 3 kg, 9 cm. For nasotracheal intubation the rule can be modified to 1,2,3/8,10,12.[6] When there is marked micrognathia or a syndrome associated with shortened trachea, the safe length is less.

It is rarely necessary to insert a tube more than 1 to 2 cm below the vocal cords, regardless of infant size. The exceptions will be when the presence of anatomic defects dictates a bypass such as a tracheal fistula or subglottic obstruction or when selective bronchial intubation is intended.

TABLE 32-1

ET Tube Diameter for Patient Weight

Weight	Tube Size
<1250 gm	2.5
1250–3000 gm	3.0
>3000 gm	3.5

10. ET tube adaptor

Several modifications of adaptors are available for use. When frequent suctioning, bronchoscopy, or installation of medications through the ET tube is anticipated, it may be helpful to replace a standard adaptor with one modified to allow entry into the tube without disconnecting it from positive pressure ventilation.

11. Stiffener (optional)
  a. Sterile stylet
    (1) Flexible and biocompatible
    (2) No detachable parts
    (3) Secured not to extend beyond bevel and side-hole of tube
  b. Ice to harden tube within its sterile container for use without stylet

12. Magill forceps (optional for nasotracheal intubation)

13. Pediatric laryngoscope with straight blade
  a. Miller blade no. 0 for babies less than 3 kg
  b. Miller blade no. 1 for babies more than 3 kg
  c. Modified blade to allow continuous flow of oxygen of 1 to 2 L/min for better maintenance of oxygenation during procedure[7]

14. Compound of benzoin tincture and cotton-tipped applicators

15. Adhesive tape: 8- to 10-cm lengths of ½ inch width tape with half the length split and one 10- to 15-cm length unsplit.

D. PRECAUTIONS (TABLE 32-2)

1. Select orotracheal route for all emergency intubations or when a bleeding diathesis is present. Reserve nasotracheal intubation for elective procedures after stabilization with orotracheal tube unless oral anatomy precludes oral intubation.

2. Prepare all equipment before starting procedure. Keep equipment ready at bedside of patients likely to require intubation.

3. Use tubes appropriately sized to minimize both trauma and airway resistance.[1]

4. Interrupt an unsuccessful attempt before compromising patient.
  a. Ventilate by bag and mask.
  b. Allow recovery between attempts.
  c. Prevent traumatic complications caused by undue haste.

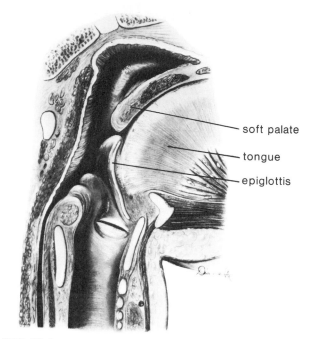

FIG. 32-1
Anatomical view of neonatal larynx. The glottis sits very close to the base of the tongue so that visualization is easiest without extending the neck.

5. Recognize anatomic differences in neonatal upper airway (Fig. 32-1).

6. Ensure visualization of larynx. This is the most important part of intubation (see Color Fig. 32-2).
  a. Have assistant maintain proper position of patient.
  b. Avoid hyperextending or rotating neck.

7. Do not use pressure or force that predisposes to trauma.
  a. Avoid using maxilla as fulcrum for laryngoscope blade.
  b. Avoid excessive external tracheal pressure.
  c. Avoid pushing tube against any obstruction.

8. Make certain all attachments are secure.
  a. Avoid obscuring the point of connection of tube and adapter with any fixation device.
  b. Secure tube carefully in position to avoid dislodgement, kinking, or movement.
    (1) Vary contact point from side to side to prevent damage to developing palate and palatal ridges.[8–10]
    (2) Note relationship of head position to in-

TABLE 32-2

Trouble-shooting Problems with Intubation

Problem	Suggested Approach for Solution
Infant's tongue gets in the way	When opening mouth, push tongue aside with finger before inserting blade.
	Keep laryngoscope blade midline or just off center away from passage for ET tube.
Copious scretion prevents visualization.	Suction prior to attempt.
	Place suction catheter in oropharynx through left side of mouth and have assistant apply suction.
Tube seems too big to fit through vocal cords.	Verify correct size for ideal patient weight.
	Decrease angle of neck extension.
	Apply traction rather than leverage to blade.
	Select next smaller size.
	Evaluate for stenosis of airway.
Vocal cords are closed.	Await spontaneous breath.
	Apply gentle pressure over suprasternal area.
	Give succinylcholine (2 mg/kg); ventilate.
Unsure of appropriate depth for insertion	Insert tube only just past vocal cords.
	Determine length of ET tube at lip (1,2,3/7,8,9 for oral tube).
	Obtain radiograph with head in neutral position and document position relative to carina and to thoracic inlet.
Hard to ventilate through tube after insertion	Verify that tube is intratracheal.
	Verify that tube is not in bronchus.
	Consider tube or airway obstruction.
Rapid appearance of swelling and crepitance over neck and anterior chest	Remove tube and evaluate for tracheal perforation.
Return of blood via ET tube in absence of lung disease	Remove tube and evaluate for perforation or trauma.
Tube slips into bronchus.	Avoid neck extension.
	Keep tape secure.
	Maintain appropriate lip-to-tip distance.
Unplanned extubation	Regularly verify correct lip-to-tip distance.
	Keep tape secure and replace as often as necessary.
	Support neck whenever moving infant.
	Avoid neck flexion or traction on tube.
	Secure hands of infant.

tratracheal depth of tube on radiograph.[2,11,12]

9. Avoid leaving ET tube unattached without some form of continuous positive airway pressure to replace the natural expiratory resistance lost in bypassing upper airway.

10. Recognize that in neonates ET tubes are more often pushed in too far because of the short distance from the glottis to the carina. Use a standardized graph or location device.[2]

   a. Illuminated tube[13]

   b. Magnetic field interference-sensing technique[14]

   c. Lighted stylet[15]

We do not recommend the technique of intentionally inserting the tube until there are no breath sounds on one side and then withdrawing until they are heard.[16] Breath sounds may be heard on both sides even though the tube is in a mainstem bronchus because a side-hole may ventilate the contralateral side. Additionally, a small chest makes side distinction difficult as sounds are well transmitted.

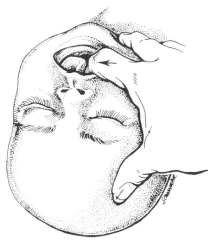

11. Recognize the association of short trachea (<15 tracheal cartilage rings) with certain syndromes: DiGeorge anolmaly, skeletal dysplasias, brevicollis, congenital rubella syndrome, interrupted aortic arch, and other congenital syndromes involving the tracheal area.[17]

12. Identify and direct prevention at factors that are most likely to contribute to spontaneous extubation.[18]
    a. Increased secretions
       (1) Necessitating more frequent suctioning
       (2) Loosening of tape
    b. Infant activity
    c. Procedures requiring repositioning infant
    d. Tube slippage

E. TECHNIQUE

Orotracheal Intubation (see Table 32-2)

1. Maintain a relaxed body posture.
   a. Sit at patient's head or
   b. Elevate bed to eye level.
2. Put on gloves.
3. With a small roll supporting the shoulders, extend infant's neck slightly, pulling chin into a "sniff" position (Fig. 32-2).
4. Clear oropharynx with gentle suctioning.
5. Empty stomach.
6. Ventilate and preoxygenate infant as indicated by clinical condition. Follow heart rate and oxygenation.

FIG. 32-3
Open the mouth and push the tongue aside with the forefinger while stabilizing the head with the thumb and other fingers of the right hand.

7. Hold handle of laryngoscope in left hand with thumb and first two fingers (Fig. 32-3).
   a. Put thumb over flat end of laryngoscope blade.
   b. Stabilize hand with remaining fingers resting on patient's cheek.
8. Open infant's mouth and depress tongue toward the left with the back of right forefinger.
   a. Steady head with rest of right hand.
   b. Avoid using blade to open mouth (Fig. 32-3).
9. While visualizing, insert laryngoscope blade in the midline until its tip is between base of tongue and epiglottis within the vallecula (Fig. 32-4). Keep laryngoscope midline or to the left side of mouth.
10. Apply traction to the laryngoscope to open mouth further and simultaneously tilt blade tip slightly to elevate epiglottis. Visualize glottis.

    It is important to use more traction than leverage on the laryngoscope blade and to use base of tongue as the pivot point, rather than maxilla (Fig. 32-5).

11. Suction if necessary.
12. Have an assistant apply gentle pressure at the suprasternal notch to open the larynx and to feel the tube pass.[19]
13. Hold tube with concave curve anterior, and pass it down right side of mouth, outside the blade, while maintaining visualization (Fig. 32-6).

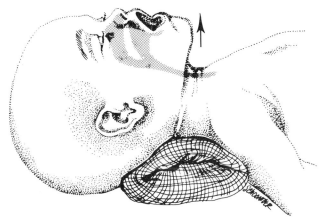

FIG. 32-2
Appropriate sniff position for intubation. Note that the neck is not hyperextended; the roll provides stabilizing support.

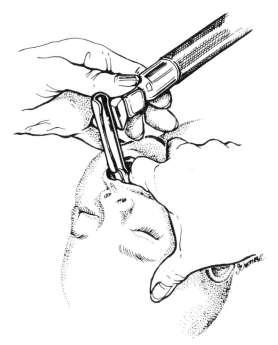

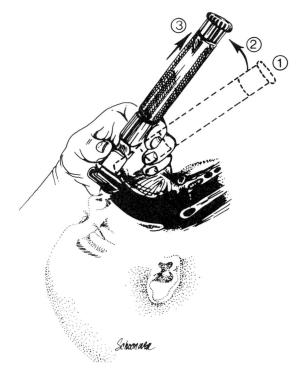

FIG. 32-4
Pass the laryngoscope carefully along the finger to the back of the oropharynx.

FIG. 32-5
With the laryngoscope at the proper depth, tilt the blade with the tongue as the fulcrum; at the same time, pull on the laryngoscope handle to move the tongue without extending the infant's neck. Use more traction than leverage.

FIG. 32-6
Visualize the glottis and pass the ET tube into the oropharynx. Keep the tube outside the curve of the laryngoscope blade for better mobility.

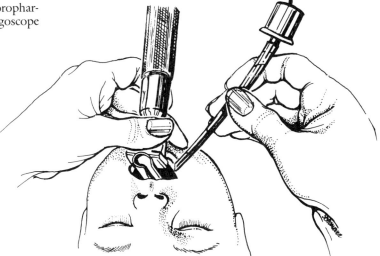

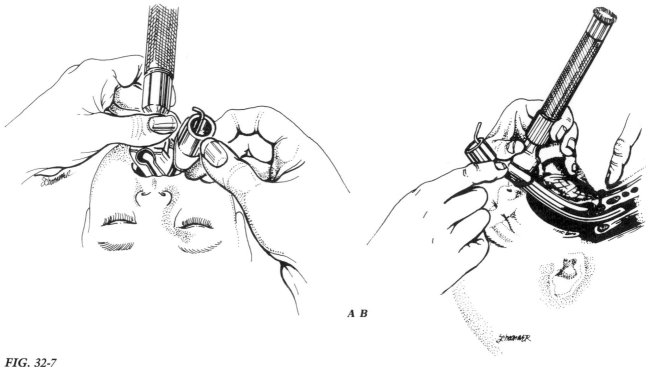

A B

FIG. 32-7
(*A*) Pass the ET tube through the glottis to the appropriately predetermined length and remove laryngoscope. (*B*) An assistant applies gentle pressure in the suprasternal notch to open the larynx and to detect when the tube passes into the trachea.

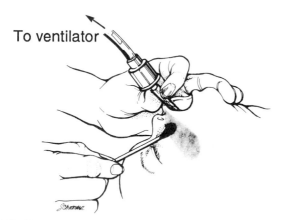

FIG. 32-8
After initially determining that the ET tube is in correct position, connect the ET tube to an artificial ventilation source. Begin fixation of the tube by painting the philtrum with tincture of benzoin and allowing it to dry.

14. As infant inhales, pass tube through cords 2 cm into trachea or just until tip is felt passing the suprasternal notch (Fig. 32-7).
15. If tube appears too large or does not pass easily
    a. Decrease angle of neck extension
    b. Apply gentle external pressure over the larynx.
    c. Wait for a spontaneous inspiration to open the cords.
16. Confirm position of tube within trachea.
    a. Auscultate for equality of breath sounds and observe chest movement.
    b. Observe respiratory wave pattern on oscilloscope to determine that artificial breath is at least as large as spontaneous breath.
    c. Verify proper lip-to-tip distance.
17. Suction ET tube with sterile catheter, following technique described in Chapter 34, Respiratory Physical Therapy, Tracheal Suctioning.
18. Attach appropriate mechanical device.
19. Readjust FIO_2 as per infant's requirements.
20. Fix tube (Figs. 32-8, 32-9).

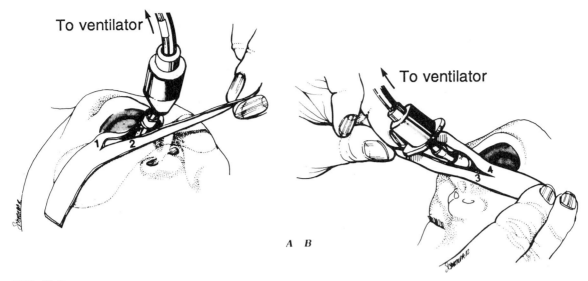

FIG. 32-9
Fixation of tube with half split tape. (*A*) First half of one split tape (*1*) encircles the tube and the other half (*2*) attaches to the upper lip. (*B*) Second split half (*3*) attaches to the upper lip while the bottom half (*4*) encircles the tube.

21. Obtain radiograph with tube in neutral position and note the lip-to-tip distance and direction of bevel (Figs. 32-10, 32-11).

> In most instances when a good tube length has been determined for any infant, reintubations at the previously established lip-to-tip length will not require radiographic confirmation unless the clinical condition warrants.

22. Cut off excess tube length to leave 2 to 4 cm outside the mouth and reattach adapter firmly.

> If a longer external length is needed, before replacing the adaptor, slip a short length of a larger ET tube around the narrower tube to prevent its kinking, i.e., a 6-cm length of 3.5 tube over a 2.5 tube.

23. Confirm lip-to-tip distance regularly.
24. Retape tube as necessary to maintain stability.

Nasotracheal Intubation

Because it is easier, most neonatologists prefer orotracheal intubation, because there are few proven advantages to nasal intubations in very small infants.[20,21] Nasotracheal tubes are helpful when a large infant is very active or has oral secretions too copious to keep tube taped in position. When anatomy precludes oral intubation or for oral surgery, nasotracheal intubation is necessary.

Premedication with succinylcholine and atropine seems to lead to shorter times for intubation with fewer negative systemic effects.[22]

1. Use sterile tube cooled in ice. If stylet is used to curve tube while it is cooling, remove it prior to nasal insertion.
2. Premedicate with atropine (20 μg/kg) and succinylcholine (2 mg/kg) just before inserting tube. Be prepared to provide assisted ventilation by bag and mask.
3. If present, maintain orotracheal tube in position at far left of the mouth, allowing continued ventilation during nasotracheal intubation. Release fixation but keep its position secure.
4. Visualize oropharynx with laryngoscope as described in previous section, taking particular care not to hyperextend neck.
5. Suction oropharynx, keeping laryngoscope in place.
6. Insert cooled tube through nostril, following natural curve of nasopharynx.
7. As tube passes into the pharynx, align the tip with

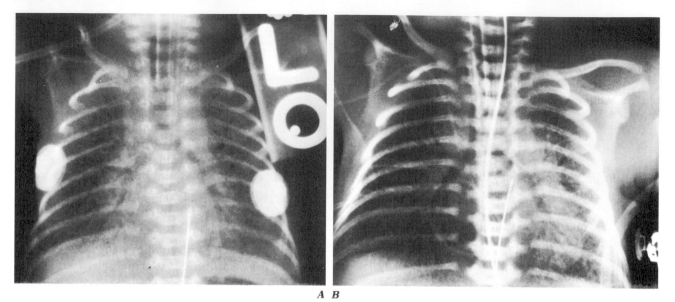

A B

FIG. 32-10
Although the carina is usually at the level of T4 on the AP supine chest radiograph, this relationship may be significantly disturbed by a number of factors, including radiographic technique (x-ray-tube position, angulation). For this reason and because the carina is usually easily visualized, as in these cases, one should directly relate the tip of the ET tube to the carina radiographically, knowing the position of the head at the time of film exposure. In both cases films were taken to verify ET tube position but demonstrated problems with other procedures. (*A*) Appropriate radiographic angle. (Note the oral gastric tube in the esophagus and not reaching the stomach.) (*B*) Slightly lordotic radiographic angle. (Note the central venous line coiled in the heart.)

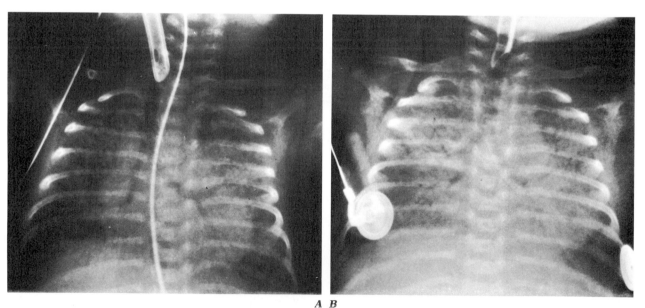

A B

FIG. 32-11
Sequential radiographs demonstrate the effect of head rotation on bevel direction. (*A*) With the head rotated to the right, the bevel appears to be directed against the tracheal wall. (*B*) The head is rotated to the left, and the bevel is now positioned properly. If the bevel is directed against the posterior tracheal wall in a spontaneously breathing infant, there may be symptoms of tracheal obstruction on expiration. Rather than turning the head to achieve satisfactory position, rotate the ET tube and retape in position.

the center of the tracheal orifice, moving infant's head as needed.

8. When tip of nasotracheal tube appears to be in direct line with glottis, have assistant carefully withdraw orotracheal tube.

9. Apply gentle pressure over suprasternal notch and advance tube through cords.

   Use of the Magill forceps is often more cumbersome than helpful in smaller infants. A Magill forceps should always be available but, in a properly positioned infant, a curved tube usually passes directly into the trachea without forceps unless the neck is too extended, flexed, or rotated.

10. Secure tube and verify position. The length of a nasotracheal tube will be about 2 cm longer than the suitable length of an orotracheal tube.

There are a number of fiberoptic devices available for use in small infants to assist in difficult nasal or oral intubations[23]

1. Fiberoptic bronchoscope (see Chap. 35, Flexible Fiberoptic Bronchoscopy) assists in determining correct tube location because intratracheal position of tip can be directly visualized.

2. Optical stylet put into place with the ET passed over it into the larynx; manipulation of rigid tube is more difficult but the resolution is high as long as secretions can be kept clear.

3. Bullard laryngoscope with fiberoptic viewing and integral forceps for manipulation of the tube is particularly useful for infants with marked microagnathia as it requires a minimal opening of 4 mm.

Elective Change of Orotracheal Tube in Intubated Patient

This procedure allows continued ventilation through a pre-established airway whenever it is necessary to change an ET tube or to place a nasotracheal tube. By maintaining the original airway as long as possible during the change, there is less need for haste and less stress to the patient. An obvious prerequisite is that the original ET tube be patent and correctly positioned in the trachea.

Rapid Replacement Method

1. Prepare equipment and patient as for initial orotracheal intubation.

2. Release tube fixation device without displacing tube.

3. Have assistant hold first ET tube in place at far left of the infant's mouth while continuing to ventilate infant.

4. Visualize glottis with laryngoscope.

5. Pass second orotracheal tube down far right of the mouth until it aligns with glottic opening.

6. When new tube is positioned for direct insertion, have assistant withdraw first tube carefully.

7. Advance new tube into position.

8. Verify position and secure tube as previously described.

Alternate Method: Insertion Over a Feeding Tube

Because of the narrow diameter of ET tubes in small infants, feeding tubes narrow enough to fit inside the ET lumen are often too flexible to stay within the trachea as the tubes are being changed. Be prepared to intubate directly should the feeding tube dislodge.

1. Prepare equipment and patient as for initial orotracheal intubation.

2. Release tube fixation device without displacing tube.

3. Select the largest feeding tube that will easily go through the current and new endotracheal tubes. Remove the flared end of feeding tube and the adaptor on the new tube.

4. Remove adaptor of currently in-place ET tube.

5. Quickly insert the feeding tube through the lumen to a depth not greater than the ET tube.

6. While holding feeding tube in place, pull ET tube out of trachea and off feeding tube.

7. Slide new ET tube over feeding tube into trachea.

8. Replace tube adaptor.

9. Verify position and secure tube as previously described.

Selective Left Endobronchial Intubation

The angles of the bronchi are such that more often than not a tube will seek the right mainstem bronchus. The exceptions will be conditions that push the left side down (left upper lobe emphysema) or that pull the right side up (marked upper lobe atelectasis or hypoplasia). Normally, successful right mainstem intubation simply requires a longer tube. Selective intubation of the left bronchus is a more difficult and dangerous procedure; therefore, following all precautions is especially important.

Place the ET tube under guidance by direct bronchoscopy or under fluoroscopy when these procedures are available without compromise to infant[24,25] (see Chap. 35).

The following procedure is a simple, indirect method based on a modification that tends to make the ET tube bend toward the left when it meets resistance at the carina.[26]

1. Cut an elliptical hole through half the diameter of ET tube 1 cm in length and 0.5 cm above the tip of the oblique distal end.
2. Perform an orotracheal intubation as above, keeping the cut hole directed toward the left lung.
3. Turn infant's head toward the right.[27]
4. While auscultating the lung fields, advance the tube to 0.5 to 1 cm below the calculated depth of the carina or until differential breath sounds are heard.
5. If breath sounds diminish on the left, withdraw the ET tube until they return.
6. Take a chest film to confirm left bronchial position.
7. Fix tube securely.
8. Reassess position frequently as tube may dislodge from one mainstem into the other.
9. Follow patient closely for particular complications of
   a. Air leak of ventilated area
   b. Stasis pneumonia of nonventilated area
   c. Dislodgement from left mainstem bronchus
   d. Ventilatory insufficiency due to significant disease in the only lung being ventilated

Nonvisualized Oral Intubation

This technique has a higher risk of complications and is less often successful than when direct visualization is used. Reserve the blind oral intubation for true emergencies in small infants when there is equipment failure (e.g., laryngoscope light) and when ventilation by mask is contraindicated (e.g., thick meconium).

1. Stand at infant's feet.
2. Carefully slide first two fingers of gloved, left hand into back of oropharynx at the base of tongue, until reaching vallecula and epiglottis. Keep fingers in the center of the tongue.
3. Using index finger, pull epiglottis forward.
4. Keep infant's head in midline.
5. With right hand, guide ET tube, without stylet, along left middle finger, which is held just above index finger.

6. Advance tube carefully just beyond fingertips.
7. Avoid pushing against any obstruction.
8. If available, have assistant press gently on trachea in suprasternal notch and report when tube passes under finger.
9. Verify position, and fix tube as previously described.

Blind Nasotracheal Intubation[28]

Blind nasotracheal intubation is often used in adults. Because a stiff tube is needed, the chance of perforation in infants is greater if a stylet is used. While an intubation under direct visualization is preferred, the presence of severe microagnathia or oral masses makes this approach valuable. It is critical not to push against any resistance.

1. Keep infant supine with neck flexed and shoulders supported by a small roll.
2. Shape a stylet so the tip of the endotracheal tube will curve anteriorly at 90 degrees. Be certain the tip of the stylet stays above the end of the ET tube. Alternately, freeze an ET tube in this configuration and remove stylet just prior to insertion.
3. Maintaining the curve in the tube anterior, insert the tube carefully through the nostril until its tip is in the oropharynx.
4. Pull the jaw forward into a sniff position with the head midline and put slight external pressure over the cricoid cartilage.
5. Advance the tube to a suitable depth unless there is any resistance.
6. Remove stylet and verify presence of exhaled humidity and equal breath sounds.

Intubation in Severe Cleft Defects

There are several possible modifications for ET tubes useful for fixation or elective intubation when there is a large cleft palate. For emergency intubations, the following modification using a standard tongue blade is usually immediately available.[29] For techniques on difficult intubation alternatives, see above.[23]

1. Open infant's mouth and lay sterile tongue blade flat across maxilla, with ends extending from corners of mouth. Have assistant hold in place.
2. Follow steps for routine intubation, using tongue blade for support of laryngoscope as necessary.
3. After intubation, fix tube to padded tongue blade.
4. Recognize that tongue thrust on tube in absence of a

normal palate may lead to extubation even without visible external lengthening of tube.

Emergency Retrograde Intubation[30]

When facial anomalies preclude other routes, retrograde intubation using a modified Seldinger technique is possible. Because the cartilaginous support of the trachea is so poor, needle puncture is far more difficult in neonates (see Chap. 33, Tracheotomy)

Equipment

1. Venous cannula with stylet, 14 or 16 gauge
2. Feeding catheter. Verify that the catheter will pass through the lumen of the angiocath.
   a. 14-gauge cannula will admit a 5 Fr feeding tube
   b. 16-gauge cannula will admit a 3.5 Fr feeding tube
3. Hemostat
4. Endotracheal tube

Technique

1. Sedate infant if possible.
2. Clean skin over cricothyroid area
3. At the level of the cricothyroid, puncture skin with cannula and stylet. Angle cannula at 45 degrees from the skin and directed toward the head.
4. Insert into lumen or trachea only until there is a give in resistance or air returns.
5. Remove the stylet.
6. Thread feeding tube through the lumen of the cannula until it can be retrieved from the nose or oropharynx.
7. Bring cephalic end of feeding tube out of the nose or mouth leaving other end well outside skin insertion.
8. While feeding tube is in place, remove the cannula from the tracheal insertion site.
9. Clamp the feeding tube at its tracheal insertion so it will not be pulled into the trachea further than desired.
10. At the upper end, slip the ET tube over the feeding tube and along its course until it has passed the proper distance into the trachea. Stabilize the ET tube.
11. Cut the feeding tube at its tracheal insertion.
12. While keeping the ET tube in place, pull the feeding tube through the ET tube.
13. Secure ET tube after verifying correct intratracheal position.

F. FIXATION TECHNIQUES

There have been many fixation devices and techniques described in the literature. None of them can prevent all accidental extubations or malpositions. We describe a simple and effective method here.[31]

1. Taping with tube sutured to elastoplast[32]
2. Drilled umbilical clamp[33]
3. Intraoral dental appliance[34]
4. Logan bow and moleskin
5. Double stick electrode disc and tape[35]

The location of the tip of an ET tube depends on the position and motion of the head and neck in addition to tube length and stability.[11,36] While paying careful attention to tube fixation, one should recognize the ease of displacement and be prepared to diagnose and correct it. One of the best means of preventing accidental extubations is by simply being aware of the depth of the tube at the level of the lips. Periodically checking this depth and repositioning with retaping as needed prevents most malpositions. Good head support and hand restraints prevent many others.

1. Prepare two 8- to 10-cm lengths of adhesive tape split half of the length and one 10- to 15-cm length without a split.
2. Paint skin adjacent to the sides of the mouth and above the lips with tincture of benzoin (Fig. 32-8).
3. Paint the endotracheal tube as it exits 1 cm outside the lips.
4. Allow to dry while holding the tube in place.
5. Tape the unsplit end of adhesive to the cheek on one side of the mouth and wrap the bottom half clockwise around the endotracheal tube just at the lip. Fold the last 2-mm end of tape on itself to leave a tab for easier removal (Fig. 32-9).
6. Secure the other half above the upper lip.
7. Repeat the procedure from the other side, reversing the direction of the taping and securing half on that side of the upper lip (Fig. 32-9).
8. Secure one end of the long tape to one cheek at the zygoma. Loop the tape around the tube and secure

the other end to a similar point on the opposite cheek.

9. Note the markings on the ET tube at the level of the lips and the tape.
10. Whenever the tape seems to be loosened from secretions, remove tape and repeat application of benzoin while holding tube at proper lip-to-tip depth.

G. PLANNED EXTUBATION

Various vasoconstrictors and anti-inflammatory medications have been recommended to reduce postextubation stridor and to improve the success of extubation. Systemically administered dexamethasone appears to have no effect in reducing acute post extubation stridor in neonates.[37] Local application of steroids directly to the vocal cords has not been well studied.

1. Perform prescribed chest physiotherapy and suctioning prior to extubation.
2. Release all fixation devices while holding tube in place.
3. Using manual ventilation, give infant a sighing inspiration, and withdrawn tube during the following exhalation.
4. Avoid suctioning during tube withdrawal, unless specifically removing foreign material from trachea.
5. Allow recovery time before suctioning oropharynx.
6. Keep the inspired gases well humidified.

> For infants intubated longer than 48 hours, we recommend the use of continuous distending airway pressure by nasal prongs until there is the return of a good cry, and therefore, good cord mobility as an assistance to successful extubation.

H. COMPLICATIONS

1. Acute trauma
   a. Tracheal or hypopharyngeal perforation[38–41]
   b. Pseudodiverticulum[42,43]
   c. Hemorrhage
   d. Laryngeal edema
   e. Mucosal necrosis[44,45] (See Color Fig. 32-3 at beginning of this book.)
   f. Injury to vocal cord
   g. Dislocation of arytenoid[46]
2. Chronic trauma[47,48]
   a. Cricoid ulceration and fibrosis

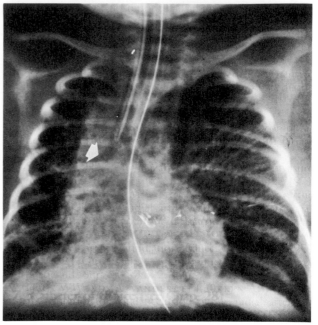

FIG. 32-12
Radiographic magnification hi-KV film (2×) demonstrating an abrupt cutoff of the right bronchus intermedius (*arrow*) due to an endobronchial granuloma with secondary volume loss at the right lung base. Although these granulomas may be due to endotracheal tube trauma, in this area they are more likely related to suction-tube injury. The ET tube is just entering the right bronchus.

   b. Stenosis of glottic or subglottic larynx or of trachea[49–53] (See Color Fig. 32-3.)
   c. Subglottic granuloma[54,55] (See Fig. 32-12 and Color Fig. 32-4 at beginning of this book)
   d. Hoarseness, stridor, wheezing
   e. Subglottic cyst[56]
   f. Tracheomegaly[57]
   g. Protrusion of laryngeal ventricle[58]
3. Interference by oral tube with oral development[8,59]
   a. Alveolar grooving
   b. Palatal grooves[60] (Fig. 32-13)
   c. Posterior cross-bites
   d. Defective dentition[10]
      (1) Enamel hypoplasia[61]
      (2) Incisor hypoplasia[62]
   e. Poor speech intelligibility

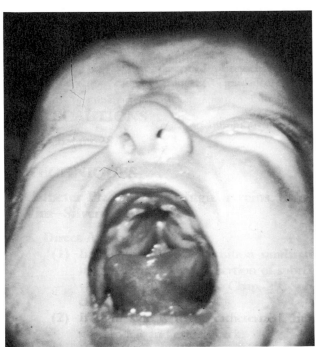

FIG. 32-13
Palatal groove after prolonged oral intubation. Such grooves may be seen after prolonged use of ET or oral gastric tubes when the normal forces of the tongue are prevented from assisting palatal development.

4. Local effects from nasal tube[63,64]
   a. Erosion of nasal septum[65]
   b. Stenosis of nasal vestibule[66] (Fig. 32-14)
   c. Nasal congestion
   d. Midfacial hypoplasia[67]
   e. Otitis media[68]
5. Systemic side-effects[69,70]
   a. Infection[71,72]
   b. Aspiration[73,74]
   c. Increased intracranial pressure[75,76]
   d. Hypoxemia
   e. Hypertension
   f. Apnea
   g. Bradycardia and cardiac arrest
6. Misplacements into esophagus or bronchus (Figs. 32-15 to 32-17)
   a. Atelectasis
   b. Pulmonary air leak
   c. Loss of tube into esophagus[77–79]
   d. Across tracheoesophageal fistula[80]
7. Displacement, accidental extubation[81]
8. Obstruction[82]
9. Kinking, proximally or distally[83]

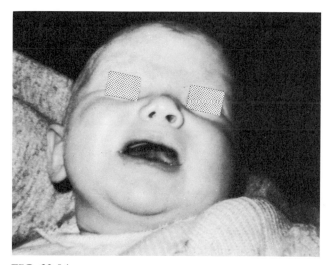

FIG. 32-14
Nasal stenosis due to nasal cartilage necrosis following an indwelling nasotracheal tube.

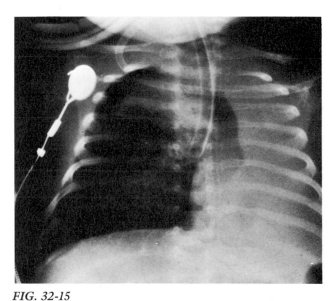

FIG. 32-15
Radiograph demonstrating an ET tube malpositioned in the bronchus intermedius, with resulting atelectasis of the right upper lobe and of the left lung. There is marked overaeration of the right middle and lower lobes but no pneumothorax as yet.

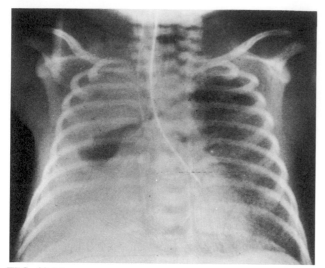

10. Unrecognized disconnection from adapter or pressure source
11. Rupture of ET tube[84]
12. Foreign body from stylet left unrecognized in airway
13. Swallowed laryngoscope light[85]
14. Post-extubation atelectasis[86]
15. Increased airway resistance increasing work of breathing.[87,88]

FIG. 32-16
Relatively uncommon malposition of an ET tube in the left bronchus with atelectasis of much of the right lung.

FIG. 32-17
(*A*) Radiograph suggesting that the endotracheal tube is in the right mainstem bronchus. Note the gaseous distension of the stomach and intestine. The wavy tube on the right is external. (*B*) In the lateral view, the same ET tube is easily seen to be in the esophagus (arrowheads) posterior to the trachea (arrows).

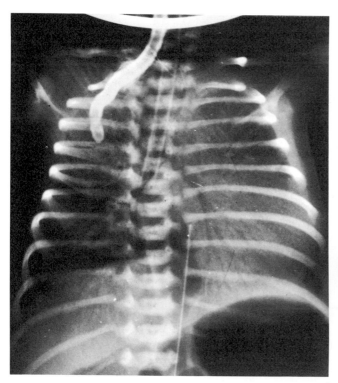

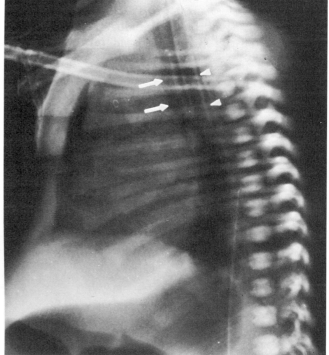

A   B

References

1. HATCH D: Tracheal tubes and connectors used in neonates—dimensions and resistance to breathing. Br J Anaesth 50:959, 1978
2. MATTILA M, HEIKEL P, SUUTARENEN T, LINDORS E: Estimation of a suitable tube length for infants and children. Acta Anaesthesiol Scand 15:239, 1971
3. LOEW A, THIBEAULT D: A new and safe method to control the depth of endotracheal intubation in neonates. Pediatrics 54:506, 1974
4. TOCHEN M: Orotracheal intubation in the newborn infant: A method for determining depth of tube insertion. J Pediatr 95:1050, 1979
5. ROOPCHAND R, ROOPNARINESINGH S, RAMSEWAK S: Instability of the tracheal tube in neonates. Anaesthesia 44:107, 1989
6. KOHELET D, GOLDBERG A, GOLDBERG M: Depth of endotracheal placement in neonates. J Pediatr 101:157, 1982
7. TODRES ID, CRONE RK: Experience with a modified laryngoscope in sick infants. Crit Care Med 9:544, 1981
8. BOICE J, KROUS H, FOLEY J: Gingival and dental complications of orotracheal intubation. JAMA 236:957, 1976
9. BISKINIS E, HERZ M: Acquired palatal groove after prolonged orotracheal intubation. J Pediatr 92:512, 1978
10. MOYLAN F, SELDIN E, SHANNON D, TODRES I: Defective primary dentition in survivors of neonatal mechanical ventilation. J Pediatr 96:106, 1980
11. KUHNS L, POZNANSKI A: Endotracheal tube position in the infant. J Pediatr 78:991, 1971
12. WOODALL D, WHITFIELD J, GRUNSTEIN M: New recommendations for endotracheal tube positioning in the newborn infant (abstr). Pediatr Res 15 (Part 2):733, 1981
13. HELLER RM, COTTON RB: Early experience with illuminated endotracheal tubes in premature and term infants. Pediatr 75:664, 1985
14. BLAYNEY M, COSTELLO S, PERLMAN M, ET AL: A new system for location of endotracheal tube in preterm and term neonates. Pediatrics 87:44, 1991
15. STEWART RD, LAROSEE A, KAPLAN RM, ILKHANIPOUR K: Correct positioning of an endotracheal tube using a flexible lighted stylet. Crit Care Med 18:97, 1990
16. BLOCH EC, OSSEY K, GINSBERG B: Tracheal intubation in children: A new method for assuring correct depth of tube placement. Anesth Analg 67:590, 1988
17. WELLS TR, WELLS AL, GALVIS DA, ET AL: Diagnostic aspects and syndromal associations of short trachea with bronchial intubation. Am J Dis Child 144:1369, 1990
18. LITTLE LA, KOENIG JC, NEWTH CJL: Factors affecting accidental extubations in neonatal and pediatric intensive care patients. Crit Care Med 18:163, 1990
19. BEDNAREK F, KUHNS L: Endotracheal tube placement in infants determined by suprasternal palpation: A new technique. Pediatrics 56:224, 1975
20. MCMILLAN DD, RADEMAKER AW, BUCHAN KA ET AL: Benefits of orotracheal and nasotracheal intubation in neonates requiring ventilatory assistance. Pediatrics 77:39, 1986
21. SPITZER A, FOX W: Post-extubation atelectasis—the role of oral versus nasal endotracheal intubation. J Pediatr 100:806, 1982
22. BARRINGTON KJ, FINER NN, ETCHES PC: Succinylcholine and atropine for premedication of the newborn infant before nasotracheal intubation: A randomized, controlled trial. Crit Care Med 17:1293, 1989
23. STOOL SE: Intubation techniques of the difficult airway. Pediatr Infect Dis J 7:154, 1988
24. GEORGESON K, VAIN N: Intubation of the left main bronchus in the newborn infant: A new technique. J Pediatr 96:920, 1980
25. MATHEW O, THACH B: Selective bronchial obstruction for treatment of bullous interstitial emphysema. J Pediatr 96:475, 1980
26. WEINTRAUB Z, OLIVEN A, WEISSMAN D, SONIS A: A new method for selective left main bronchus intubation in premature infants. J Pediatr Surg 25:604, 1990
27. SIVASUBRAMANIAN K: Technique of selective intubation of the left bronchus in newborn infants. J Pediatr 94:479, 1979
28. WILLIAMSON R: Blind nasal intubation of an apneic neonate. Anesthesiology 69(4):633, 1988
29. ZAWISTOWSKA J, MENZEL M, WYTYCZAK M: Difficulties and modifications of intubation technique in infants with labial, alveolar and palatal clefts. Anaesthesia Resuscitation and Intensive Therapy 1:211, 1973
30. COOPER CM, MURRAY-WILSON A: Retrograde intubation. Management of a 4.8-kg, 5 month infant. Anaesthesia 42:1197, 1987
31. BROWN MS: Prevention of accidental extubation in newborns. Am J Dis Child 142:1240, 1988
32. GREGORY G: Respiratory care of newborn infants. Pediatr Clin North Am 19:311, 1972
33. CUSSEL G, LEVY L, THOMPSON R: A method of securing orotracheal tubes in neonatal respiratory care. Pediatrics 53:266, 1974
34. EHRENBERG A, NOWAK AJ: Appliance for stabilizing orogastric and orotracheal tubes in infants. Crit Care Med 12:669, 1984
35. RICHARDS S: A method for securing pediatric endotracheal tubes. Anesth Analg 60:224, 1981
36. HEINONEN J, TAMMISTO T, TAKKI S: Effect of the Trendelenburg tilt and other procedures on the position of endotracheal tubes. Lancet 1:850, 1969
37. TELLEZ DW, GALVIS AG, STORGION SA, ET AL: Dexamethasone in the prevention of postextubation stridor in children. J Pediatr 118:289, 1991
38. SERLIN S, DAILY W: Tracheal perforation in the neo-

nate: A complication of endotracheal intubation. J Pediatr 85:596, 1975

39. SCHILD J, WUILLOUD A, KOLLBERG H, BOSSI E: Tracheal perforation as a complication of nasotracheal intubation in a neonate. J Pediatr 88:631, 1976

40. FINER N, STEWART A, ULAN O: Tracheal perforation in the neonate: Treatment with a cuffed endotracheal tube. J Pediatr 89:510, 1976

41. MOLLITT DL, SCHULLINGER JN, SANTULLI TV: Selective management of iatrogenic esophageal perforation in the newborn. J Pediatr Srug 16:989, 1981

42. GIRDANY B, SIEBER W, OSMAN M: Traumatic pseudodiverticulums of the pharynx in newborn infants. N Engl J Med 280:237, 1969

43. PRAMANIK, AK, SHARMA S, WOOD BP: Traumatic hypopharyngeal pseudodiverticulum. Am J Dis Child 143:95, 1989

44. JOSHI V, MANDAVIA S, STERN L, WIGLESWORTH F: Acute lesions induced by endotracheal intubation. Occurrence in the upper respiratory tract of newborn infants with respiratory distress syndrome. Am J Dis Child 124:646, 1972

45. FISK G, DEBAKER W: Mucosal changes in the trachea and main bronchi of newborn infants after naso-tracheal intubation. Anaesth Intensive Care 3:209, 1975

46. ROBERTS D, MCQUINN T, BECKERMAN RC: Neonatal arytenoid dislocation. Pediatrics 81:580, 1988

47. FAN LL, FLYNN JW, PATHAK DR: Risk factors predicting laryngeal injury in intubated neonates. Crit Care Med: 11:431, 1983

48. GOULD SJ, HOWARD S: The histopathology of the larynx in the neonate following endotracheal intubation. J Pathol 146:301, 1985

49. COTTON RT: Prevention and management of laryngeal stenosis in infants and children. J Pediatr Surg 20:845, 1985

50. JONES R, BODNAR A, JOHNSON D: Subglottic stenosis in newborn intensive care unit graduates. Am J Dis Child 135:367, 1981

51. PAPSIDERO M, PASHLEY N: Acquired stenosis of the upper airway in neonates. Ann Otol Rhinol Laryngol 89:512, 1980

52. O'NEILL JA: Experience with iatrogenic laryngeal and tracheal stenoses. J Pediatr Surg 19:235, 1984

53. SHERMAN JM, LOWITT S, STEPHENSON C, IRONSON G: Factors influencing acquired subglottic stenosis in infants. J Pediatr 109:322, 1986

54. STRIKER T, STOOL S, DOWNES J: Prolonged nasotracheal intubations in infants and children. Arch Otolaryngol 85:210, 1967

55. GRYLACK LJ, ANDERSON KD: Diagnosis and treatment of traumatic granuloma in tracheobronchial tree of newborn with history of chronic intubation. J Pediatr Surg 19:200, 1984

56. COURIEL J, PHELAN P: Subglottic cysts: A complication of neonatal endotracheal intubation? Pediatrics 68:103, 1981

57. PALMER J, SCHIDLOW D, WOLFSON D, ET AL: Tracheomegaly: A finding in two children who survived prolonged intubation and mechanical ventilation for hyaline membrane disease (abstr). Pediatr Res 13 (Part 2):539, 1979

58. SEID A, MILLET D, COTTON R: Protrusin of the laryngeal ventricle in a pediatric patient following nasotracheal tube intubation. Otolaryngol Head Neck Surg 87:199, 1979

59. ANGELOS GM, SMITH DR, JORGENSON R, SWEENEY EA: Oral complications associated with neonatal oral tracheal intubation: a critical review. Pediatr Dent 11:133, 1989

60. MOLTENI RA, BUMSTEAD DH: Development and severity of palatal grooves in orally intubated newborns: Am J Dis Child 140:357, 1986

61. SEOW WK, HUMPHRYS C, TUDEHOPE DE: Increased prevalence of developmental dental defects in low birth weight, prematurely born children: A controlled study. Pediatr Dent 9:221, 1987

62. KOPRA DE, CREIGHTON PR, BUCKWALD S, ET AL: The oral effects of neonatal intubation. J Dent Res 67:165, 1988

63. BAXTER R, JOHNSON J, GOETZMAN B, HACKEL A: Cosmetic nasal deformities complicating prolonged nasotracheal intubation in critically ill newborn infants. Pediatrics 55:884, 1975

64. GOWDAR K, BULL M, SCHREINER R, LEMONS J, GRESHAM EL: Nasal deformities in neonates. Their occurrence in those treated with nasal continuous positive airway prssure and nasal endotracheal tubes. Am J Dis Child 134:954, 1980

65. PETTETT G, MERENSTEIN G: Nasal erosion with nasotracheal intubation. J Pediatr 87:149, 1975

66. JUNG A, THOMAS G: Stricture of the nasal vestibule: A complication of nasotracheal intubation in newborn infants. J Pediatr 85:412, 1974

67. ROTSCHILD A, DISON PJ, CHITAYAT D, SOLIMANO A: Midfacial hypoplasia associated with long-term intubation for bronchopulmonary dysplasia. Am J Dis Child 144:1302, 1990.

68. HALAC E, INDIVERI DR, OBERGÓN RJ, CASAÑAS M: Complication of nasal endotracheal intubation. J Pediatr 103:166, 1983

69. KELLY MA, FINER NN: Nasotracheal intubation in the neonate: Physiologic responses and effects of atropine and pancuronium. J Pediatr 105:303, 1984

70. MARSHALL TA, DEEDER R, PAI S, ET AL: Physiologic changes associated with endotracheal intubation in preterm infants. Crit Care Med 12:501, 1984

71. DEUTSCHMAN CS, WILTON P, SINOW J, ET AL: Paranasal sinusitis associated wtih nasotracheal intubation: A frequently unrecognized and treatable source of sepsis. Crit Care Med 14:111, 1986

72. HARRIS H, WIRTSCHAFFER D, CASSADY G: Endotraheal intubation and its relationship to bacterial colo-

nization and systemic infection of newborn infants. Pediatrics 58:816, 1976

73. GOITEIN KJ, REIN AJ, GORNSTEIN A: Incidence of aspiration in endotracheally intubated infants and children. Crit Care Med 12:19, 1984

74. BROWNING DH, GRAVES SA: Incidence of aspiration with endotracheal tubes in children. J Pediatr 103:583, 1983

75. FRIESON RH, HONDA AT, THIEME RE: Changes in anterior fontanel pressure in preterm neonates during tracheal intubation. Anesth Analg 66(9):874, 1987.

76. RAJU T, VIDYASAGAR D, TORRES C, ET AL: Intracranial pressure during intubation and anesthesia in infants. J Pediatr 96:860, 1980

77. ABRAHAMS N, GOLDACRE M, REYNOLDS E: Removal of swallowed neonatal endotracheal tube. Lancet ii 2:135, 1970

78. STOOL S, JOHNSON D, ROSENFELD P: Unintentional esophageal intubation in the newborn. Pediatrics 48:299, 1971

79. LABABIDI Z, BLAND H, JAMES E: Retrieval of an endotracheal tube from the esophagus. J Pediatr 93:1025, 1978

80. BUCHINO JJ, KEENAN WJ, PLETSCH JB, ET AL: Malpositioning of the endotracheal tube in infants with tracheoesophageal fistula. J Pediatr 109:524, 1986

81. TODRES ID, DEBROS F, KRAMER SS, ET AL: Endotracheal tube displacement in the newborn infant. J Pediatr 89:126, 1976

82. REDDING GJ, FAN L, COTTON EK, BROOKS JG: Partial obstruction of endotracheal tubes in children: Incidence, etiology and significance. Crit Care Med 7:227, 1979

83. GOTTSCHALK S, SCHUTH C, QUINBY G JR: A complication of tracheal intubation: Distal kinking of the tube. J Pediatr 92:161, 1978

84. SPEAR RM, SAUDER RA, NICHOLS DG: Endotracheal tube rupture, accidental extubation, and tracheal avulsion: Three airway catastrophes associated with significant decrease in peak pressure. Crit Care Med 17:701, 1989

85. NAUMOVSKI L, SCHAFFER K. FLEISHER B: Ingestion of a laryngoscope light bulb during delivery room resuscitation. Pediatrics 87:581, 1991

86. WYMAN ML, KUHNS LR: Lobar opacification of the lung after tracheal extubation in neonates. J Pediatr 91:109, 1977

87. LESOUEF PN, ENGLAND SJ, BRYAN AC: Total resistance of the respiratory system in preterm infants with and without endotracheal tube. J Pediatr 104:18, 1984

88. PÉREZ FONTÁN JJ, HELDT GP, GREGORY GA: Resistance and inertia of endotracheal tubes used in infants during periodic flow. Crit Care Med 13:1052, 1985

33 *Tracheotomy*

Kenneth M. Grundfast
Mary Ann Fletcher

A. INDICATIONS

1. Upper airway obstruction when endotracheal (ET) tube is inappropriate or impossible (see Chap. 32)
   a. Laryngeal stenosis
   b. Congenital anomalies of pharynx or larynx (e.g., hemangioma, macroglossia, web, cyst, vascular ring, tracheal hypoplasia)
   c. Bilateral vocal cord paralysis[1]
2. Anticipation of prolonged need for artificial airway
   a. Anatomic anomaly surgically irreparable
   b. Repeatedly failed extubation despite appropriate medical therapy

   There may be a role for a cricoid split procedure rather than tracheotomy in selected patients who fail extubation after maximal medical therapy.[2-4]

   c. Unalterable abnormality of central ventilatory drive
   d. Permanent paralysis of diaphragm
   e. Prolonged requirement for assisted ventilation

   There is no critical duration for neonates after which an ET tube should be switched to a tracheostomy. Because complications from tracheotomy are so frequent in neonates, prolonged intubation with an ET tube is often a more successful therapy, particularly in tiny premature infants where recovery from pulmonary disease is expected and complications from ET tubes are relatively infrequent. Guidelines for older patients are rarely directly applicable.

3. Need for extraordinary pulmonary toilet
4. Adjunct to craniofacial surgery

B. CONTRAINDICATIONS

1. Anatomic abnormality, making trachea surgically inaccessible
2. Anatomic obstruction of distal trachea not relievable by tracheostomy (Fig. 33-1)

3. Severe tracheomalacia, in which natural expiratory resistance provided by glottis is essential in maintaining airway
4. Lack of expertise in caring for tracheotomy patients

   Transfer to a facility with experienced staff may be indicated as the risk of postoperative complications is particularly high in neonates.

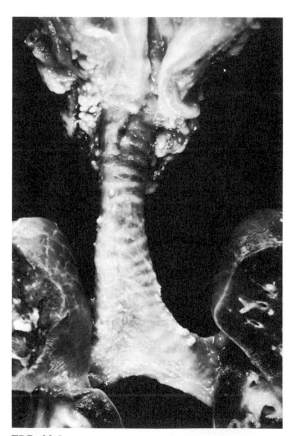

FIG. 33-1
Congenitally fused tracheal rings. Because the tracheal obstruction is distal to a tracheotomy site, a tracheotomy would not relieve the symptoms.

Surgical Tracheotomy

C. EQUIPMENT FOR SURGICAL TRACHEOTOMY

1. Cup with antiseptic solution
2. Gauze swabs
3. Standard pediatric tracheotomy set
   a. Drapes
   b. Scalpel
   c. Small, curved hemostats
   d. Senn retractors
   e. Nonabsorbable sutures (3-0 or 4-0) on small, curved needles
   f. Scissors
      (1) Small Mayo
      (2) Iris
   g. Gauze dressings
   h. Wide umbilical (webbed) twill tape
4. Neonatal tracheostomy tube (Fig. 33-2)
   a. Soft, pliable, nonreactive
   b. Non-cuffed
   c. Easy to clean and maintain
   d. Sized for patient's tracheal diameter and length

   e. External flange small enough for patient's neck or modified
   f. External adapter for respiratory equipment

D. PRECAUTIONS

1. Recognize anatomical differences of neonatal larynx compared to adult (Fig. 33-3).
   a. Increased mobility of head and neck articulations
   b. Increased mobility of trachea
   c. More cephalad larynx
   d. Trachea relatively deeper to skin
   e. More anterior relation of innominate artery and left innominate vein
   f. Enlarged thymus
   g. Passage of trachea into superior mediastinum at a deeper level
   h. Soft cartilages; thyroid cartilage least palpable element
2. Correct any remediable medical conditions prior to procedure unless relief of airway obstruction is urgent.
3. Avoid obstructing view of field by drapes. Anesthesiologist must be able to visualize neck during surgery.

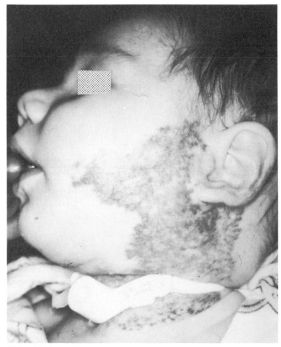

FIG. 33-2
Shiley neonatal tracheostomy tube.

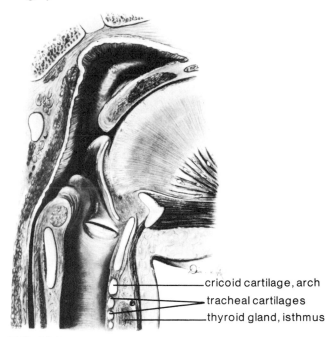

— cricoid cartilage, arch
— tracheal cartilages
— thyroid gland, isthmus

FIG. 33-3
Sagittal section. Larynx lies more cephalad than in adult. Note the proximity of the thyroid isthmus to the tracheal rings. (Drawing contributed by John Bosma, M.D.)

4. Carefully maintain landmarks during procedure.
   a. Remove nasogastric tube or esophageal stethoscope prior to beginning dissection to avoid mistakenly identifying esophagus as trachea.
   b. Repeatedly palpate structures to verify tracheal location.
5. Keep stay sutures in place to facilitate reinsertion until tract has been established.
6. Observe for aerophagia after recovery from tracheotomy, and remove excess swallowed air as needed.
7. If necessary, modify tracheotomy tube by paring and smoothing inferior portion to prevent pressure on skin.[5]

E. TECHNIQUE[6–9]

1. Prepare infant as for major surgical procedure, using general anesthesia and orotracheal intubation.
2. Monitor infant carefully, and follow all steps necessary to maintain homeostasis (see Part I, Preparation and Support).

3. Position and restrain infant (Fig. 33-4).
   a. Firm roll under shoulders without hyperextending neck
   b. Symphysis menti and suprasternal notch in same sagittal plane
4. Cleanse skin as for major surgical procedure (see Chap. 4, Aseptic Preparation).
5. Scrub; put on gown, mask, and gloves.
6. Drape infant to maintain visualization of head and neck.
7. Identify larynx and trachea by palpation (Fig. 33-5). Palpate trachea after each layer is incised throughout procedure to ensure its location.
8. Make a 1.5-cm horizontal incision 1 to 1.5 cm above sternal notch (Fig. 33-6).
9. Separate subcutaneous layers, removing any fat pad as necessary, and identify facial layers. Grasp fascia with hemostats, and pull outward. Open with scissors in midline.
10. Retract isthmus of thyroid superiorly. Identify vessels and thymus. Use only essential dissection, keeping surrounding tissue as intact as possible to lessen future air dissection.

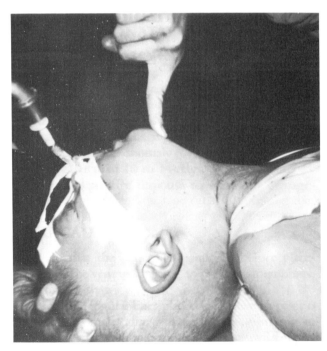

FIG. 33-4
Positioning an infant with too much extension for tracheotomy. The neck should not be as hyperextended as in this case because the incision may then be too low and lead to retraction of the stoma into the thorax.

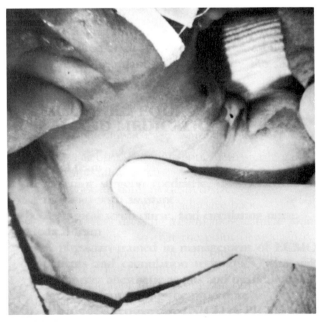

FIG. 33-5
Palpation of cricoid, thyroid, and tracheal cartilages, which will not be as firm as in an adult, and are, therefore, harder to distinguish.

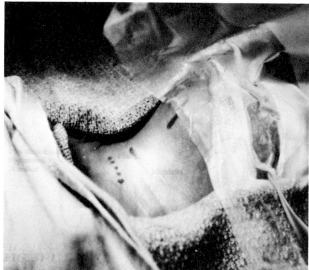

FIG. 33-6
Line of incision (dotted) 1–1.5 cm above the sternal notch (solid lower line).

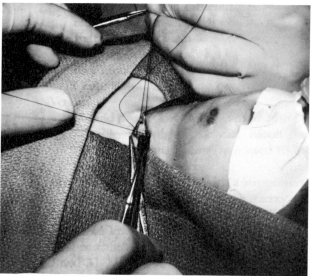

FIG. 33-7
Placement of stay sutures through the tracheal wall.

11. Place two stay sutures 1 to 2 mm from midline in tracheal wall. Label left and right (Fig. 33-7).
12. Make vertical incision into trachea between stay sutures through the 2nd, 3rd, and 4th tracheal rings (Figs. 33-8, 33-9).

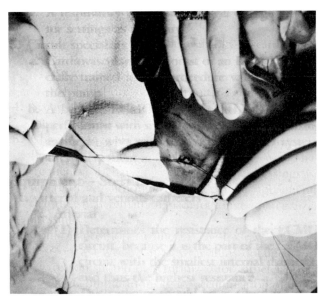

FIG. 33-8
Traction on stay sutures elevates the trachea for incision. Note how the anesthesiologist maintains visualization of procedure.

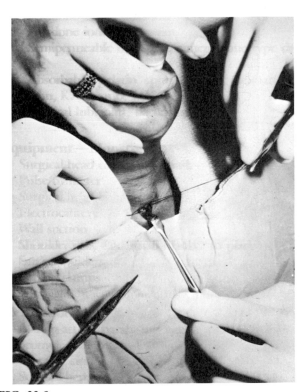

FIG. 33-9
Incision through the second, third, and fourth tracheal rings. Stay sutures are retracting the cartilages to maintain the opening. The anesthesiologist will now retract ET tube as tracheostomy tube is inserted.

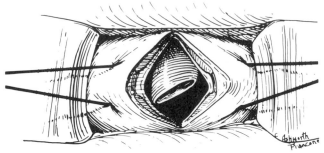

FIG. 33-10
Artistic conception of view through tracheal incision with the tip of the ET tube visible. Stay sutures hold cartilages open.

There is some concern that the type of incision may affect the future growth of the trachea. In developing animals, a transverse tracheal incision without incising cartilage appeared to cause less growth deformation.[10] This technique is well described in infants.[6,11]

13. Withdraw orotracheal tube to level just above incision (Fig. 33-10).
14. Putting traction on stay sutures to open trachea, grasp internal end of tracheostomy tube with curved arterial forceps and insert into tracheal lumen.

15. Remove shoulder roll to allow normal neck positioning and flexion.
16. Ventilate through tracheostomy tube, and auscult both sides of chest to verify position of tube.
17. When tracheostomy tube appears to be in position by auscultation, remove orotracheal tube.
18. If needed, place sutures in both ends of skin incision, without constricting opening. Leave stay sutures in place until tract has developed (Fig. 33-11).
19. Tie tube in place around neck with twill tape loose enough to admit one finger with neck in a neutral position (Fig. 33-12).
20. Obtain anteroposterior and lateral chest radiographs to determine position of tube and exclude pulmonary air leak.

F. POSTOPERATIVE MANAGEMENT[9,12]

1. Provide 24-hour supervision.
2. Keep orotracheal intubation equipment available.
3. Keep sterile, appropriately sized tracheostomy tube and small, curved forceps at bedside.
4. Keep sterile suction apparatus available. Suction as needed to maintain tube patency.

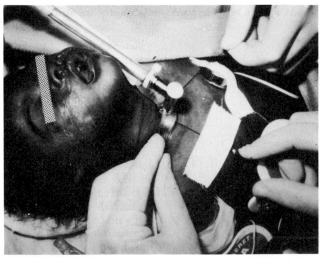
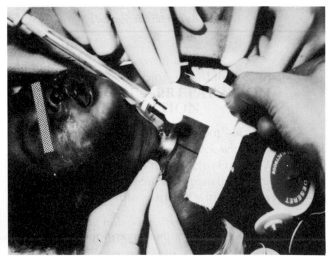

A   B

FIG. 33-11
Fixation of stay sutures. As soon as the position of the tracheostomy tube is confirmed and stomal ventilation started, the tube may be fixed. Equal tension is kept on the stay sutures during taping. (*A*) Right suture is marked to avoid confusion in future replacement. (*B*) Taping of the left suture with the stoma kept midline.

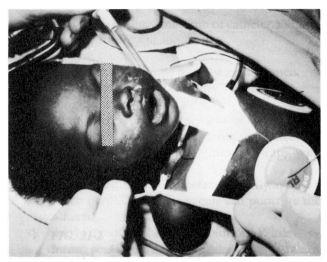

FIG. 33-12
Tying of webbed twill tape loose enough to admit one finger in a neutral neck position.

5. Provide air or oxygen as required that is warmed close to body temperature at 100% relative humidity.
6. Check external position of tube frequently. Auscultate to verify correct intratracheal position and patency.
7. Clean skin area around tracheostomy daily.
8. Notify surgeon immediately if any further subcutaneous air or bleeding develops.
9. Obtain culture of secretions if there is any increase or change in character.

G. REPLACEMENT OF DISLODGED TUBE PRIOR TO TRACT FORMATION (5–7 DAYS)

1. Pull on stay sutures.
2. Use sterile, curved forceps to grasp end of sterile tracheostomy tube, and replace into trachea between stay sutures.
3. If tracheostomy tube does not pass easily, thread a sterile feeding tube through the tube and then into the stoma to serve as a guide wire for the tracheostomy tube.
4. Obtain radiographs to verify position.
5. Consider immediate oral intubation.
   a. If tube is not easily inserted, or
   b. If there is any emphysema or bleeding

Emergency Tracheotomy[9]
Emergency tracheotomy by surgical incision is particularly dangerous in neonates. It is appropriate to attempt an emergency tracheotomy only after unsuccessful attempts at oral or nasal intubation, employing alternative methods as suggested in Chap. 32.

1. Put on sterile gloves. Cleanse anterior neck with iodophor surgical prep. Blot excess.
2. Extend neck with roll under shoulders.
3. Palpate landmarks and locate cricothyroid membrane.

   The membrane is very small and difficult to distinguish in neonates. Locate the cricothyroid junction and avoid critical vascular structures off midline.

4. Attach a 3-ml syringe to a 14-gauge intravascular cannula with stylet.
5. While aspirating, insert through cricothyroid membrane in the midline.

   Because the cartilages are so pliable in neonates, it is difficult to penetrate the anterior membranes without collapsing the airway and penetrating posteriorly as well. It may be helpful to make a small, midline incision through the skin one finger breadth above the suprasternal notch to ease insertion.

6. As soon as air is aspirated, remove syringe and stylet, while advancing cannula into trachea.
7. Attach cannula to 3-mm endotracheal tube adaptor to provide artificial ventilation until permanent airway is established.

H. COMPLICATIONS

Many complications relating to tracheotomy are an indirect result of associated conditions, particularly when chronic lung disease or airway pathology exist.

1. Air leaks
   a. Subcutaneous emphysema (Limited subcutaneous emphysema within 1 cm of the tracheostomy is usual for first 48 hours.)[13]
   b. Pneumomediastinum[14,15–17]
   c. Pneumothorax[14,17–20]
   d. Pneumoperitoneum
2. Extubation out of tracheostomy

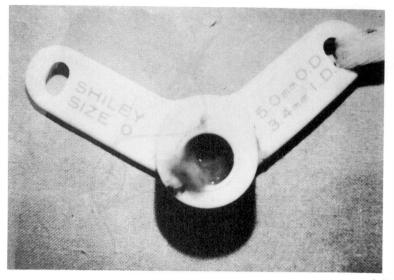
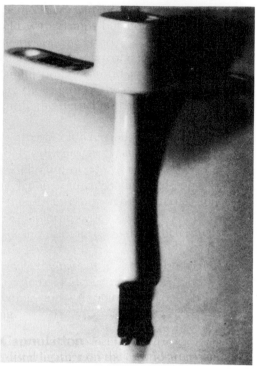

A B

FIG. 33-13
Total obstructions of tracheostomy tubes. (*A*) Mucous plug incompletely suctioned. (*B*) Dry mucous plug pushed deeper by a suction catheter.

FIG. 33-14
Erosion granulation tissue (*open arrow*) distal to tracheal stoma (*closed arrow*).

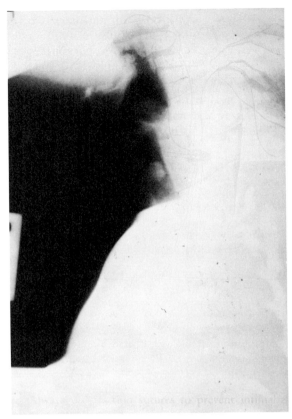

FIG. 33-15
Polyp of trachea at tracheotomy site on lateral radiograph.

3. Displacement[14]
   a. Mainstem bronchus
   b. Pretracheal region or false tract
4. Obstruction[13]
   a. Mucus plug (Fig. 33-13)
   b. Crusting
5. Aspiration
   a. Excess gagging postoperatively
   b. Associated loss of control of adductor laryngeal muscles
6. Aerophagia[21]
7. Hemorrhage[14]
   a. Intraoperative
      (1) Anomalous vessel
      (2) More anterior position of innominate vessels
      (3) Transection of thyroid[22]
   b. Erosion of adjacent vessel

8. Tracheoesophageal fistula
   a. Iatrogenic when emergency incision done without orotracheal tube in place
   b. Acquired from erosion[23]
9. Tracheal erosion (Fig. 33-14)
10. Breakdown on tissue around tracheostomy[5]
11. Granulation tissue[24,25]
    a. Ring
    b. Polyp (Fig. 33-15)[16,26,27]
12. Stenosis from scarring ring[28,25]
13. Difficulty in decannulation due to laryngeal abductor muscle failure[24]
14. Fused vocal cords due to loss of abductor[16]
15. Tracheomalacia[16,29]
    a. Generalized
    b. Localized at stoma
16. Inverted tracheal cartilage[16]
17. Epidermal ingrowth, causing tracheal obstruction
18. Infection at site[14]
19. Thermal instability due to inappropriate temperature of airway support
20. Fluid overload or dried secretions due to inappropriate humidification

References

1. GRUNDFAST KM, HARLEY E: Vocal cord paralysis. Otolaryngol Clin North Am. 22:569, 1989
2. FRANKEL LR, ANAS NG, PERKIN RM, ET AL: Use of the anterior cricoid split operation in infants with acquired subglottic stenosis. Crit Care Med 12:395, 1984
3. GRUNDFAST KM, COFFMAN AC, MILMOE G: Anterior cricoid split: A simple surgical procedure and a potentially complicated care problem. Ann Otol Rhinol Laryngol 94:445, 1985
4. SEID AB, CANTY TG: The anterior cricoid split procedure for the management of subglottic stenosis in infants and children. J Pediatr Surg 20:388, 1985
5. ROTHFIELD RE, PETRUZZELLI GJ, STOOL SE: Neonatal tracheotomy tube modification. Otolaryngol Head Neck Surg 103:133, 1990
6. LYNN HB, VANHEERDEN JA: Tracheostomy in infants. Surg Clin North Am 53:945, 1973
7. WHITE JJ, HALLER JA JR: An improved technique for tracheostomy in infants and children. Medical Times 101:120, 1973
8. DOUGLAS GS, HOSKINS D, STOOL SE: Tracheotomy in pediatric airway management. Pediatr Ann 5:509, 1976

9. STOOL SE, EAVEY RD: Tracheotomy. In Bluestone CD, Stool SE, Scheetz MD (eds): Pediatric Otoloryngology, 2nd ed. Philadelphia: WB Saunders, 1990, p 1226.

10. MENDEZ-PICON G, EHRLICH FE, SALZBERG AM: The effect of tracheostomy incisions on tracheal growth. J Pediatr Surg 11:681, 1976

11. HEROY JH, MACDONALD MG, MAZZI E, RISEMBERG HM: Airway management in the premature infant. Ann Otol Rhinol Laryngol 87:53, 1978

12. CROCKER D: Management of tracheostomy. Pediatrics 46:286, 1970

13. HAWKINS DB, WILLIAMS EH: Tracheostomy in infants and young children. Laryngoscope 86:331, 1976

14. ROGERS LA: Complications of tracheostomy. South Med J 62:1496, 1969

15. SCHMIDT GB, BENNETT EJ, DALAL RY: Death precipitated by tracheostomy in a child. JAMA 231:277, 1975

16. GAUDET PT, PEERLESS A, SASAKI CT, KIRCHNER JA: Pediatric tracheostomy and associated complications. Laryngoscope 88:1633, 1978

17. BIFANO E, CLARK D, PINCUS L: Tracheostomy and decannulation in neonates. Pediatr Res 14 (Part 2):591, 1980

18. RABUZZI DD, REED GF: Intrathoracic complications following tracheotomy in children. Laryngoscope 81:939, 1971

19. COHEN SR, EAVEY RD, DESMOND MS, MAY BC: Endoscopy and tracheotomy in the neonatal period: A 10-year review, 1967–1976. Ann Otol Rhinol Laryngol 86:577, 1977

20. GIBSON R, BYRNE JE: Tracheotomy in neonates. Laryngoscope 82:643, 1972

21. ROSNAGLE RS, YANAGISAWA E: Aerophagia. An unrecognized complication of tracheotomy. Arch Otolaryngol 89:537, 1969

22. TSCHANG TP, CRAMER S: Massive hemorrhage from perforated thyroid complicating tracheostomy. Report of two cases. Arch Otolaryngol 103:557, 1977

23. APLIN CE, SMITH M, HARRISON R, RICHARDSON CJ: Acquired tracheoesophageal fistula in a premature infant. J Pediatr 91:983, 1977

24. BROMBERG D, TURTZ MG: Tracheal granulation: A complication of pediatric tracheotomy. Ann Otol Rhinol Laryngol 86:631, 1977

25. SASAKI CT, GAUDET PT, PEERLESS A: Tracheostomy decannulation. Am J Dis Child 132:266, 1978

26. PAHOR AL: Tracheal polyp complicating tracheostomy in an infant. Ear Nose Throat J 56:249, 1977

27. FILSTON HC, JOHNSON DG, CRUMRINE RS: Infant tracheostomy. Am J Dis Child 132:1177, 1978

28. RODGERS BM, ROOKS JJ, TALBERT JL: Pediatric tracheostomy: Long term evaluation. J Pediatr Surg 14:258, 1979

29. MURPHY DA, POPKIN J: Tracheal collapse in tracheostomized infants: Resistance in reference to flow rates in a variety of tracheostomy tubes. J Pediatr Surg 6:314, 1971

34 Respiratory Physical Therapy

Mary Ann Fletcher

This chapter outlines a number of discrete techniques, each with its own risks and benefits. When these techniques are applied in combinations appropriate to individual patient needs, an effective physiotherapy regimen should result. The blanket application of "chest physiotherapy" to all intubated patients is not recommended. Therapy applied without consideration of physiologic cost and benefit may do more harm than good. For most infants, attention to position and maintenance of lung volume will eliminate need for more intensive and stressful therapies such as percussion and cough simulation. An understanding of the physiologic effects of various components of chest physiotherapy is helpful in determining which therapy, if any, will benefit each patient.[1]

> The term "chest physiotherapy" is often used incorrectly to connote only the percussion component. To clarify meaning, we encourage use of the term "respiratory physical therapy" to encompass all aspects of mechanical techniques as well as breathing modifications.

Postural Drainage

A. INDICATIONS

> Every body position provides drainage from some area of the lung. Unless there is attention to repositioning, a neonate may remain in virtually the same position for prolonged periods. If the sick infant is kept on his back, only the anterior segments of the upper lobes will be drained with progressively decreasing ventilation to the lower lobes.

1. Prevention
   a. Changes in ventilation/perfusion secondary to gravitational forces acting over prolonged time in immobile patient[2,3]
   b. Spillage of infectious material from an affected area to a clear area
   c. Aspiration of stomach contents
   d. Postextubation atelectasis[4,5]
2. Treatment
   a. Accumulated secretions[6]
   b. Aspiration
3. Splinting of chest wall to decrease ventilation to one hemithorax

   > Because chest wall compliance contributes to overall pulmonary compliance in neonates, restricting free movement of one hemithorax will decrease relative ventilation to that side with an increase in ventilation to the nonrestricted, and, therefore, more compliant side.

   a. To encourage ventilation away from affected lung
      (1) Unilateral interstitial emphysema[7]
      (2) Lobar emphysema
      (3) Bronchopleural fistula
   b. To encourage ventilation toward affected lung: atelectasis
4. Adjunct to other components of respiratory physiotherapy for maintenance of bronchial hygiene
5. Augmentation of pleural drainage by thoracostomy tube or decrease in flow to bronchopleural fistula

B. CONTRAINDICATIONS

> Note that the presence of thoracostomy tubes or umbilical catheters is not a contraindication to positional changes as long as care is taken to prevent their dislodging. In most instances in which abdominal positioning may be contraindicated, the infant can be supported to avoid pressure on the abdomen or hips.

1. Head-down positioning
   a. Infants least able to withstand increases in intracranial pressure
      (1) Premature infants less than 1250 gm
      (2) Recent intracranial hemorrhage

     (3) Brain edema
     (4) Untreated hydrocephalus
  b. Immediately after feeding
2. Abdominal positioning without support
  a. In period immediately after abdominal surgery
  b. In anteriorly located thoracoabdominal malformations (e.g., omphalocele)
  c. With abdominal distention, in which abdominal contents compromise diaphragmatic movement
  d. In congenitally dislocated hip

C. Equipment

1. Folded cloth blankets
2. Sand bag
3. Padded infant or doll seat
4. Wedge
  a. 30-60-90-degree triangle
  b. Prop for mattress or infant

D. PRECAUTIONS

1. Secure therapeutic and monitoring equipment to allow optimal positioning of infant.
2. Avoid head-down positions immediately after feedings or in infants with gastroesophageal reflux.

3. In selecting positions favorable for draining an affected area, take care to prevent atelectasis and stasis in other regions of lung.
4. Avoid positions that will cause significant respiratory compromise; monitor effects of various positions.
  a. Flat or head down on the abdomen when there is abdominal distention. Keep hips flexed so knees support weight rather than abdomen.
  b. Dependent positioning of normal side when there is contralateral lung disease or diaphragmatic weakness
  c. Sitting up without head support causing airway obstruction
5. Consider need for flexion of hips and shoulders to encourage fetal posture.
6. Use head and neck roll to keep head in neutral position.
  a. Maintain optimum airway.
  b. Prevent plagiocephaly.

E. TECHNIQUE

1. Select positions appropriate for infant's condition and the type of respiratory care being given (Fig. 34-1; Plate 34-1).

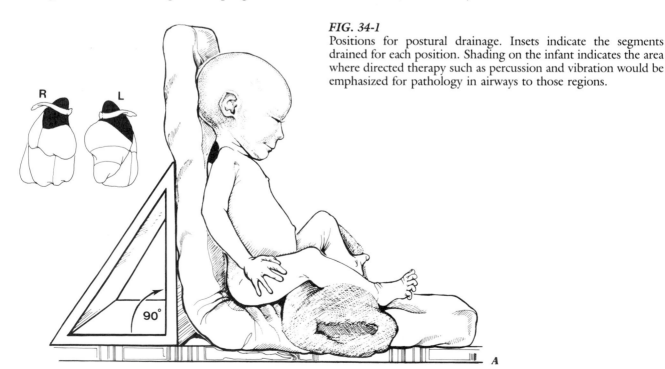

FIG. 34-1
Positions for postural drainage. Insets indicate the segments drained for each position. Shading on the infant indicates the area where directed therapy such as percussion and vibration would be emphasized for pathology in airways to those regions.

R   L

90°

A

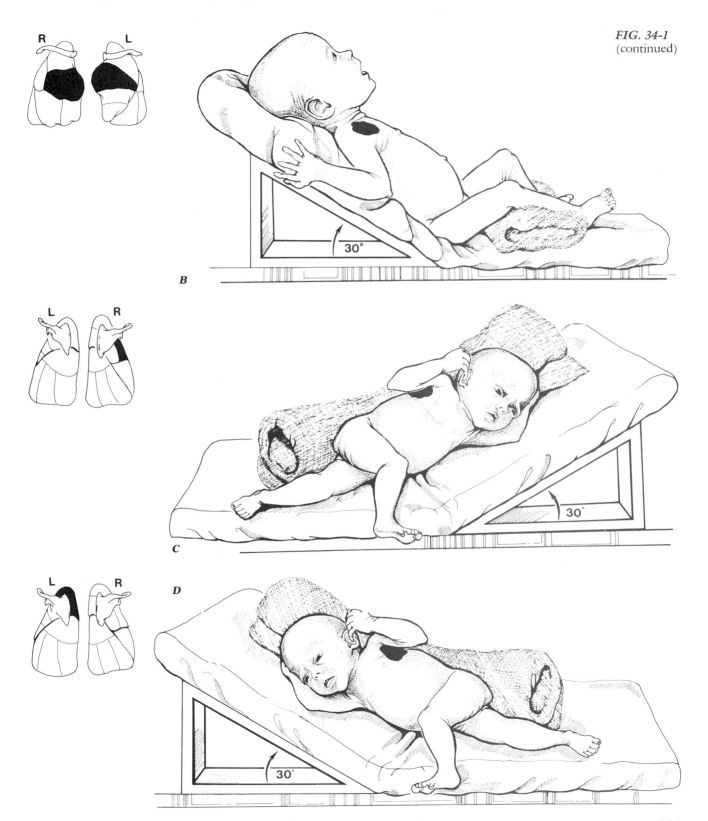

FIG. 34-1
(continued)

B

C

D

FIG. 34-1
(continued)

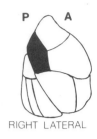

RIGHT LATERAL

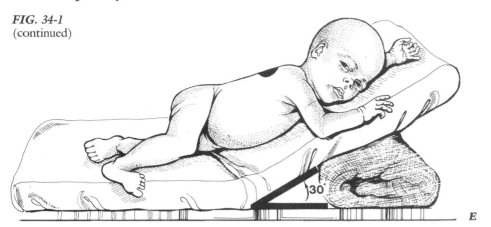

30°

E

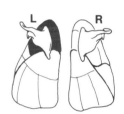

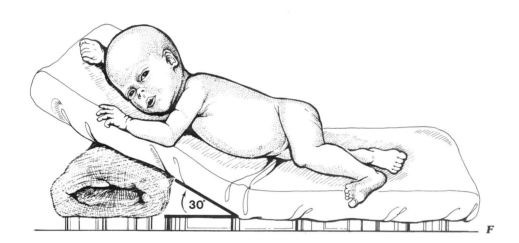

30°

F

G

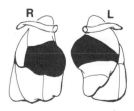

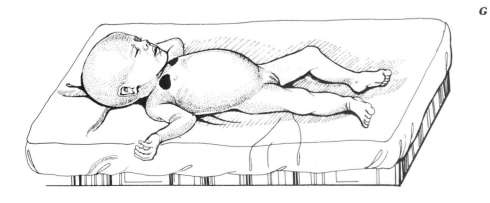

FIG. 34-1
(continued)

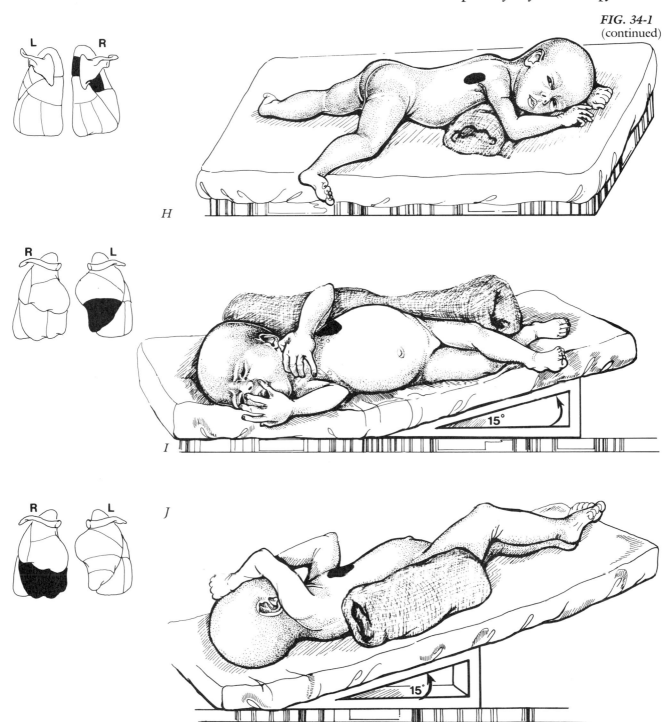

H

I

J

FIG. 34-1
(continued)

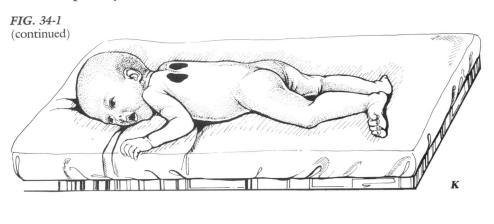
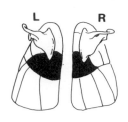

K

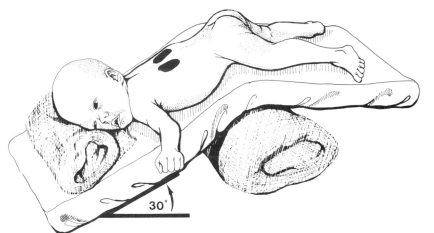
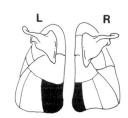

30°

L

M

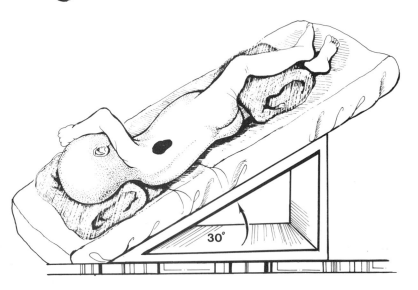
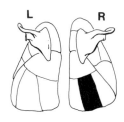

30°

FIG. 34-1
(continued)

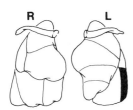

ANTERIOR

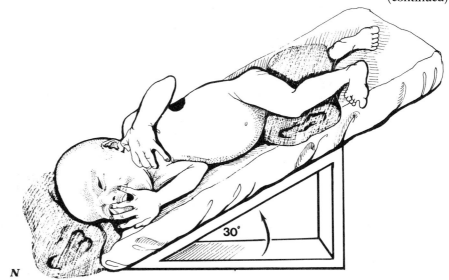

N

O

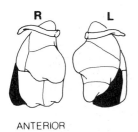

ANTERIOR

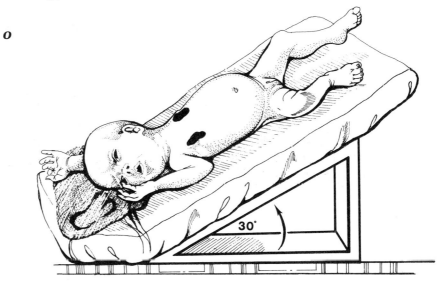

2. Determine duration for each position.
   a. For preventive care of immobile infant, change position every 1 to 2 hours.
   b. During a respiratory treatment, change position throughout treatment, e.g., during vibration or percussion.
3. Establish sequence for positions.
   a. Facilitate rotation of monitoring or therapeutic equipment
   b. Note positions and timing on bedside chart.
      (1) Allows all care givers to know in what position to place infant at a specific time or after procedure that changed position (e.g., radiograph)
      (2) Guarantees full range of positioning throughout timed sequence
4. Start position sequence as illustrated in Figure 34-1 and Plate 34-1.
5. Prop infant well to maintain position without compromise to diaphragm or airway.
6. Monitor effect of each position change.
   a. Therapeutic and monitoring equipment
   b. Infant's airway
   c. Constriction of respiratory excursions
   d. Cardiovascular system
   e. Pulmonary function (blood gas deterioration, increased tachypnea, etc.)
      (1) Unilateral lung disease with normal lung dependent
      (2) Abdominal compression restricting diaphragmatic excursion
   f. Flexion posturing rather than extension

F. COMPLICATIONS

1. Dislodging vital support equipment: endotracheal (ET) tube, chest tube, umbilical catheter
2. Increased intracranial pressure
3. Respiratory compromise
   a. Diaphragmatic compression[8]
   b. Splinting
4. Spillage of purulent material
5. Aspiration
6. Apnea from airway obstruction

Vibration

A. INDICATIONS

To thin and mobilize secretions toward large airways, where suctioning or cough will remove them

> Mucus is a thixotropic substance with the property of liquefaction upon shaking. Theoretically, application of vibration thins mucus and allows better mobility.

B. CONTRAINDICATIONS

1. Increased irritability, causing respiratory compromise during procedure
2. Absence of thick secretions
3. Significant pulmonary interstitial emphysema

C. EQUIPMENT

1. Monitor for ECG and respiratory rate
2. Continuous blood-gas or saturation monitor[9]
3. Mechanical vibrator (commercial or toothbrush)
   a. Battery-operated with no electrical leakage
   b. Soft surface for patient contact
   c. Clean for each patient.

> Many commercial "percussors" are really using vibration instead. High frequency chest oscillation applied by means of an oscillator jacket for a period of up to 30 minutes has been demonstrated to be effective in adults.[10]

D. PRECAUTIONS

1. Use only battery-operated, electrically safe vibrators.
2. Do not apply vibrator directly to broken or very immature skin.

> Vibrations will be transmitted if the therapist's finger is held on the patient's chest and the vibrator applied to the finger rather than directly to skin. This application is more often relaxing and less stressful to the patient.

3. Modify treatment if infant is stressed by procedure.[9]
   a. Stop if indications are not present.
   b. Apply gentler vibratory force by interposing pad or finger.

c. Keep away from bones and nonpulmonary viscera.

d. Modify FIO_2 as indicated by oxymetry.

E. TECHNIQUE

Mechanical Vibrator

1. Interpose fingers or soft pad between vibrator and skin.
2. With infant in various drainage positions, apply vibrator over region of drainage for 2 to 3 minutes in each area (see Fig. 34-1).
3. Coordinate vibration with exhalation.
   a. Apply pressure to compress chest in direction of bronchial drainage for underlying segments.
   b. Time with ventilator, or
   c. Have assistant perform manual ventilation during procedure and apply vibration with pressure at end of sigh with inflation hold.

Hand Vibration

1. On exhalation or after a mechanical inspiration, with wrist held taut, apply quick vibratory compression of chest in direction of bronchial drainage for underlying segment.
2. Stop compression and vibration during inhalation.

Finish procedure with suctioning and either sigh with inflation hold or mask IPEP (see section on Intermittent Positive Expiratory Pressure in this chapter).

F. COMPLICATIONS

1. Hypoxemia
2. Bruising
3. Periosteal reaction to ribs[11]

Percussion

A. INDICATIONS

To loosen abnormal secretions within the tracheobronchial tree[6,12]

   a. Secretory (late) phase of respiratory distress syndrome[13]
   b. Aspiration

c. Secretory lobar pneumonia after 24 hours on antibiotics

d. Prevention of postextubation atelectasis[4,5]

B. CONTRAINDICATIONS

1. Absence of abnormal secretions
2. Significant pulmonary interstitial emphysema
3. Pulmonary hemorrhage
4. Abscess, empyema, or localized pneumonia prior to medical sterilization by antibiotics
5. Increased intracranial pressure
6. Recent intracranial hemorrhage
7. Rib fractures or recent thoracotomy that is painful
8. Bleeding diathesis
9. Critical hypoxemia
10. Extreme immaturity
11. Unstable cardiorespiratory status

C. EQUIPMENT

1. Monitoring devices
   a. Cardiorespiratory monitor
   b. Continuous blood-gas monitor
2. Cupping device

   There have been a number of devices designed to replace the hand for percussion. In cupping the neonatal chest, it is difficult to achieve an effective air column with finger positioning. Few, if any, of these devices have been tested as to efficacy in neonates, and most are used because of ease and availability to the percussor. Most "percussors" operate more like vibrators and do not really generate a column of air.

   a. Soft neonatal face mask with adapter occluded by plunger of 10-ml plastic syringe (Fig. 34-2).
   b. Pneumatically operated percussion device specifically designed for use in neonates

D. PRECAUTIONS

1. Use only in patients considered stable or large enough to receive more benefit than stress from this procedure.
2. Secure vital support and monitoring equipment to prevent dislodging during procedure.
3. Use only wrist action in manual cupping to avoid

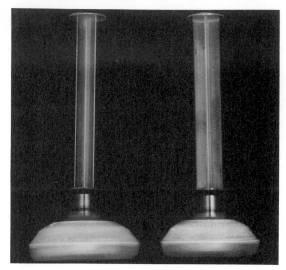

FIG. 34-2
Readily available modification of soft neonatal face masks for effective cupping device.

exerting excessive pressure on the chest. (There should be no residual marks.)

4. Use only cupping devices that have truly soft edges and deliver a column of air under pressure.
5. Avoid cupping over recent incision, fractures, the liver, the spleen, heart, and vertebrae.
6. Stop or modify treatment if there is any deterioration of oxygenation, or if infant resists manipulation.[9]

E. TECHNIQUE

Cupping

It is the column of air created by cupping the hand that transmits the pressure to lungs. Direct pressure from contact of the hand or a cupping device is not thought to be the therapeutic pressure.

1. With infant in prescribed drainage positions, perform cupping over region being drained (see Fig. 34-1).
2. Flex wrist and percuss at rate of 180 to 240 beats/min (3–4 beats/sec).
3. With pneumatically operated device, hold device against chest, exerting mild pressure.

Contact-Heel Percussion[12]

1. Position infant in appropriate drainage positions, particularly for posterior and anterior basal segments.
2. During expiration apply pressure to the area of percussion, using the thenar–hypothenar eminences in slight apposition.
3. Use rate of 40 compressions/min.
4. With each beat, compress chest wall 1 to 2 cm.
5. Continue in each area for 5 to 10 minutes.

F. COMPLICATIONS

The rate of complications is minimized if patient is manually ventilated during procedure by assistant who monitors both the airway and the pressure delivered. Because compression tends to decrease ventilation, pressures higher than required at rest may be needed to replace lung volume.

1. Patient resists mechanical ventilation.
   a. Increased oxygen consumption with hypoxemia
   b. Increased intrathoracic pressure or barotrauma, leading to pulmonary air leaks
   c. Extubation
2. Hypoxemia
3. Bruising
4. Rib fractures
5. Hematoma of liver or spleen (Fig. 34-3)
6. Atelectasis
   a. Pain induced by procedure

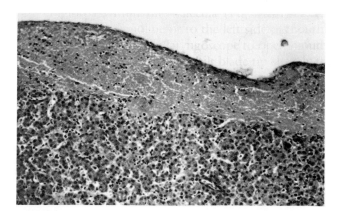

FIG. 34-3
Subcapsular hematoma of liver possibly caused by overzealous chest percussion.

b. Compressive effects of percussion on compliant chest

c. Mucus plugging of larger airways

Intermittent Positive Expiratory Pressure (IPEP)

A. INDICATIONS

1. To replace a natural sigh mechanism, the absence of which leads to microatelectasis
   a. Immaturity
   b. Neurologic disease or depression
2. As an adjunct to other components of respiratory physiotherapy in replacing lung volume lost after suctioning or chest wall compression[14]
3. To encourage deeper tidal volume in tachypneic infant breathing shallowly
4. To open compliant, collapsed airways
5. To prevent postextubation atelectasis
6. To restore decreased resting lung volume to normal

B. CONTRAINDICATIONS

1. Pulmonary air leaks
2. Emphysema with air trapping not due to airway collapse and not amenable to treatment with distending airway pressure
3. Gastric feeding less than 2 hours earlier

C. EQUIPMENT

1. Soft face mask
2. IPEP device to create continuous positive pressure
   a. Carden valve* (Fig. 34-4)
   b. Must be lightweight without appreciable dead space
   c. Should not require two hands for application of total system
3. Blended oxygen/air source
4. Manometer (Fig. 34-5)

D. PRECAUTIONS

1. Use soft mask that will provide close fit without pressure to face.

*Carden valve is available from Dupaco, 2620 Temple Heights Drive, Oceanside, CA, 92056.

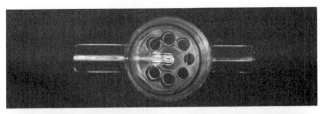

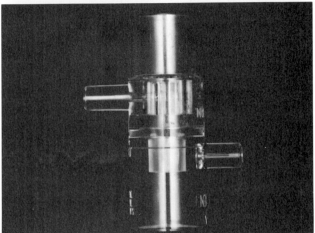

FIG. 34-4
Carden valve for generating continuous positive pressure at level commensurate with gas flow rate into it. Views on end and in profile show gas and pressure portals as well as internal resistance that creates pressure.

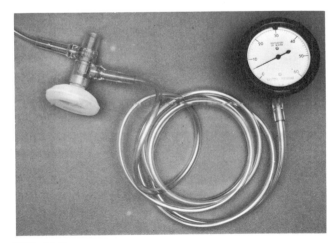

FIG. 34-5
Assembled equipment for intermittent positive expiratory pressure by mask with a manometer and blended oxygen source connected to a lightweight Carden valve.

2. Use mask of appropriate size that covers nose and mouth, but not eyes.
3. Keep jaw held forward in sniff position to hold nasopharynx open.
4. Schedule treatment before gastric feedings and empty stomach of air after treatment.
5. Apply only if response is positive.

E. TECHNIQUE

1. Position infant.
   a. Sitting up (support head and chest with free hand), or
   b. Reclining
2. Apply mask to nose and mouth with first two fingers while holding jaw forward with remaining fingers.
3. Apply for prescribed therapy.
   a. Pressures of 5 to 10 cm H_2O
   b. Duration of 5 minutes
4. Evaluate efficacy.
   a. Positive effect
      (1) Patient relaxation
      (2) Slowing of tachypnea
      (3) Deeper inspiration with wider chest wall excursions (increased tidal volume)
      (4) Decreased retractions
      (5) Improved oxygenation
      (6) Improved pulmonary compliance
   b. Negative effect
      (1) Fighting
      (2) Increased retractions
      (3) Apnea
      (4) Hypoxia
      (5) Gastric distention
         (a) Reposition jaw into more of a sniff position to decrease air entry into esophagus.
         (b) Suction stomach after treatment.
5. Lower pressure if negative effect is observed.

F. COMPLICATIONS

1. Pneumothorax
2. Unrecognized aspiration
3. Increased intracranial pressure
4. Gastric distention from swallowed air

Sigh with Inflation Hold

A. INDICATIONS

1. To replace lung volume lost after suctioning or chest compression (vibration, percussion), particularly in an intubated infant.[15]
2. To allow longer inspiratory time for re-expansion of areas of atelectasis
   a. Lower peak inspiratory pressure
   b. No overexpansion of normal areas
3. As adjunct in cough simulation therapy (see Cough Simulation)
4. To replace natural sigh missing in immature or depressed infant who does not cry vigorously and is at risk for loss of FRC over time

B. CONTRAINDICATIONS

1. Pulmonary air leaks
   a. Interstitial pulmonary emphysema
   b. Uncontrolled pneumothorax, pneumomediastinum
2. Localized emphysema
3. Generalized air trapping with overdistention

C. EQUIPMENT

1. Ventilation bag with manometer
2. Mask or ET tube
3. Cardiorespiratory monitor
4. Continuous blood-gas monitor

D. PRECAUTIONS

1. Do not apply too much pressure to cause overexpansion or apnea.
2. Apply at rate that does not change infant's ventilatory pattern.
   a. Prevent apnea from decreased CO_2 in spontaneously ventilating infant.
   b. Use similar rate as machine in artificially ventilated infant.

E. TECHNIQUE

1. Determine by observation the positive pressure required by hand ventilation to deliver a tidal volume appropriate for the infant.

a. Normal lung = 15 to 20 cm H_2O
b. Noncompliant lung = 25 to 35 cm H_2O
c. Reasonable chest-wall excursion

2. For spontaneously ventilating infant with or without ET tube, apply and hold positive pressure
   a. Every fifth breath
   b. For 1 to 2 seconds of held pressure
3. For infant on ventilator, apply and hold positive pressure
   a. Every tenth breath
   b. 5 to 10 cm H_2O pressure above peak mechanical pressure
   c. For 1 to 2 seconds
4. Combine with other components of respiratory physical therapy
   a. In cough simulation with suctioning
   b. After chest compression
      (1) Vibration with compression
      (2) Percussion
5. Omit sighs if infant spontaneously cries vigorously and deeply.
6. Omit or modify if infant resists ventilation.
7. Decrease pressure applied or intermittent rate if infant hypoventilates or becomes apneic.
8. Follow effect on oxygenation and vary FIO_2 accordingly.

F. COMPLICATIONS

1. Pulmonary air leak
2. Apnea from overdistention or hyperventilation
3. Hypoxia
4. Hyperoxia

Cough Simulation

Augmentation or replacement of cough mechanism in the presence of copious secretions

A. INDICATIONS

1. Protection of lung against aspiration
2. Help in propelling secretions or other material upwardly through airways
   a. Intubated infant
   b. Immature infant
   c. Neurologically weakened or impaired infant

d. Integral part of physiotherapy directed at mobilization of secretions

B. CONTRAINDICATIONS

1. Presence of normal cough mechanism
2. Rib fractures
3. Pulmonary interstitial emphysema
4. Pulmonary hemorrhage during active bleeding
5. Presence of contraindications to vibration and chest compression
6. Recent full gastric feeding
7. Acute intracranial hemorrhage
8. Extreme immaturity or other conditions in which aggressive handling could be too stressful

C. COMPONENTS OF EFFECTIVE COUGH MECHANISM IN SUCCESSION

1. Deep inspiratory effort
2. Held inspiration to allow peripheral diffusion of gas
3. Tight closure of glottis
4. Strong contraction of abdominal and thoracic muscles to increase intrathoracic pressure
5. Rapid opening of glottis

D. EQUIPMENT

1. Bag for positive pressure ventilation by hand
   a. Manometer
   b. ET tube or mask
2. Suction equipment
3. Cardiorespiratory monitor
4. Continuous blood-gas monitor

E. PRECAUTIONS

1. Use only peak inspiratory pressures that are in range of peak mechanical pressure for the infant.
2. Avoid compression of ribs over liver, spleen, heart, or recent thoracotomy.
3. Do not use where abrupt increases in intracranial pressure are deleterious.
4. Reserve this treatment for infants in whom normal suctioning fails to clear inspissated tracheobronchial secretions.

F. TECHNIQUE

Requires two persons (one to apply the sigh and one to apply the compression)

1. Complete other components of respiratory physical therapy as prescribed.
   a. Postural drainage
   b. Vibration
   c. Percussion

   Because the normal components of the cough mechanism are incomplete, the cough that occurs during deep tracheal suctioning is irritative and rarely effective and secretions may not be brought as close to the suction catheter as needed for removal.

2. Position infant in supine, head-down, or neutral, flat position.
3. Apply sigh with inflation hold for 1 to 2 seconds at 5 cm H_2O pressure higher than normal peak inspiratory pressure.
4. On release of inspiration hold, with both hands apply quick chest compression of 1 to 2 cm displacement over lower chest. Compress in direction of bronchial drainage, toward trachea.
5. Suction airway.
6. Ventilate infant after suctioning until stable.
7. Repeat, with suctioning as indicated for audible or palpable airway secretions.
8. Apply sigh with inflation hold at end of cough simulation therapy.

G. COMPLICATIONS

1. Rib fractures
2. Pulmonary air leak
3. Hematoma of underlying viscera
4. Acute increase in venous blood pressure

Tracheal Suctioning

Suctioning of the nose, mouth, and pharynx is potentially quite traumatic in neonates. The same equipment, precautions, and complications apply as for tracheal suctioning. When properly used, bulb syringes are as effective for oral and nasal clearance as suction catheters and cause fewer side effects.[16] Always suction an ET tube before suctioning the mouth; suction the mouth before the nose.

When continuous suctioning of the mouth is required in infants who will accept a pacifier, a sump device may be made by the following simple adaptation of commonly available equipment[17]: Cut extra side holes in a standard suction tube. Cut 2–3 holes in the nipple of the pacifier. Insert the tube into an open-ended pacifier and tie it securely with umbilical tie tape to make airtight seal. Make certain tube coils within pacifier and does not protrude from holes. Allow infant to suck on pacifier with catheter attached to continuous suction.

A. INDICATIONS

1. To clear tracheobronchial airway of secretions (Fig. 34-6)
2. To keep artificial airway patent
3. To obtain material for analysis or culture

B. RELATIVE CONTRAINDICATIONS

1. Recent surgery in the area
2. Extreme reactive bradycardia
3. Pulmonary hemorrhage

C. EQUIPMENT

Sterile

1. Saline for instillation into airway
2. Saline or water for irrigation of catheter
3. Gloves
4. Suction catheters
   a. Available safety features
      (1) Markings at measured intervals
      (2) Microscopically smooth surface
      (3) Multiple side holes in different planes
      (4) Large bore hole for occlusion to initiate vacuum
      (5) No more than half the inside diameter of artificial airway
         (a) Use 8 Fr for ET tube > 3.5 mm.
         (b) Use 5 Fr for ET tube < 3.5 mm.
   b. Ideal but not readily available features
      (1) Air cushion around tip to minimize contact with mucosa[18]
      (2) Curved at end to facilitate selective bronchial suctioning when indicated[19]

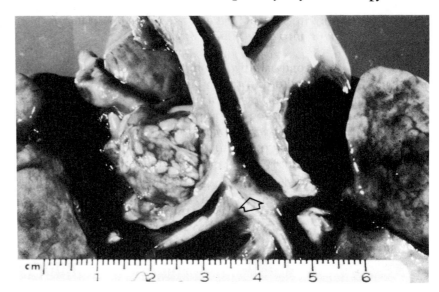

FIG. 34-6
Excessive secretions occluding the left mainstem bronchus evident on posterior opening of trachea at autopsy.

5. Modified endotracheal tube adaptor that allows passage of suction catheter without disconnecting tube from ventilator*[20-22]
6. Vacuum source
   a. Pressure set just high enough to move secretions into suction catheter
   b. Mechanically controlled pressure source

   Pressure generated by oral suction on mucus extractors can be extremely variable and dangerously high.[23]

Unsterile
1. Adjustable vacuum source with specimen trap, tubing, and pressure gauge
2. Ventilatory device as indicated
   a. Manometer
   b. Warmed, humidified oxygen at controlled level
   c. Bag with positive end-expiratory pressure (PEEP) device

D. PRECAUTIONS

1. When feasible, use two people when suctioning airways to minimize risk of patient compromise and complications and to shorten time of procedure.

*Novometrix C/S Suction Adaptor, Novometric Medical Systems, Inc., Wallingford, CT 06492

2. Determine for each patient if it is better to continue mechanical ventilation during the suctioning or to use a sigh with inflation hold after suctioning. Consider effect of interruption of ventilator therapy and loss of lung volume with each catheter passage.
3. Allow patient to recover between passages of catheter.
4. Stabilize head and airway to prevent tube dislodgement.
5. Assess secretions by auscultation and palpation to determine frequency for suctioning.
   a. Avoid unnecessary suctioning just to follow a schedule.
   b. Schedule prophylactic suctioning for tube patency only as often as needed to maintain it.
   c. Consider increase in monitored airway resistance as indication for suctioning.[24]
6. Readjust humidification as indicated by character and volume of secretions.
7. Avoid inadvertent suction during insertion of catheter.
8. Use lowest vacuum pressure effective in clearing secretions within a few seconds.
9. Do not insert catheter as far as it will go or until reflex cough occurs. Use prescribed length. Do not suction if catheter is inserted too far.

Just touching the catheter to the tracheal wall may cause trauma. This is very fragile tissue and should be treated as such.

10. Limit time of insertion and suctioning to least time required to remove secretions.

E. TECHNIQUE FOR INTUBATED PATIENTS

1. For artificial airways, use sterile technique with one sterile gloved hand and one free hand.
2. When possible, monitor oxygenation continuously.

   A suction pressure of 52 mm Hg applied to an airway for 15 seconds decreases the mean PO_2 from 72 to 43 mm Hg.[25]

3. Monitor heart rate continuously.
4. It is usually best to remove infant from ventilator and have second person perform assisted ventilation manually, using following guidelines adjusted to individual needs.
   a. FIO_2 set at or up to 10% higher than baseline
      (1) Monitor oxygenation; adjust FIO_2 to prevent swings in oxygenation.
      (2) Evaluate effect of procedure.
   b. Peak inspiratory pressure as on ventilator or up to 10 cm H_2O higher
   c. Continuous distending airway pressures same as on ventilator
   d. Respiratory rate 40 to 60 breaths per minute, applying an inspiratory hold intermittently

   When there is a high risk of pulmonary air leak as in the presence of significant interstitial emphysema, it may be safer to use a technique of rapid manual ventilation at lower peak pressure instead of sighing with a prolonged inspiratory pressure. In other cases, in which loss of lung volume with suctioning is of greater concern, use sigh with a hold on inflation at a rate similar to ventilator. With suctioning, there is a loss of lung volume with a decrease in compliance. The adverse effect persists for a significant time when mechanical ventilation at the same settings is used during and after the suction procedure.

5. Determine length of ET tube plus adapter and note on suction catheter as limit of depth of insertion.

6. Set vacuum at lowest level to achieve removal of secretions.

   The level of vacuum required depends on a number of variables, including
      a. Air-tightness of system and fluctuations in generated vacuum pressures
      b. Accuracy of manometer
      c. Diameter of catheter (smaller catheter, higher pressure)
      d. Thickness and tenacity of secretions

7. Holding catheter in one hand, moisten tip with water or saline. Note appropriateness of suction level by rate of liquid uptake. Adjust pressure with free hand.
8. Open artificial airway with free hand.
   a. Detach from bag; hold oxygen near end of tube, or
   b. Open suction port of specialized ET tube adapter.
9. With free hand, stabilize airway. Pass catheter down airway to depth limit noted for the patient's ET tube. Do not apply vacuum during insertion (i.e., keep suction-control port open).
10. Close proximal suction-control port and withdraw catheter.
11. Limit time for insertion and removal to 15 to 20 seconds.
12. Reattach ET tube to bag and ventilate for 10 to 15 breaths or until patient is stable.
    a. Note oxygenation.
    b. Note heart rate.
    c. Note chest excursions.
13. If secretions are thick or tenacious, instill 0.25 ml of saline into ET tube and continue ventilation.
14. Clear catheter with sterile water.
15. Repeat process until airway is clear. If suctioning of a mainstem bronchus is indicated (persistent lobar atelectasis or foreign body), place patient in following positions[19,26,27]
    a. Head midline or to left: catheter tends to enter right mainstem bronchus
    b. Patient turned to left, head turned to right: catheter tends to enter left mainstem bronchus

F. COMPLICATIONS

1. Extubation
2. Hypoxia[25]

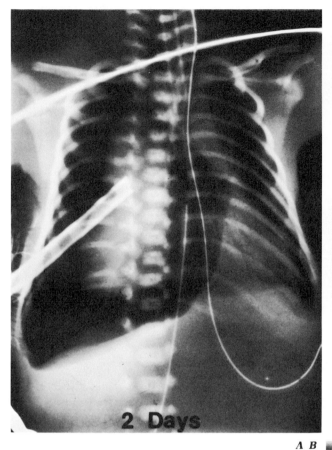

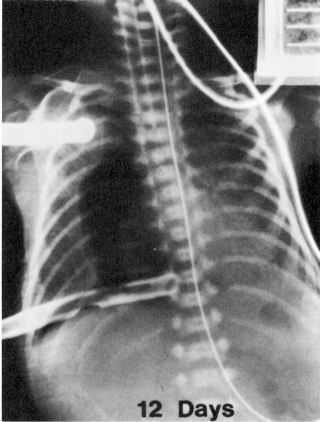

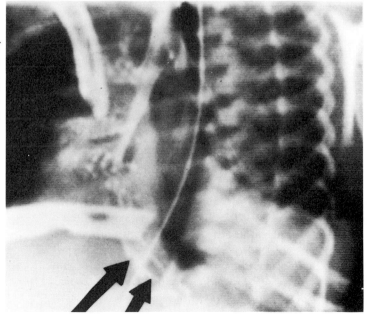

Λ B
C

FIG. 34-7
Three radiographs from same patient with perforation of bronchus from suction catheter. (*A*) Tension pneumothorax on the right side immediately after suctioning at 2 days of age. (*B*) At day 21 the pulmonary air leak remains; chest tubes demonstrated continuous bubbling pattern. (*C*) A bronchogram demonstrates a bronchopleural fistula from the right lower lobe with contrast in the pleural space (*arrows*).

3. Cardiovascular effect
    a. Arrhythmias[28,29]
        (1) Bradycardia
        (2) Premature ventricular contractions
        (3) Arrest[30]
    b. Hypotension
4. Increased intracranial pressure[31]
5. Apnea
6. Loss of lung volume
    a. Local atelectasis[32]
    b. Decreased compliance
    c. Hypoxia
7. Trauma[18]
    a. Tracheal erosion
    b. Perforation of trachea/bronchi and pulmonary air leak[33–35] (Fig. 34-7)
    c. Hemorrhage
    d. Perforation of esophagus (see Fig. 38-2)[35–37]
8. Endobronchial granuloma
    a. Airway obstruction
    b. Atelectasis
9. Infection
    a. Contamination
    b. Bacteremia[38]

References

1. SELSBY D, JONES JG: Some physiological and clinical aspects of chest physiotherapy. Br J Anaesth 64:621, 1990

2. MARTIN W, HERRELL N, RUBIN D, FANAROFF A: Effect of supine and prone position on arterial oxygen tension in the preterm infant. Pediatrics 63:528, 1979

3. WAGAMAN MJ, SHUTACK JG, MOOMJIAN AS ET AL: Improved oxygenation and lung compliance with prone positioning of neonates. J Pediatr 94:787, 1979

4. WYMAN ML, KUHNS LR: Lobar opacification of the lung after tracheal extubation in neonates. J Pediatr 91:109, 1977

5. FINER NN, MORIARTEY RR, BOYD J, ET AL: Postextubation atelectasis: A retrospective review and a prospective controlled study. J Pediatr 94:110, 1979

6. ETCHES P, SCOTT B: Chest physiotherapy in the newborn: Effect on secretion removed. Pediatrics 62:713, 1978

7. COHEN RS, SMITH DW, STEVENSON, DK, ET AL: Lateral decubitus position as therapy for persistent focal pulmonary interstitial emphysema in neonates: A preliminary report. J Pediatr 104:441, 1984

8. SPAHR R, MACDONALD H, MUELLER-HEUBACH E: The effect of the knee-chest position on oxygenation and blood pressure in the sick neonate (abstr). Pediatr Res 13(Part 2):506, 1979

9. HERALA M, GISLASON T: Chest physiotherapy. Evaluation by transcutaneous blood gas monitoring. Chest 93(4):800, 1988

10. FREITAG L, BREMME J, SCHROER M: High frequency oscillation for respiratory physiotherapy. Br J Anaesth 63:44S, 1989

11. WOOD BP: Infant ribs: Generalized periosteal reaction resulting from vibrator chest physiotherapy. Radiology 162:811, 1987

12. FINER NN, BOYD J: Chest physiotherapy in the neonate: A controlled study. Pediatrics 61:282, 1978

13. TUDEHOPE D, BAGLEY C: Techniques of physiotherapy in intubated babies with respiratory distress syndrome. Aust Paediatr J 16:226, 1980

14. TYRELL JC, HILLER EJ, MARTIN J: Face mask physiotherapy in cystic fibrosis. Arch Dis Child 61:598, 1986

15. HALLOWAY R, ADAMS EB, DESAI SD, THAMBIRAN A: Effect of chest physiotherapy on blood gases of neonates treated by intermittent positive pressure respiration. Thorax 24:421, 1969

16. COHEN-ADDAD N, CHATTERJEE M, BAUTISTA A: Intrapartum suctioning of meconium: comparative efficacy of bulb syringe and DeLee catheter. J Perinatol 7:111, 1987

17. HUDDART SN, GORNALL P: Oral suction in infants. J Pediatr Surg 26:666, 1991

18. SACHNER MA, LANDA JF, GREENELTCH N, ROBINSON MJ: Pathogenesis and prevention of tracheobronchial damage with suction procedures. Chest 64:284, 1973

19. BUSH GH: Tracheobronchial suction in infants and children. Br J Anaesth 35:322, 1963

20. CABAL L, DEVASKAR S, PLAJSTEK C, ET AL: An improved technique for airway suctioning (abstr). Pediatr Res 13 (Part 2):532, 1979

21. GUNDERSON LP, MCPHEE AJ, DONOVAN EF: Partially ventilated endotracheal suction. Am J Dis Child 140:462, 1986

22. MAYHALL CG: The Trach Care closed tracheal suctioning system: A new medical device to permit tracheal suctioning without interruption of ventilatory assistance. Infect Control Hosp Epidemiol 9:125, 1988

23. WATKINSON M, RAO JN: Endotracheal suction techniques in the neonate: Arch Dis Child 61:1147, 1986

24. PRENDIVILLE A, THOMSON A, SILVERMAN M: Effect of tracheobronchial suction on respiratory resistance in intubated preterm babies. Arch Dis Child 61:1178 1986

25. FOX WW, SCHWARTZ J, SHAFFER T: Pulmonary physiotherapy in neonates: Physiologic changes and respiratory management. J Pediatr 92:977, 1978

26. FEWELL J, ARRINGTON R, SEIBERT J: The effect of head position and angle of tracheal bifurcation on bronchus

catheterization in the intubated neonate. Pediatrics 64:318, 1979

27. SALEM M, WONG A, MATHRUBHUTAM M, ET AL: Evaluation of selective bronchial suctioning techniques used for infants and children. Anesthesiology 48:379, 1978

28. SHIM C, FINE N, FERNANDEZ R, WILLIAMS MH JR: Cardiac arrhythmias resulting from tracheal suctioning. Ann Intern Med 71:1149, 1969

29. CALDWELL CC, LEVKOFF AH, PUROHIT DM: Paroxysmal supraventricular tachycardia in a neonate. Clin Pediatr 16:579, 1977

30. KEOWN KK: Cardiac arrest during therapeutic tracheal suctioning. Anesth Analg (Cleve) 39:568, 1960

31. PERIMAN JM, VOLPE JJ: Suctioning in the preterm infant: Effects on cerebral blood flow velocity, intracranial pressure and arterial blood pressure. Pediatrics 72:329, 1982

32. BRANDSTATER B, MUALLEM M: Atelectasis following tracheal suction in infants. Anesthesiology 31:468, 1969

33. ANDERSON KD, CHANDRA R: Pneumothorax secondary to perforation of sequential bronchi by suction catheters. J Pediatr Surg 11:687, 1976

34. VAUGHAN RS, MENKE JA, GIACOIA GP: Pneumothorax: A complication of endotracheal tube suctioning. J Pediatr 92:633, 1978

35. CLARK TA, COEN RW, FELDMAN B, PAPILE L: Esophageal perforations in premature infants and comments on the diagnosis. Am J Dis Child 134:367, 1980

36. BAR-MOOR J, SIMON K: Another complication of continuous upper pouch suction in esophageal atresia. J Pediatr Surg 16:730, 1981

37. NAGARAJI H, MULLEN P, GROFF D, ET AL: Iatrogenic perforation of the esophagus in premature infants. Surgery 86:583, 1980

38. STORM W: Transient bacteremia following endotracheal suctioning in ventilated newborns. Pediatrics 65:487, 1980

PLATE 34-1
Positions for postural drainage. Inserts indicate the segments drained for each position. Shading on the infant indicates the area where directed therapy such as percussion and vibration would be emphasized for pathology in airways to those regions.

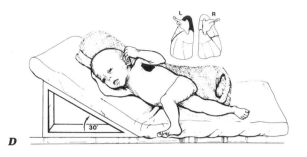

D

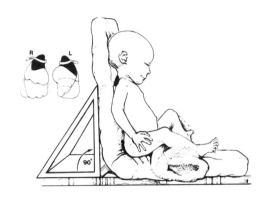

A

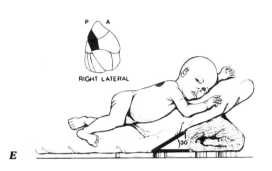

E

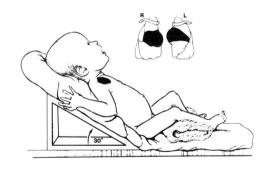

B

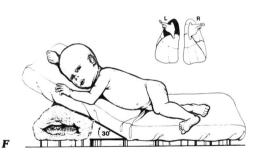

F

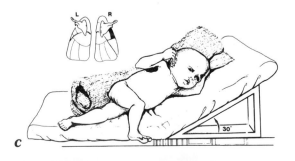

C

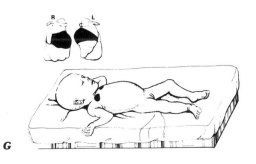

G

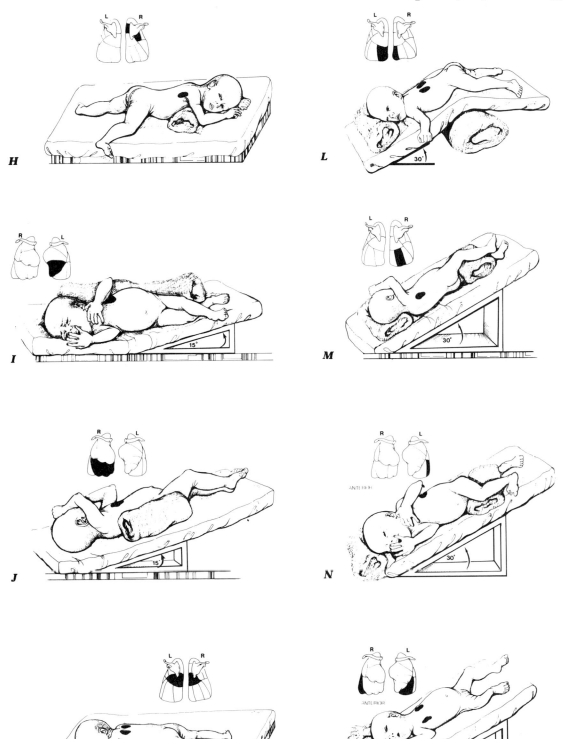

H

I

J

K

L

M

N

O

35 *Flexible Fiberoptic Bronchoscopy*

H. Joel Schmidt*†
Robert J. Fink

A. INDICATIONS[1-6]

1. Confirm endotracheal (ET) tube placement.[7]
2. Bronchoscopically aided intubation of different airways
3. Visualize tone of unanesthetized hypopharynx.
4. Diagnose airway diseases (Table 35-1).[8-10]
   a. Malformations
   b. Causes of abnormal phonation
   c. Reasons for failed extubation
   d. Acute pathology
   e. Foreign body
5. Obtain direct bronchoalveolar specimens.
6. Lavage atelectatic lobes.

B. CONTRAINDICTIONS

1. Severe thrombocytopenia
2. Unresponsive hypoxemia
3. Extreme ventilator dependence
4. Diameter of nares or artificial airway limits size and passage of bronchoscope (Table 35-2).

   Soft cartilage allows for the passage of a bronchoscope that is somewhat larger than the nasal orifice.

5. The cricoid diameter is not dilatable and can limit access to the lower airway.

   The cricoid diameter in millimeters can be approximated by dividing the gestational age in weeks by 10 and adding 0.5. For example, an appropriately grown infant at 30 weeks gestation would have a cricoid diameter of 30/10 + 0.5 or 3.5 mm and would allow the passage of a scope size no greater than this.

C. PRECAUTIONS

1. Keep patient NPO for 4 to 6 hours, and evacuate the gastric contents to decrease the risk of aspiration.

---

*Major, U.S. Army.

†The opinions contained herein are those of the author and are not to be considered as the official views of the Department of the Army or Defense.

2. Monitor the patient throughout the procedure and until stable.
3. Have an attendant observe the patient and the monitors while the bronchoscopist attends to the procedure.
4. Assume that an infant cannot ventilate around a 3.5 mm flexible bronchoscope and limit the time of airway obstruction.
5. Avoid excessive sedation that would decrease respiratory drive.
6. Maintain full visualization while advancing the scope. If the field is obscured, clear the secretions before advancing the scope.
7. Withdraw the bronchoscope slowly to prevent trauma.

TABLE 35-1

Diagnoses that Can Be Aided by Flexible Laryngoscopy/Bronchoscopy

Area	Diagnosis
Larynx	Laryngomalacia
	Cyst
	Hemangioma
	Cleft
	Vocal cord paralysis
Trachea	Subglottic stenosis
	Congenital
	Acquired
	Tracheomalacia
	Granuloma
	Complete tracheal rings
	Tracheo-esophageal fistula
	Vascular rings
Bronchi to alveoli	Edema
	Infection
	Aspiration
	Mucous plugging
	Hemoptysis

TABLE 35-2
Minimal Airway Size for Flexible Bronchoscope

Scope Outer Diameter (mm)	ET Tube Size	Tracheostomy Tube Size
<1.8	2.5	00
2.2–2.4	3.0	00
2.5–2.7	3.5	0
3.5–3.6	4.5	2

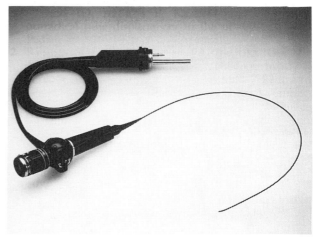

FIG. 35-1
Pediatric flexible fiberoptic bronchoscope, Olympus Model BF-N20. (Photo provided by Olympus Corporation.)

8. If topical anesthesia is used on the oropharynx, keep the patient NPO for at least 30 minutes after the procedure.
9. In unstable patients not already intubated, electively intubate with the largest possible ET tube.
10. Use plastic specimen traps for sample collection to prevent alveolar macrophage adherence to glass.

D. EQUIPMENT

1. Supplemental oxygen
2. Suction apparatus with two suction lines.
3. Cardiorespiratory monitor
4. Pulse oximeter
5. Universal precaution apparel including goggles (see Chap. 4, Aseptic Preparation).
6. Flexible fiberoptic bronchoscope (Table 35-3, Fig. 35-1)
7. Swivel adapter with port (if using ET tube) (Fig. 35-2)
8. Plastic specimen traps
9. Light source with at least a 250 watt lamp

TABLE 35-3
Selected Pediatric Flexible Fiberoptic Bronchoscopes

Type	Outer Diameter (mm)	Suction Size (mm)	Distal Flexion Capability	Indications
Neonatal*	1.8, 2.3, and 2.4	none	no	visual diagnosis via artificial airway
	2.2	none	yes	visual diagnosis to include segmental bronchi via any route
	2.5	0.5	no	visual diagnosis via artificial airway plus lavage capabilities
	2.7	none	yes	same as for 2.2 mm
Pediatric	3.5† and 3.6*	1.2	yes	diagnosis, treatment, and sampling in 30+ week normally sized infant via the nose or an artificial airway

*Olympus Corporation, Medical Instrument Division, 4 Nevada Dr., Lake Success, New York 11042
†Pentax, Precision Instrument Corporation, 30 Ramland Road, Orangeburg, NY 10962-269

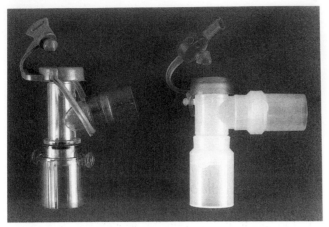

Fig. 35-2
Examples of Swivel airway adapters (*right*, Marquest Medical Products, Inc., Englewood, CO 80112, Model # 178800; *left*, Mallinckrodt Critical Care, Division of Mallinckrodt, Inc., 73 Quaker Road, Glens Falls, New York 12801, Cat.#85882)

A 400–500 watt source is preferred, particularly for the smaller scopes because of the smaller light fiber bundles.

10. Medicines
    a. 4% cardiac lidocaine diluted to 1% with non-bacteriostatic saline
    b. 2% xylocaine jelly for nasal route
    c. Sterile, water-soluble lubrication jelly for ET tube route.
    d. Drugs needed for CPR readily available.
11. Preservative-free 0.9% saline solution for lavage
12. Ventilation bag, mask, and laryngoscope with appropriately sized ET tubes

E. TECHNIQUE: TRANSNASAL LARYNGOSCOPY[8]

1. Prepare the patient as outlined in Precautions.
2. Place the patient supine on the examination table under a warming unit, or in incubator with the bronchoscopist at the patient's head.
3. Position the patient as for endotracheal intubation with a towel roll under the neck and shoulders (Fig. 32-2).
4. Gently restrain or swaddle the patient. See Chapter 3, Restraint.

5. Instill 1 ml of 1% lidocaine solution into the larger nostril.
6. Select a bronchoscope with distal flexion capabilities and a diameter no more than the size of the nares.
7. Lubricate the tip of the scope with 2% xylocaine jelly.
8. Hold the flexible bronchoscope as in Figure 35-3.
9. Slowly advance the scope through the nose with the guiding hand stabilized by the last two fingers on the patient's cheek.
10. Guide the scope through the largest passage (usually between the middle and inferior turbinates, and the septum).
11. Once through the nose, visualize the larynx by slightly flexing the bronchoscope tip anteriorly.

    The plane of flexion can be rotated by rolling the shaft of the flexible bronchoscope between the thumb and two fingers of the hand guiding the scope through the patient's nose.

12. When the laryngoscopy is complete, withdraw the scope slowly.

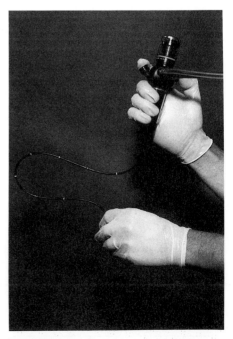

FIG. 35-3
Holding the flexible fiberoptic bronchoscope.

F. TECHNIQUE: TRANSNASAL BRONCHOSCOPY

1. Visualize the larynx as above, using an appropriately sized flexible bronchoscope with suction and distal flexion capability (see section B, 4-5).
2. Instill 0.5 to 1 ml of 1% lidocaine on the larynx through the suction channel and wait 1 to 2 minutes.
3. Decisively pass the tip between the cords while simultaneously flexing posteriorly so as to end up at least two centimeters below the cords.

   Passing the cords slowly can cause unnecessary damage to the cords if the patient should cough as the cords are passed.

4. Guide the scope down the trachea by feeding it through fingers. Stay in the middle of the trachea so as not to cause abrasions to the mucosa.
5. Once in the trachea apply more topical anesthesia as necessary to control coughing.
6. Sequentially examine the airways. Steer by flexing the tip and rotating the shaft of the flexible scope.

   It is best to view the normal segments first and then progress to the areas in question.

7. Instill air or oxygen via the suction channel to assist in insufflating atelectatic areas, using a flow rate of 1 L/min and occluding the suction port for half-second periods.
8. In those infants unable to breath around the scope, withdraw the scope often enough to allow ventilation.
9. Slowly withdraw the flexible bronchoscope while visualizing the field.

   The sub-glottic space is best viewed while withdrawing from the trachea.

G. TECHNIQUE: BRONCHOSCOPY VIA ARTIFICIAL AIRWAY[11]

1. Restrain the infant, keeping the neck in the neutral position as for usual ventilator support.
2. Select a bronchoscope with an outer diameter at least 0.8 mm smaller than the inner diameter of the artificial airway to allow easy passage while maintaining some ventilation of the infant.
3. Attach a swivel adapter with a suction port (Fig. 35-2) to the ET tube in place.

4. Suction the artificial airway with a suction catheter prior to passing the flexible scope.
5. Lubricate the tip of the scope with a small quantity of sterile, water-soluble lubricant. Pass the scope through the ET or tracheostomy tube until the airway comes into view.
6. Examine the airways as above.
7. Verify the position of artificial airway as the scope is withdrawn.[7]

H. TECHNIQUE: BRONCHOALVEOLAR LAVAGE

1. Use a flexible bronchoscope with a suction channel.
2. Visualize the airway as described above.
3. Place a suction trap on the suction adapter of the scope.
4. Gently wedge the tip of the bronchoscope in the affected bronchus.
5. While interrupting the suction to the scope, instill nonbacteriostatic saline through the suction port into the isolated airway.

   Use volumes of 5 ml for infants less than 3 kg, and 10 or 15 ml for larger infants.

6. Apply suction to the scope and retrieve as much of the instilled volume as possible.

   About half of the volume instilled can be suctioned back into the trap. Brief repeated suctioning is recommended over prolonged suction because the airway is less likely to collapse, and prolonged suctioning can produce atelectasis by degassing the alveoli.

7. Process specimens
   a. Use plastic containers to decrease alveolar macrophage adherence.
   b. Process as quickly as possible. See Table 35-4 for helpful tests.
8. For therapeutic lavage, perform multiple small volume lavages to the affected area.

I. TECHNIQUE: ET TUBE PLACEMENT

1. Perform flexible bronchoscopy as in G above.
2. Select the smaller flexible bronchoscope.
3. Identify the carina, taking care not to confuse the right upper lobe/bronchus intermedius branching with the mainstem carina.[7]

TABLE 35-4

Helpful Tests for Bronchoalveolar Lavage Sample

Test Category	Type of Test
Stains	Acid-fast stain
	Gram stain
	KOH stain
	Lipid laden macrophage quantitation
	Pneumocystis stains
	Vegetable cell wall stain
	Wright's stain
Cultures	Bacterial
	Fungal
	Mycobacterial
	Mycoplasma
	Viral
Antigen testing	Herpes simplex
	Influenza
	Legionella
	RSV

---

4. Position the tip of the endotracheal tube at least 1 cm above the carina.

J. TECHNIQUE: BRONCHOSCOPIC NASOTRACHEAL INTUBATION

1. Select the proper sized ET tube (see Section B, 4–5).

   A 4.0 ET tube can be inserted over a 3.6 mm bronchoscope, but it will not be possible to reinsert the bronchoscope.

2. Lubricate and pass the bronchoscope through the ET tube, pulling the tube all the way up the shaft of the scope. Remove the lubricant from the shaft.
3. Under direct visualization advance the bronchoscope to the carina. See Section F above.
4. Advance the ET tube over the shaft using a twisting motion on the tube. Additional lubrication to the outside of the ET tube may be necessary at the nose.
5. Once the tube is below the cords, hold it in place and withdraw the scope until the tube tip comes into view. Advance both to the proper position above the carina.
6. Hold the tube firmly at the nose and remove the scope.

7. Secure the tube (see Chap. 32, Tracheal Intubation).
8. Recheck the tube position as above.

K. COMPLICATIONS

1. Hypoxia
   a. Obstructed airway
   b. Mobilized secretions or saline left after lavage
2. Bradycardia from vagal stimulation due to inadequate topical anesthesia
3. Laryngospasm/bronchospasm secondary to mechanical stimulation to an area with inadequate topical anesthesia
4. Infections
   a. Spread of infectious material following lavage
   b. Bacterial endocarditis

   Prophylax patients with congenital heart disease.

   c. Introduction of pathogens from upper airway
5. Pneumothorax from excessive gas insufflation or lavage
6. Bleeding
   a. Epistaxis
   b. Friable mucosa or mucosal abrasions
7. Laryngeal trauma

References

1. FAN LL, SPARKS LM, DULINSKI JP: Applications of an ultrathin flexible bronchoscope for neonatal and pediatric airway problems. Chest 89:673, 1986
2. NUSSBAUM E. Flexible fiberoptic bronchoscopy and laryngoscopy in children under 2 years of age: Diagnostic and therapeutic applications of a new pediatric flexible fiberoptic bronchoscope. Crit Care Med 10:770, 1982
3. WOOD R: Clinical applications of ultrathin flexible bronchoscopes. Pediatr Pulmonol 1:244, 1985
4. WOOD RE: Spelunking in the pediatric airways: Explorations with the flexible fiberoptic bronchoscope. Pediatr Clin North Am 31:785, 1984
5. WOOD RE, FINK RJ: Applications of flexible fiberoptic bronchoscopes in infants and children. Chest 73:737, 1978
6. WOOD RE, POSTMA D: Endoscopy of the airway in infants and children. J Pediatr 112:1, 1988
7. VIGNESWARAN R, WHITFIELD JM: The use of a new ultra-thin fiberoptic bronchoscope to determine en-

dotracheal tube position in the sick newborn infant. 80:174, 1981

8. FAN LL, FLYNN JW: Laryngoscopy in neonates and infants: Experience with the flexible fiberoptic bronchoscope. Laryngoscope 91:451, 1981

9. MILLER RW, WOO P, KELLMAN RK, SLAGLE TS: Tracheobronchial abnormalities in infants with bronchopulmonary dysplasia. J Pediatr 111:779, 1987

10. COLOMBO JL, HALLBERG TK: Recurrent aspiration in children: Lipid-laden alveolar macrophage quantitation. Pediatr Pulmonol 3:86, 1987

11. SHINWELL ES, HIGGINS RD, AUTEN RL, SHAPIRO DL: Fiberoptic bronchoscopy in the treatment of intubated neonates. Am J Dis Child 143:1064, 1989

Part 7
Tube Placement

36 Thoracostomy Tubes

Mary Ann Fletcher
Martin Raymond Eichelberger

Drainage of air or fluid accumulations in the thorax is an important procedure in neonatal units, often performed as an emergency. Physicians who assume the primary responsibility for inserting and caring for chest tubes must recognize that complications in insertion and maintenance occur regularly. Anticipating potential need, keeping appropriate equipment available, and using proper anatomical approaches helps to lessen difficulties. Once a chest tube is in place, proper functioning requires continued assessment.

A. INDICATIONS

1. Evacuation of pneumothorax
   a. Tension
   b. Lung collapse with ventilation/perfusion abnormality
   c. Bronchopleural fistula
2. Evacuation of large pleural fluid collections
   a. Postoperative hemothorax
   b. Empyema
   c. Chylothorax
3. Extrapleural drainage after surgical repair of esophagus

B. CONTRAINDICATIONS

1. Smaller air or fluid collection without significant symptoms
2. Spontaneous pneumothorax that, in the absence of lung disease, is likely to resolve without intervention

C. EQUIPMENT

Sterile

1. General all purpose tray with No. 15 surgical blade and curved hemostats
2. Gloves
3. Surgical drapes
4. Transillumination device with sterile glove to cover tip

5. Thoracostomy tube: Techniques of insertion differ with each type. See original references for description of technique variations.[1,2]
   a. Straight polyvinylchloride (PVC) tube with or without trocar, 8 to 10 Fr
   b. Pigtail
      (1) PVC with pigtail at 90 degree angle to shaft[1]
         (a) 8 to 10 Fr
         (b) total length 10 cm
         (c) insertion with or without trocar
      (2) Polyurethane modified vascular catheter with pigtail in same plane as shaft[2]
         (a) 8.5 Fr
         (b) total length 15 cm
         (c) insertion guide wire and dilator for insertion by Seldinger technique
6. Evacuation device (select one)
   a. Infant thoracostomy tube set: There are several commercially available units appropriate for infants (Fig. 36-1).
      (1) Evacuation rate[3]
         (a) With single tube, capacity depends on level of water in chamber (cm H_2O).
         (b) With multiple tubes, capacity also depends on applied vacuum.
      (2) Negative pressure of 20 cm H_2O evacuates more than 4 liters air/minute in experimental setting.[3]
         (a) Appropriate starting point for most infants with lung disease on ventilators (10–15 cm H_2O)
         (b) Potentially inadequate for bronchopleural fistula
         (c) Excessive and potentially harmful in changing intrapulmonary airflow in presence of smaller pleural leak (use 10 cm H_2O)

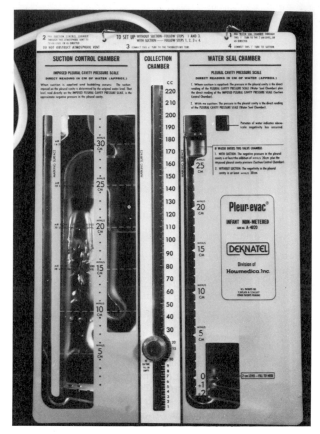

FIG. 36-1
One model of an underwater drainage system demonstrating the three necessary chambers. Systems now are compact and easy to set up and read. This system is set at 22 cm H_2O as would be necessary only for a rapid rate of air accumulation.

> Measured rates across bronchopleural fistulas in infants have indicated ranges from 30 to 600 ml/min.[4] If suction pressure is too high, gas flow to alveoli may be diverted across a fistula. The pressure and flow applied to the endotracheal tube also directly influences flow across a fistula.[5] Because there are many interactive factors in how much air might have to be evacuated, there can be no single best suction level for all patients; the most effective, least harmful level has to be determined for each situation.

    b. Heimlich one-way flutter valve[6,7] (Bard-Parker) (Fig. 36-2)
        (1) Temporary substitute for underwater seal
            (a) Useful during transport or delivery-room care

            (b) Less effective without suction
                1) With rapid intrapleural accumulation
                2) In debilitated infants who cannot generate enough pressure on exhalation to force intrapleural air through valve
        (2) Ineffective in presence of fluid when valve remains open
    c. Bottles connected in-line with appropriate adapters and connecting tubing (Fig. 36-3)
        (1) Underwater seal bottle
        (2) Vacuum breaker bottle
        (3) Overflow bottle
  7. Nonabsorbable suture on small cutting needle, 4.0
  8. Cotton-tipped applicators
  9. Semipermeable transparent dressing
 10. Antibiotic ointment
 11. Petroleum gauze

Unsterile
1. Tincture of benzoin
2. $\frac{1}{2}$-inch adhesive tape
3. Towel roll

D. FACTORS INFLUENCING EFFICIENCY OF AIR EVACUATION

1. Contiguity of air to chest-tube portals that are patent
    a. In supine infant, air accumulates in the medial, anterior, or inferior hemithorax, making low, anterior location for tip of tube ideal for evacuation.[8]
    b. Negative pressure on chest tube may draw tissue into side portals and occlude them.
2. Rate of air accumulation proportional to
    a. Airway flow and pressure

> Dennis and associates demonstrated in experimental rabbits that a positive end-expiratory pressure (PEEP) level above 6 cm H_2O resulted in greater air leak than peak inspiratory pressure (PIP), up to 30 cm H_2O PIP.[9]

    b. Size of fistula or tear
    c. Infant position

> If the affected side is the dependent hemithorax, and therefore is splinted, there is a lower rate of

FIG. 36-2
Heimlich valve.

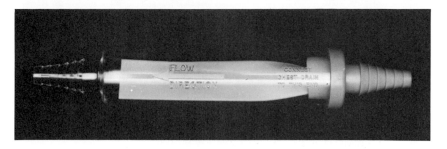

air leak than if the affected side is not dependent or is elevated.[10]

3. Rate of evacuation
  a. directly proportional to
    (1) Internal radius of chest tube(r^4)
    (2) Pressure gradient across tube (P)
      (a) Suction pressure applied

The negative pressure applied may affect intrapleural pressure only in the immediate vicinity of the tip of the tube.[3]

      (b) Positive intrathoracic pressure during exhalation, spontaneous or mechanical

  b. inversely proportional to length of tube (l) and viscosity (h)

Poiseuille's law regarding flow across a tube:
$$F = \frac{DP\pi r^4}{8hl}$$

(F = flow; DP = pressure gradient; r = radius; h = viscosity, l = length)

E. PRECAUTIONS

1. Anticipate which infant is at risk to develop pulmonary air leak, and keep equipment for diagnosis and emergency evacuation at hand.[11–15]

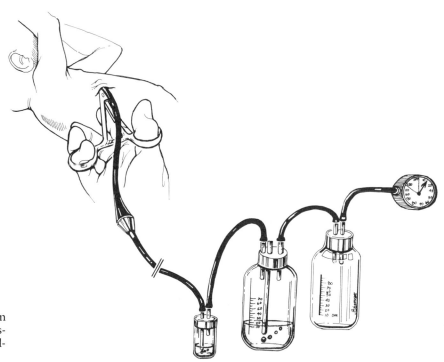

FIG. 36-3
An underwater collection system demonstrating the basic elements necessary for collecting air or fluid without allowing return leakage into chest tube.

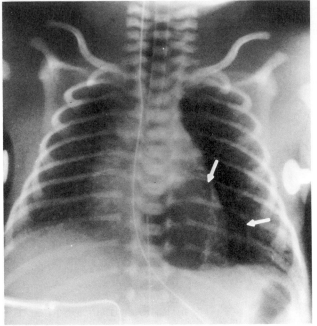
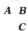
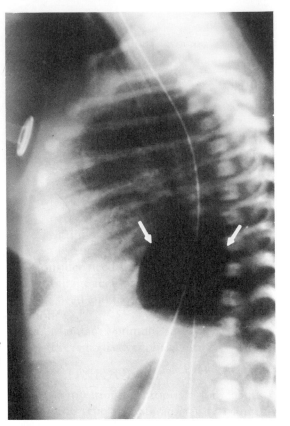

A B
C

FIG. 36-4

Sequential radiographs. (*A*) An AP radiograph demonstrating a cystic lucency at the left base behind the heart that resembles the artifact caused by taking a film through the hole in the top of an incubator. Note also the coarse, irregular lucencies of interstitial emphysema (PIE) in the left lung. (*B*) Lateral film showing the lucency to be real (*arrows*) and, in this case, a pneumomediastinum located most probably in the left inferior pulmonary ligament. (*C*) PIE or air in the pulmonary ligament are often harbingers of impending pneumothorax, in this case, a tension pneumothorax. Note low position of ET tube.

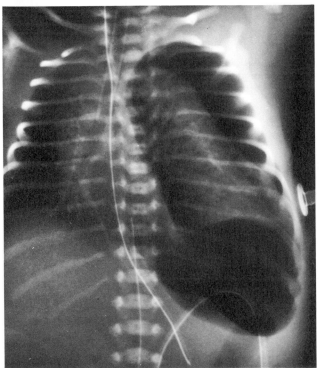

2. Recognize that transillumination may be misleading.[16,17]
   a. True positive
      (1) Follows shape of thoracic cavity (not corona of light source)
      (2) Varies with respiration and position
      (3) Has larger area compared to corona of light at another, normal site
   b. False-positive
      (1) Subcutaneous edema
      (2) Subcutaneous air
      (3) Extrapleural air not in contact with pleural space
   c. False-negative
      (1) Thick chest wall
      (2) Darkly pigmented skin
      (3) Area over air accumulation obscured by dressing or monitor probe
      (4) Weak light because of fiberoptic deterioration or voltage turned too low
      (5) Room too light
      (6) Abnormal color vision in observer
3. Distinguish pleural air collections from skin folds, thymus, Mach effect, artifacts, or other nonpleural, intrathoracic air collections on radiograph (Figs. 36-4 to 36-7).[8,18,19]

4. Select the appropriate insertion site (Figs. 36-8, 36-9).

   Allen recommends insertion of the thoracostomy tube in the anterior–superior portion of the chest wall, first to third intercostal space at the midclavicular line, to ensure anterior placement of the chest tube tip.[20] While an anterior insertion may be appropriate for the right-angled pigtail tube used by Allen et al, a properly placed lateral tube will have its tip anterior but, more important, will not leave a more visible scar on the anterior chest (see Fig. 36-20, page 327).

   a. Reduces complications
   b. Facilitates insertion of thoracostomy tube into appropriate position
      (1) Anterior–medial tip for air collections
      (2) Posterior tip for fluid accumulation
5. Use a tunnel approach across two rib spaces rather than from skin directly into pleural space. The tunnel will help prevent atmospheric air from entering through insertion site, particularly after removal of tube (Fig. 36-10, A, B).
6. While inserting the chest tube, allow some air to remain within pleural space as protective buffer between lung and chest wall.[21]

FIG. 36-5
Radiographic artifact of cystic lucency behind the heart (*arrows*) caused by taking film through top of incubator. The lateral film was negative, therefore excluding a cystic pulmonary lesion or air in the pulmonary ligament.

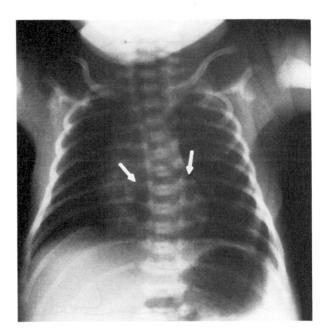

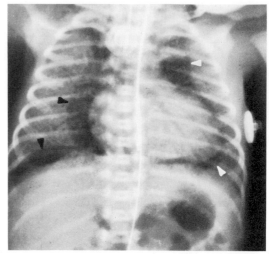

A
B C

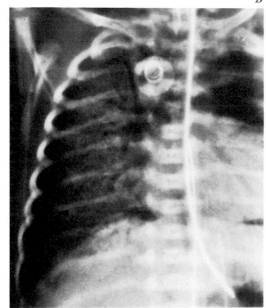 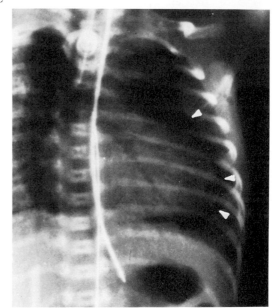

FIG. 36-6
(*A*) AP radiograph demonstrates ventral air over the hemidiaphragms and around the heart (*white and black arrowheads*). The sometimes difficult question of pneumothorax versus pneumomediastinum is answered by the decubitus films. (*B*) The left lateral decubitus radiograph (right side up) shows that the right-sided gas is a pneumothorax (*black arrowheads*). (*C*) The right decubitus film indicates that the adventitial air fails to come up over the lung and is located in the mediastinum (*white arrowheads*). This important distinction is made obvious by the decubitus radiographs.

FIG. 36-7

(A) On this AP supine film, there is a line that parallels the chest wall (*arrowheads*), which suggests the presence of a pneumothorax. (B) This left decubitus film (right side up) confirms this line to be a skin fold, negative for air. When there is a question of potential adventitial air or of the anatomic location of real adventitial air, a decubitus film with the side in question up is the most important radiographic study.

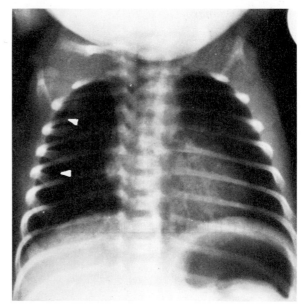

A
B

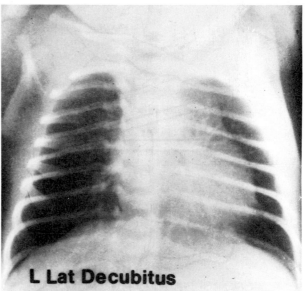

FIG. 36-8

Anterior versus posterior position of the tube for drainage of air or fluid. As air collects anteromedially in the supine neonate, the posterior tip is less appropriate.

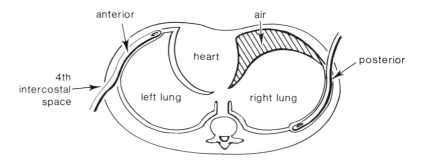

FIG. 36-9
Sequential radiographs in patient with right pneumothorax. An air collection in supine neonates (*A*) is most effectively treated with an anteromedial chest tube (*B* and *C*). The medial extension is falsely exaggerated by the slight right posterior oblique position of the chest. Pulling this tube back might put the side holes outside the pleural space. There is a pneumomediastinum, most evident on the lateral view, not drained by the pleural tube. Note the nuchal air on all three films.

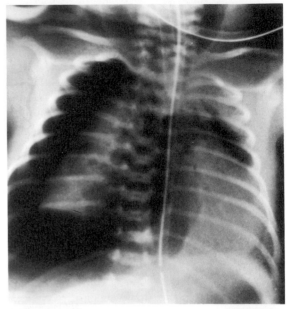

A
B C

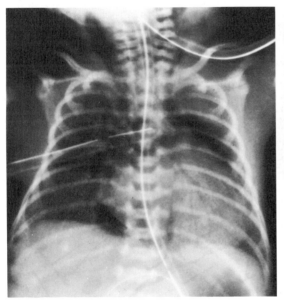

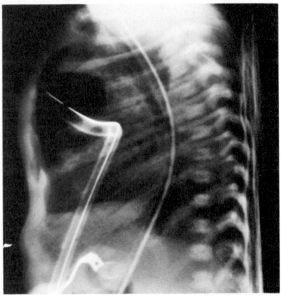

a. Use emergency evacuation only to reverse critical patient compromise. Remove air only until vital signs are stable.

b. Position infant so point of entry is the most elevated area of chest.
(1) Allows air to rise and to provide protective buffer
(2) Aids in directing tip anteriorly toward apex of thorax

7. Consider the possibility that a rapid, complete evacuation may cause an abrupt increase in mean arterial blood pressure and cerebral blood velocity to undesirable, supranormal levels.[22]

8. Avoid positioning infant in lateral decubitus position for any longer than necessary with "normal" lung dependent, thereby further compromising ventilation.

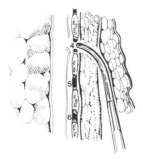

FIG. 36-10
Chest wall in cross section. A thoracostomy tube should enter the pleural space through a tunnel under the skin across at least one rib space to minimize the potential for outside air to gain entry into the pleural cavity.

9. To prevent laceration of lung parenchyma, avoid inserting needles beyond parietal pleura for diagnostic or emergency taps. Use a straight clamp perpendicular to needle shaft to limit depth of penetration (Fig. 36-11).

10. Do not use purse-string suturing of incision site because resulting scars tend to pucker[23] (Fig. 36-20).

11. Recognize that air leaks are likely to persist after initial evacuation in the presence of continuing lung disease or positive-pressure ventilation.

    In their series, Bhatia et al[24] noted that only 50% of the patients resolved their air leaks within the first 4 days after chest tube placement, and 83% resolved after 7 days.

    a. Continue to watch for patency of chest tube (Fig. 36-12).
    b. Verify that tube position remains correct.
    c. Modify positive pressure ventilator patterns to minimize risk for further air leaks.[14]
       (1) Decrease inspiratory time.
       (2) Decrease mean airway pressure.
    d. Position infant with the side of pleural gas leak dependent.[10]

F. TECHNIQUE

Insertion of Anterior Tube for Pneumothorax

1. Determine location of air collection.
   a. Physical examination

   Auscultation of the small neonatal chest may be misleading because the breath sounds normally

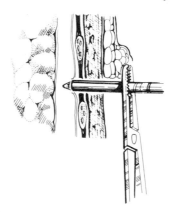

FIG. 36-11
Chest wall in cross section. If there is need to use a needle or trocar to enter the pleural space, its depth of penetration should be limited by a perpendicular clamp.

are bronchotubular and may be relatively well transmitted across an air-filled hemithorax. Also, shift of point of maximal impulse (PMI) toward the other side is unusual in the presence of noncompliant lungs. Physical findings of acute abdominal distention, irritability, and cyanosis or a change in transthoracic impedance suggest an air leak but not its location.[25,26] Supplementary diagnostic procedures are usually necessary.

   b. Transillumination[16]
   c. Radiograph[8,18,27]
   d. Comparative thermography: Temperature on the affected side may be 0.3 to 0.5°C lower than on the unaffected side.[28]

2. Artificially ventilate infant as required. The majority of infants with a pneumothorax requiring a chest tube also need ventilatory support.

3. Monitor vital signs. Move any electrodes from operative site to alternative monitoring areas.

4. Position infant with affected side elevated 60 to 75 degrees off the bed and support back with towel roll. Secure arm across the head, with shoulder internally rotated and extended (Fig. 36-13, A).

   This position is very important as it allows air to rise to the point of entry into the thoracic cavity, outlines the latissimus dorsi muscle, and encourages the correct anterior direction of the tube.

5. Prepare the skin with an iodophor antiseptic over

FIG. 36-12

Evaluation of a chest tube: flow chart to determine how well a chest tube is evacuating pleural air leak and when tube should be removed.

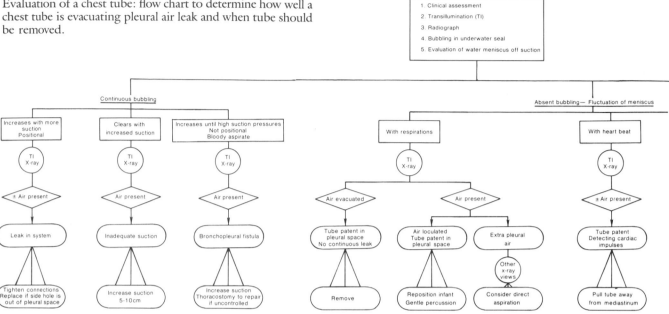

entire lateral portion of chest to the midclavicular line. Blot excess antiseptic and allow skin to dry.

6. Drape surgical area from 3rd to 8th ribs and from latissimus dorsi muscle to midclavicular line (Fig. 36-10, B). Using transparent aperture drape allows continued visualization of landmarks.

7. Locate essential landmarks (Fig. 36-10, C).
   a. Nipple and 5th intercostal spaces
   b. Midaxillary line
   c. Skin incision site in the 6th or 7th intercostal space at midaxillary line
   d. Pleural entry site at point midway between midaxillary and anterior axillary lines in the 4th or 5th intercostal space. Keep well away from breast tissue.

8. Remove trocar from tube.

   We do not recommend using a trocar during tube insertion because of greater likelihood for lung perforation. Dissection to the pleura should be done as described here with puncture of the pleura by forceps, not by the trocar. Should a trocar be used after dissecting to the pleura, there should be a straight clamp perpendicular to the

shaft at 1 to 1.5 cm from its tip to keep the tube from penetrating too deeply (Fig. 36-11).

9. Estimate length for intrathoracic portion of tube (skin incision site to midclavicle).

10. Infiltrate skin at incision site, with 0.125 to 0.25 ml of 1% lidocaine if infant is not anesthetized.

11. Using No. 15 blade, make incision through skin the same length as chest tube diameter or no more than 0.75 cm (Fig. 36-13, C).

12. Use curved mosquito hemostat for blunt dissection to 4th interspace over the top of the 5th rib (Fig. 36-14, D).
   a. Hold free index finger as a mark of the 4th rib at the end of the tunnel.
   b. Make tunnel only as wide as tube and forceps tip.

13. Puncture pleura over top of rib by applying pressure on tips of forceps with index finger (Fig. 36-13, E).
   a. Keep tip from plunging too deeply into pleural space.
   b. Listen for rush of air indicating pleural penetration.

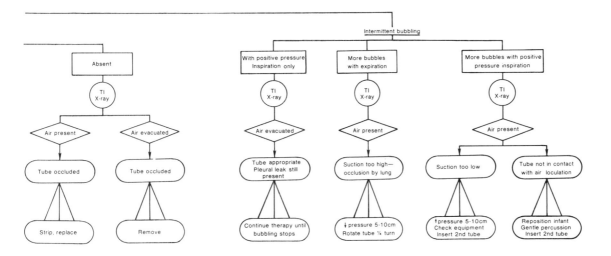

c. After puncturing pleura, open hemostat just wide enough to admit chest tube.

14. Leaving hemostat in place, thread tube between opened tips to the predetermined depth (Fig. 36-10, F).
    a. Alternately, insert closed tips of mosquito hemostat into side port of tube to its end and direct tube through tunnel.[29]
    b. Direct chest tube cephalad toward apex of thorax (midclavicle), and advance tip to midclavicular line, ensuring that side holes are within pleural space.
    c. Observe for humidity or bubbling in chest tube to verify intrapleural location.
15. Connect tube to vacuum drainage system, and observe fluctuations of meniscus and pattern of bubbling (Fig. 36-12). Avoid putting tension on tube.
16. Secure chest tube to skin with suture (Fig. 36-14).
    a. Use one suture to close end of skin incision and make airtight seal with chest tube. Tie ends of suture around tube in alternating directions without constricting tube.

Because using a traditional purse-string suture to secure the tube leaves an unsightly scar, we do not recommend it. Unless skin incision has been made unnecessarily long, a single suture is usually sufficient.

    b. Apply tincture of benzoin to chest tube near chest wall and to skin several centimeters below incision. When tacky, encircle tube with a 2-inch length of tape, leaving tab posterior (Fig. 36-14, B).
    c. Place suture through skin and tab of tape to stabilize chest tube in straight position (Fig. 36-14, B).
    d. Alternatively, secure tube with tape bridge (Fig. 36-15).
17. Apply antibiotic ointment or petroleum gauze around skin incision. Cover with small semiporous transparent dressing.

It is important not to cover wound with a heavy dressing, which restricts chest wall movement, obscures tube position, and makes transillumination more difficult. If position of tube is in doubt, secure with temporary tape bridge before

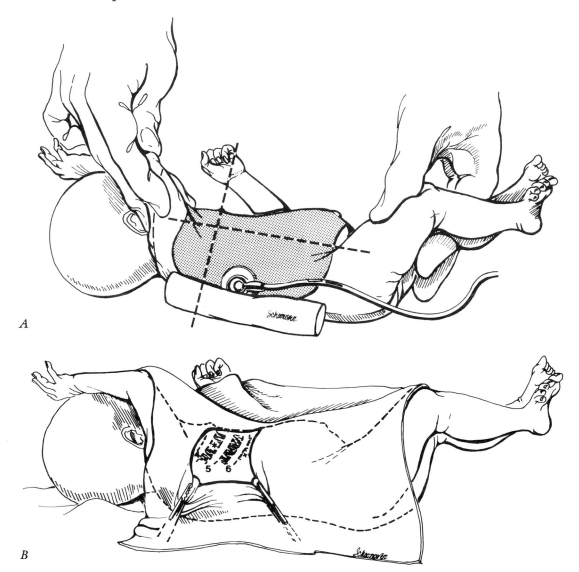

A

B

FIG. 36-13

Insertion of a soft chest tube. (*A*) Position the infant with back support so the point of tube entry will be highest. Fix arm over the head without externally rotating it. Note the midaxillary (MA) line and the line from the nipple through the fourth intercostal space (ICS). The shaded area represents antiseptic skin prep. (*B*) Drape so head of the infant is visible (x, point of incision in sixth ICS; *, point of entry into chest in fourth ICS). (*C*) Same landmarks without the drape, showing the incision in the sixth ICS in the MA line with entry into the chest at the intersection of the nipple line and the MA line. (*D*) Spreading a narrow tunnel with the curve of the hemostat up. (*E*) Turning the hemostat to puncture into the pleura in the fourth ICS. (*F*) With the index finger marking the fourth ICS puncture site, the tube is passed along the tunnel into the pleural space. The tube may be threaded through the blades of the hemostat or a closed hemostat may be inserted into the tube and used to direct it through the tunnel. It is important to keep the site of pleural entry marked.

FIG. 36-13
(*continued*)

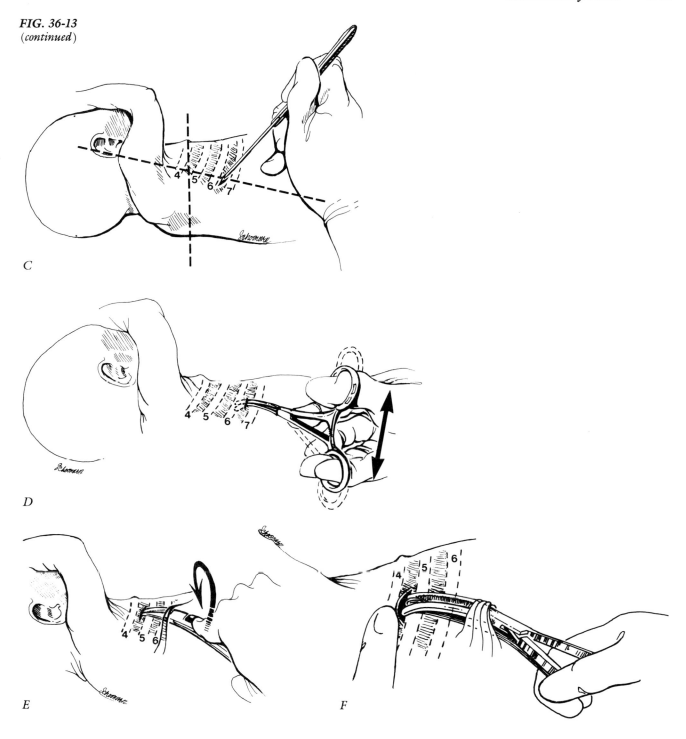

C

D

E   F

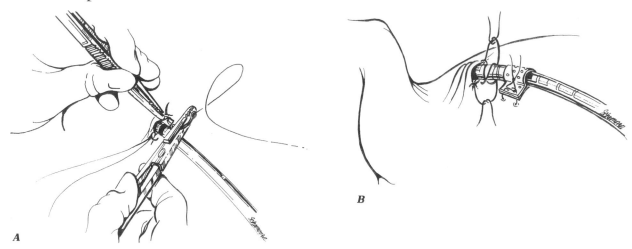

A   *B*

FIG. 36-14
Securing a chest tube. (*A*) Make the incision site airtight with the tube. Do not use a purse string around the incision, because it forms a puckered scar. The initial incision should be made small enough to require only a single suture. (*B*) After painting the tube and skin with benzoin, encircle the suture around the tube or attach a bandage and suture it to the skin.

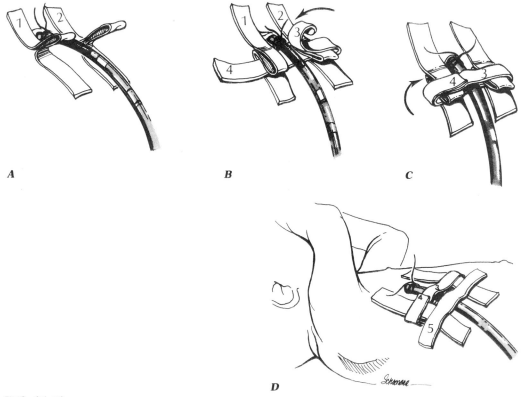

A   *B*   *C*

D

FIG. 36-15
Tape bridge. (*A*) Two tape towers. (*B* and *C*) Bridge under the tube and towers overlapping on top. (*D*) Additional cross tape to keep the chest tube flat without kinking.

TABLE 36-1

Clues to Thoracostomy Perforation of Lung

Bleeding from ET tube
Continuous bubbling in underwater seal
Hemothorax
Return of blood from chest tube
Increased density around tip of tube on radiograph
Persistent pneumothorax despite satisfactory position on frontal view
Tube lying neither anterior nor posterior to lung on lateral view
Tube positioned in fissure

TABLE 36-2

Clues to Thoracostomy Tube Positioned in Fissure

Major interlobar fissure
  Frontal View: upper medial hemithorax
  Lateral View: oblique course posterior and upward
Minor fissure (on right)
  Horizontal course toward medial side of lung

---

covering with dressing until proper position is confirmed.

18. Verify proper positioning of tube.
    a. Anteroposterior and lateral radiographs[30–32]

    Both views are recommended to detect anterior course of tube. See Tables 36-1 and 36-2 for radiographic clues on malpositions.

    b. Pattern of bubbling (Fig. 36-12)
19. Strip tube if meniscus stops fluctuating or as air evacuation decreases. Take extreme care not to dislodge tube by holding tube firmly with one hand close to chest wall.

Insertion of Posterior Tube for Fluid Accumulation

The technique is similar to that for an anteriorly positioned tube with the following differences.

1. Position infant supine, elevating the affected side by 15 to 30 degrees from the table. Secure the arm over the head. (Fig. 36-16)
2. Prepare skin over lateral portion of hemithorax from anterior to posterior axillary line.
3. Make skin incision of 0.5 to 0.75 cm in length, just behind the anterior axillary line in the 6th intercostal space and following direction of rib.
4. Using blunt dissection, tunnel posteriorly and enter the pleura.
   a. Over the top of the 6th rib for a high posterior tube
   b. Along the top of the 7th rib (in the same intercostal space) for a low posterior tube tip

   Take care to enter pleura over the top of a rib to avoid the vessels that run under the inferior surface.

5. As directed before, insert tube only deeply enough to place side holes within pleural space.
6. Collect drainage material for culture, chemical analysis, and volume.

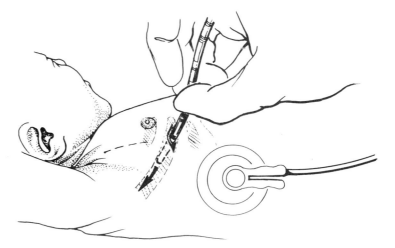

FIG. 36-16
Insertion of a posterior chest tube. With the infant supine, the incision is in or just below the anterior axillary line with the tube entry into the pleura more posteriorly after tunneling along an intercostal space. Take care to enter pleural space over the top of a rib.

7. Connect to underwater seal drainage system that includes a specimen trap.
8. Strip tube regularly.
9. Monitor and correct any imbalance caused by loss of fluid, electrolytes, protein, fats, or lymphocytes.

Removal of Thoracostomy Tube

1. Ascertain that tube is no longer functioning or needed.
   a. Evaluate as suggested in Figure 36-12.
   b. Leave chest tube to water seal without suction for 2 to 12 hours. Do not clamp tube.
      (1) Transilluminate to detect reaccumulation.
      (2) Obtain x-ray film.
   c. Document absence of significant drainage.
2. Assemble equipment.
   a. Antiseptic solution
   b. Sterile gloves
   c. Scissors
   d. Forceps
   e. Petroleum gauze cut and compressed to 2-cm diameter.
   f. Gauze pads 2 × 2
   g. 1-inch tape
3. Cleanse skin in area of chest tube with antiseptic.
4. Release tape and suture holding tube in place. Leave wound suture intact if skin is not inflamed.
5. Palpate pleural entry site and hold finger over it to prevent air entering chest as tube is withdrawn and until gauze is applied. After removing tube, approximate wound edges and place petroleum gauze over incision. Keep pressure on pleural wound until dressing is in place.
6. Cover petroleum gauze with dry, sterile gauze. Limit taping to as small an area as possible so transillumination will be possible.
7. Remove sutures when healing is complete.

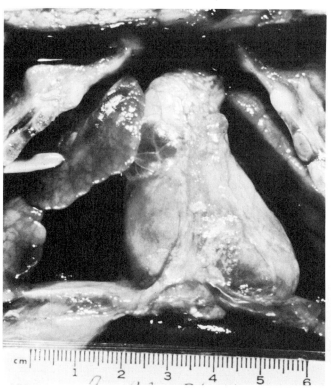 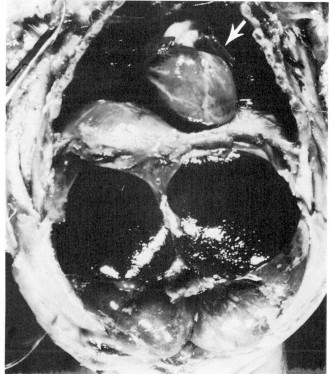

A B

FIG. 36-17
Postmortem examination of infants who died with uncontrolled air leaks. (*A*) Perforation of the right superior lobe by a chest tube inserted without a trocar, demonstrating that virtually any tube can penetrate into the lung. (*B*) Perforation of the left upper lobe by a chest tube (*arrow*).

G. COMPLICATIONS

1. Misdiagnosis with inappropriate placement
2. Burn from transillumination devices[33,34]
3. Trauma
   a. Lung laceration or perforation[21,35–38] (Fig. 36-17)
   b. Perforation and hemorrhage of major vessel (axillary, pulmonary, intercostal, internal mammary)[20,39] (Fig. 36-18)
   c. Puncture of viscus within path of tube (Fig. 36-19)
   d. Residual scarring[23] (Fig. 36-20)
   e. Damage to breast tissue[23]
   f. Chylothorax[40]
4. Nerve damage
   a. Horner's syndrome caused by pressure from tip of right-sided, posterior chest tube near 2nd thoracic ganglion at 1st thoracic intervertebral space[41]
   b. Diaphragmatic paralysis or eventration from phrenic nerve injury[42–44]
5. Misplacement of tube
   a. Tube outside pleural cavity in subcutaneous placement (Fig. 36-21)
   b. Side hole outside pleural space (Fig. 36-22)
   c. Tip across anterior mediastinum (Fig. 36-23)
6. Equipment malfunction
   a. Blockage of tube by proteinaceous or hemorrhagic material
   b. Leak in evacuation system, usually at connection sites
   c. Inappropriate suction pressures[45,46] (Fig. 36-14)
      (1) Excessive pressure
         (a) Aggravation of leak across bronchopleural fistula
         (b) Interference with gas exchange
         (c) Suction of lung parenchyma against holes of tube
      (2) Inadequate pressure with reaccumulation
7. Infection
   a. Cellulitis
   b. Inoculation of pleura with skin organisms including *Candida*[47]
8. Subcutaneous emphysema secondary to leak of tension pneumothorax through pleural opening
9. Aortic obstruction with posterior tube[48]
10. Loss of contents of pleural fluid
    a. Water, electrolytes, and protein (effusion)
    b. Lymphocytes and chylomicrons (chylothorax)

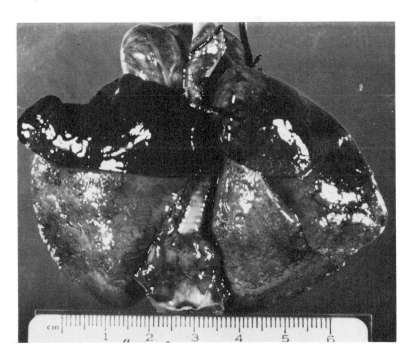

FIG. 36-18
Posterior view of thoracic organs. Traumatic hemorrhage of the left upper lobe due to perforation by a thoracostomy tube.

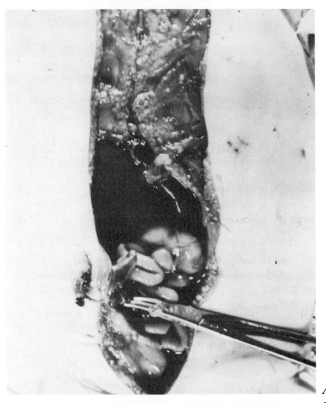

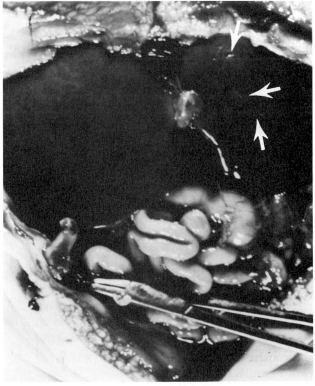

A
B

FIG. 36-19
Postmortem examination of an infant with bilateral pneumothorax, pneumomediastinum, and pneumoperitoneum secondary to pulmonary air leaks. Attempted needle aspirations, as seen by multiple skin puncture sites, (*A*) of the pneumomediastinum and pneumothorax resulted in needle punctures of the liver (*arrows, B*) with peritoneal hemorrhage.

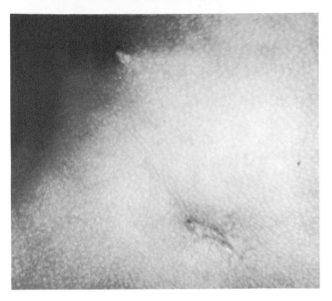

FIG. 36-20
Scar from thoracostomy insertion, emphasizing the importance of avoiding the breast area. Massage of a healed wound with cocoa butter helps break down adhesions that lead to dimpling at the scar.

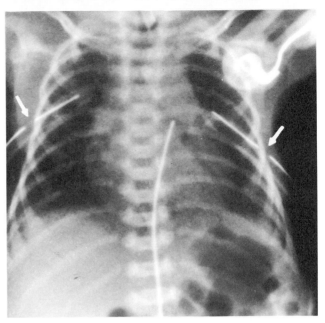

FIG. 36-22
The side holes of both thoracostomy tubes are outside the pleural space on this radiograph.

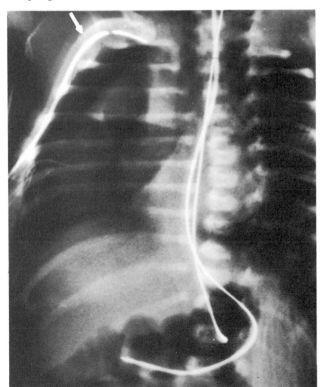

FIG. 36-21
The thoracostomy tube is completely outside the pleural space on this slightly oblique chest film. Note that the long feeding tube is not in an appropriate position for transpyloric feeding. Indwelling tubes may dislodge when other emergency procedures are performed.

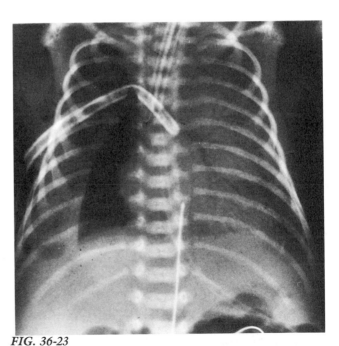

FIG. 36-23
The tip of the thoracostomy tube has been advanced too far medially and is kinked against the mediastinum. Withdrawing the tube 1 or 2 cm would improve drainage at the medial pneumothorax. Note the endotracheal tube tip in the right mainstem bronchus.

Emergency Evacuation of Air Leaks

Emergency evacuation should provide relief to the patient without iatrogenic trauma. The following techniques using modified equipment are less traumatic than using straight needles or scalp-vein sets.

We suggest using an anterior approach for emergency evacuation because of less interference while preparing lateral site for indwelling tubes.

Tubes used for emergency evacuation require suction pressures as high as 30 to 60 cm H_2O to overcome the resistance of their small diameters.[49] This requirement and their tendency to occlude make these cannulas unreliable for continuous drainage of a significant air leak.

A. INDICATIONS

Temporary evacuation of life-threatening air accumulations while preparing for permanent tube placement

B. CONTRAINDICATIONS

1. When patient's vital signs are stable enough to allow permanent thoracostomy tube instead
2. When air collection is likely to resolve spontaneously without patient compromise

Use of Presassembled Teflon Needle and Stopcock

A. EQUIPMENT

1. Preassembled device*[50,51] (Fig. 36-24)
   a. 18-gauge radiopaque Teflon cannula with two side holes near end hole
   b. Stainless-steel stylet
   c. Latex seal over cannula end
   d. Flexible, clear, plastic tubing
   e. Three-way stopcock, closed to cannula
2. 20-ml syringe
3. Antiseptic solution: iodophor
4. Petroleum gauze and tape
5. Sterile gloves

B. TECHNIQUE

1. Prepare skin of appropriate anterior hemithorax with antiseptic.

*M.D.I., Inc.

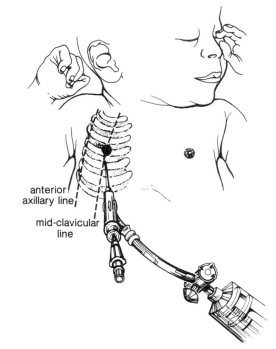

FIG. 36-24
Preassembled evacuation device (M.D.I., Inc.). The point of insertion here is anterior to that for an indwelling tube to allow evacuation while a thoracostomy tube is inserted more laterally. It is important to place the cannula well below the breast tissue.

2. Insert needle at point that is
   a. 45-degree angle to skin, directed cephalad
   b. In 4th to 5th intercostal space, just over top of 5th or 6th rib, well below breast
   c. In midclavicular line (Fig. 36-25, A)
3. As needle enters pleural space, decrease angle to approximately 15 degrees from horizontal, and advance cannula while removing stylet. Avoid excessive insertion depth of stylet. Latex seal will keep system closed after stylet is out (Fig. 36-25, B).
4. Aspirate air into syringe attached to three-way stopcock, and evacuate via open position.
5. Continue evacuation while preparing for permanent tube placement if patient's condition warrants or until leak stops.
6. Cover insertion site with petroleum gauze and small dressing after procedure.

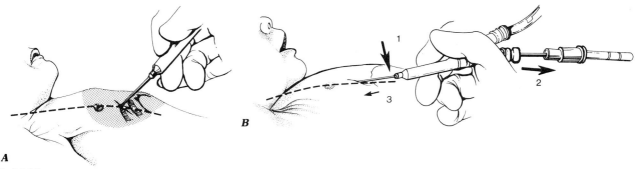

FIG. 36-25

Emergency evacuation with preassembled device or vascular cannula. (*A*) Puncture the skin and enter the pleura at a 45-degree angle over the top of a rib. (*B*) Bring the cannula close to the chest wall (*1*) and withdraw the stylet (*2*) while advancing the cannula (*3*).

Use of Angiocatheter

A. EQUIPMENT

1. Sterile gloves
2. Antiseptic solution
3. 18- to 20-gauge angiocatheter
4. IV extension tubing
5. Three-way stopcock
6. 20-ml syringe

B. TECHNIQUE

1. Prepare skin of appropriate hemithorax with antiseptic.
2. Connect male end of three-way stopcock to female end of IV extension tubing. Connect syringe to three-way stopcock.
3. Insert angiocatheter at point that is
   a. 45-degree angle to skin, directed cephalad
   b. In 4th to 5th intercostal space, just over top of rib, well below breast tissue
   c. In midclavicular line (see Figs. 36-24, 36-25, A)
4. As angiocatheter enters pleural space, decrease angle to 15 degrees above chest wall, and slide cannula in while removing stylet (see Fig. 36-25, B).
5. Attach male end of IV extension tubing to angiocatheter, open stopcock, and evacuate air with syringe.
6. Continue evacuation as patient's condition warrants while preparing for permanent tube placement.
7. Cover insertion site with petroleum gauze and small dressing after procedure.

Diagnostic Tap of Pleural Fluid

Follow procedure as for insertion of posterior chest tube with the following differences.

1. Use preassembled device or angiocath, 20 gauge.
2. Position patient without elevating side of fluid collection. It will be necessary to turn affected side down only if quantity of fluid is small.
3. Select insertion site in anterior or midaxillary lines below breast tissue for diffuse pleural collections. Direct catheter posteriorly after penetrating into pleural space.
4. Keep system closed to prevent leakage of air into pleural space.

Anterior Mediastinal Drainage

The majority of mediastinal air collections cause only mild symptoms and are not under enough tension to require drainage. Their presence often precedes tension pneumothorax in the presence of lung disease and positive-pressure ventilation.

Posterior mediastinal tube insertion as described in the literature[52] is rarely required.

A. INDICATIONS

1. Significant air accumulation with physiological compromise[53]
   a. Increased intracranial pressure[54]

    b. Poor cardiac output because of impeded venous return

    c. Critical interference with artificial ventilation

       (1) Competition with lungs for thoracic volume

       (2) Negative effect on pulmonary compliance

2. Drainage of fluid

    a. Mediastinitis after esophageal perforation

    b. Postoperative

B. CONTRAINDICATIONS

None absolute

C. EQUIPMENT

1. Transillumination device with sterile transparent bag to cover tip

2. Antiseptic for skin preparation

3. Sterile gauze pads

4. Sterile aperture drapes

5. Surgical gloves

6. No. 11 surgical blade

7. Local anesthetic, as required

8. Curved mosquito hemostat

9. Drainage tube (see equipment for Emergency Evacuation of Air Leaks)

    a. 10 Fr, soft thoracostomy tube

    b. Preassembled, closed drainage system*[50,51] (see Fig 36-25)

    c. Intravenous cannula system

       (1) 14- to 16-gauge angiocatheter with extra side holes cut near tip

       (2) IV extension tubing

       (3) Three-way stopcock

10. 10- to 20-ml syringe

11. $1/2$-inch adhesive tape

12. 4-0 nonabsorbable suture on small cutting needle with needle holder

13. Connecting tubing and underwater suction device for indwelling tube

D. PRECAUTIONS AND COMPLICATIONS

The problems encountered in evacuating material from the mediastinum are similar to those encountered in placement of chest tubes. In contrast to tension pneu-

*M.D.I., Inc.

mothorax, mediastinal collections tend to accumulate more gradually. For this reason, careful preparation of the patient and use of sterile technique are possible and essential. Refer to E and G at the beginning of this chapter for precautions and complications.

E. TECHNIQUE

Drainage for longer than 12 hours normally dictates placing a 10 to 12 Fr tube by direct dissection because smaller tubes occlude so readily. Select indwelling tubes only in the presence of significant lung disease or mediastinitis, where continued accumulations are anticipated. Remove the tubes as soon as possible because of the risks for infection.

Soft Mediastinal Tube Insertion

1. Follow sterile technique throughout.

2. Monitor infant for vital signs and oxygenation

3. Determine by transillumination or radiograph the region of maximal mediastinal air accumulation (Fig. 36-26).

4. Cover tip of transillumination light with sterile, clear, plastic bag for use after skin preparation.

5. Cleanse skin with antiseptic.

6. Drape patient with aperture drape and without obscuring infant.

7. If infant is alert, infiltrate insertion site with 0.25 ml local anesthetic.

8. With No. 11 blade, make small stab wound through skin at subxiphoid.

9. Using curved mosquito hemostat, dissect in the midline at 30-degree angle to chest wall in cephalad direction until entering mediastinal space. The mediastinum under tension should bulge downward.

10. Insert soft chest tube into dissected tunnel and direct tube cephalad and toward area of maximal transillumination.

11. Observe tube for air rush or condensation while completing insertion. If loculations are evident, break them up with blunt dissection.

12. Connect to closed drainage system at vacuum of 5 cm H_2O, and increase to 10 cm H_2O if necessary.

    Accumulation in mediastinum is usually relatively slow; therefore, lower suction pressures are effective.

    a. Use low pressure to keep tube side holes patent while clearing air collection.

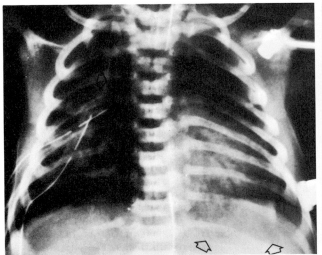
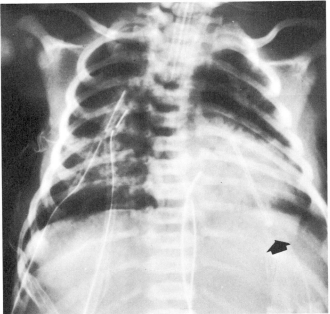
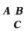
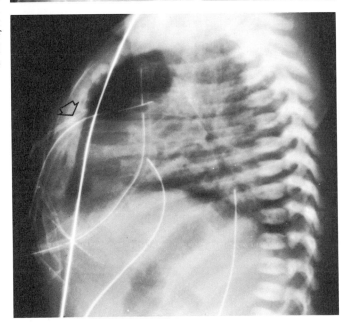

A B
C

FIG. 36-26
Sequential radiographs. (*A*) Tension pneumomediastinum (*open arrows*). A mediastinal collection this massive is unusual. (*B*) Successful drainage tube (*closed arrow*). (*C*) The apparent slipping of the mediastinal cannula (*arrow*) is an artifact of patient rotation on this lateral view. There is still mediastinal air superiorly, but there was no patient compromise at this time.

b. Monitor efficacy by radiograph and transillumination (Fig. 36-26).

13. Secure tube with suture, and tape as for thoracostomy tubes.

14. If drainage stops with significant accumulation still evident on transillumination or radiograph
   a. Verify that accumulation is in mediastinum by lateral decubitus and lateral radiographs.
   b. Verify tube position on radiographs.
   c. Rotate tube.
   d. Aspirate, but do not irrigate, tube; reattach to continuous drainage.
   e. Change position of infant to move air toward tube.

Temporary Mediastinal Drainage with Intravenous Cannula

1. Assemble equipment and prepare patient as for insertion by mediastinal dissection.
2. Make a small stab wound in subxiphoid notch.

   Mediastinal air under tension should be located in this area, pushing the liver and heart away.

3. Insert cannula with stylet at 45-degree angle to chest wall in cephalad direction.
4. As soon as cannula passes through skin, lower cannula to 30 degrees from skin.
5. Remove stylet, and attach connecting tubing, stopcock, and syringe.
6. Advance cannula into mediastinal space cephalad and medially but toward area of maximal transillumination. Aspirate while advancing, and monitor cardiac tracing. Stop insertion if there is resistance, blood, or arrhythmia.
7. Secure cannula in effective position, and attach IV extension tubing to underwater drainage system with suction pressure of 10 cm H_2O. The smaller cannula will require higher suction pressures unless the air accumulates slowly. Because air loculates within the mediastinum and the side holes occlude easily, small catheters are rarely effective for anything other than acute relief of tension. Remove cannula as soon as possible.

References

1. JUNG AL, NELSON J, JENKINS MB, HODSON WA: Clinical evaluation of a new chest tube used in neonates. Clin Pediatr 30:85, 1991
2. LAWLESS S, ORR R, KILLIAN A, ET AL: New pigtail catheter for pleural drainage in pediatric patients. Crit Care Med 17:173, 1989
3. ROTHBERG AD, MARKS KH, MAISELS MJ: Understanding the Pleurevac. Pediatrics 67:482, 1981
4. GONZALEZ F, HARRIS T, BLACK P, RICHARDSON P: Decreased gas flow through pneumothoraces in neonates receiving high-frequency jet versus conventional ventilation. J Pediatr 110:464, 1987
5. POWNER DJ, CLINE D, RODMAN GH: Effect of chest-tube suction on gas flow through a bronchopleural fistula. Crit Care Med 13:99, 1985
6. HEIMLICH HJ: Valve drainage of the pleural cavity. Diseases of the Chest 53:282, 1968
7. LACKEY DA, UKRAINSKI CT, TABER P: The management of tension pneumothorax in the neonate using the Heimlich flutter valve. J Pediatr 84:438, 1974
8. MOSCOWITZ PS, GRISCOM NT: The medial pneumothorax. Radiology 120:143, 1976
9. DENNIS J, EIGEN H, BALLANTINE T, GROSFELD J: The relationship between peak inspiratory pressure and positive end expiratory pressure on the volume of air lost through a bronchopleural fistula. J Pediatr Surg 15:971, 1980
10. ZIDULKA A, BRAIDY TF, RISSI MC, SHINER RJ: Position may stop pneumothorax progression in dogs. Am Rev Respir Dis 126:51, 1982
11. OGATA ES, GREGORY GA, KITTERMAN JA, ET AL: Pneumothorax in the respiratory distress syndrome: Incidence and effect on vital signs, blood gases, and pH. Pediatrics 58:177, 1976
12. MADANSKY DL, LAWSON EE, CHERNICK V, TAEUSCH WH: Pneumothorax and other forms of pulmonary air leak in newborns. Am Rev Respir Dis 120:729, 1979
13. MONIN P, VERT P: Pneumothorax. Clin Perinatol 5, No. 2:335, 1978
14. PRIMHAK RA: Factors associated with pulmonary air leak in premature infants receiving mechanical ventilation. J Pediatr 102:764, 1983
15. RYAN CA, BARRINGTON KJ, PHILLIPS HJ, FINER NN: Contralateral pneumothoraces in the newborn: Incidence and predisposing factors. Pediatrics 79:417, 1987
16. KUHNS LR, BEDNAREK FJ, WYMAN ML: Diagnosis of pneumothroax or pneumomediastinum in the neonate by transillumination. Pediatrics 56:355, 1975
17. WYMAN ML, KUHNS LR: Accuracy of transillumination in the recognition of pneumothorax and pneumomediastinum in the neonate. Clin Pediatr 16:323, 1977
18. FLETCHER BD: Medial herniation of the parietal pleura: A useful sign of pneumothorax in supine neonates. AJR 130:369, 1978

19. Albelda SM, Gefter WB, Kelley MA, et al: Ventilator-induced subpleural air cysts: Clinical, radiographic, and pathologic significance. Am Rev Respir Dis 127:360, 1983

20. Allen RW, Jung AL, Lester PD: Effectiveness of chest tube evacuation of pneumothorax in neonates. J Pediatr 99:629, 1981

21. Gangitano E, Pomerance J, Gans S: Successful surgical repair of iatrogenic lung perforation in a neonate. J Pediatr Surg 16:70, 1981

22. Batton DG, Hellmann J, Nardis EE: Effect of pneumothorax-induced systemic blood pressure alterations on the cerebral circulation in newborn dogs. Pediatrics 74:350, 1984

23. Cartlidge PHT, Fox PE, Rutter N: The scars of newborn intensive care. Early Hum Dev 21:1, 1990

24. Bhatia J, Mathew OP: Resolution of pneumothorax in neonates. Crit Care Med 13:417, 1985

25. Merenstein GB, Dougherty K, Lewis A: Early detection of pneumothorax by oscilloscope monitor in the newborn infant. J Pediatr 80:98, 1972

26. Noack G. Freyschuss V: The early detection of pneumothorax with transthoracic impedance in newborn infants. Acta Paediatr Scand 66:677, 1977

27. Swischuk LE: Two lesser known but useful signs of neonatal pneumothorax. AJR 127:623, 1976

28. Stein RT, Kuhns LR, Wall PM, et al: Experimental pneumothorax detected by thermography. Pediatrics 64:310, 1979

29. Mehrabani D, Kopelman AE: Chest tube insertion: A simplified technique. Pediatrics 83:784, 1989

30. Mauer JR, Friedman PJ, Wing VW: Thoracostomy tube in an interlobar fissure: Radiologic recognition of a potential problem. AJR 139:1155, 1981

31. Strife JL, Smith P, Dunbar JS, Steven JM: Chest tube perforation of the lung in premature infants: radiographic recognition. AJR 141:73, 1983

32. Bowen A, Zarabi M: Radiographic clues to chest tube perforation of neonatal lung. Am J Perinatol 2:43, 1985

33. Kuhns LR, Wyman ML, Roloff DW: A caution about using photoillumination devices. Pediatrics 57:975, 1976

34. McArtor RD, Saunders BS: Iatrogenic second-degree burn caused by a transilluminator. Pediatrics 63:422, 1979

35. Wilson AJ, Krous HF: Lung perforation during chest tube placement in the stiff lung syndrome. J Pediatr Surg 9:213, 1974

36. Moessinger AC, Driscoll JM, Wigger HJ: High incidence of lung perforation by chest tube in neonatal pneumothorax. J Pediatr 92:635, 1978

37. Sacks LM: Lung perforation by chest tubes. J Pediatr 94:341, 1979

38. Banagle RC, Outerbridge EW, Aranda JV: Lung perforation: A complication of chest tube insertion in neonatal pneumothorax. J Pediatr 94:973, 1979

39. Jung A, Minton S, Roan Y: Pulmonary hemorrhage secondary to chest tube placement for pneumothorax in neonates. Clin Pediatr (Phila) 19:624, 1980

40. Kumar SP, Belik J: Chylothorax—a complication of chest tube placement in a neonate. Crit Care Med 12:411, 1984

41. Rosegger H, Fritsch G: Horner's syndrome after treatment of tension pneumothorax with tube thoracostomy in a newborn infant. Eur J Pediatr 133:67, 1980

42. Ayalon A, Anner H, Moghilner M, Schiller M: Eventration of the diaphragm due to phrenic nerve injury by intercostal drainage. J Pediatr Surg 14:473, 1981.

43. Marinelli P, Ortiz A, Alden ER: Acquired eventration of the diaphragm: A complication of chest tube placement in neonatal pneumothorax. Pediatr 67:552, 1981

44. Phillips A, Rowe J, Raye J: Acute diaphragmatic paralysis after chest tube placement in a neonate: AJR 136:824, 1981

45. Yeh TF, Pildes RS, Salem MR: Treatment of persistent tension pneumothorax in a neonate by selective bronchial intubation. Anesthesiology 49:37, 1978

46. Grosfeld JL, Lemons JL, Ballantine TVN, Schreiner RL: Emergency thoracostomy for acquired bronchopleural fistula in the premature infant with respiratory distress. J Pediatr Surg 15:416, 1980

47. Faix RG, Naglie RA, Barr M: Intrapleural inoculation of Candida in an infant with congenital cutaneous candidiasis. Am J Perinatol 3:119, 1986

48. Gooding C, Kerlan R Jr, Brasch R: Partial aortic obstruction produced by a thoracostomy tube. J Pediatr 98:471, 1981

49. Ragosta KG, Fuhrman BP, Howland DF: Flow characteristics of thoracotomy tubes used in infants. Crit Care Med 18:662, 1990

50. Fox WW, Eavey RD, Shaffer TH: A closed system device for diagnosis and evaluation of neonatal pneumothoraces. Crit Care Med 6:376, 1978

51. Shutack JG, Wageman MJ, Moomjian AS, et al: A new device for diagnosis and treatment of neonatal pneumothorax. Pediatrics 63:252, 1979

52. Purohit DM, Lorenzo RL, Smith CE, Bradford BF: Bronchial laceration in a newborn with persistent posterior pneumomediastinum. J Pediatr Surg 20:82, 1985

53. Moore JT, Wayne ER, Hanson J: Malignant pneumomediastinum: Successful tube mediastinostomy in the neonate. Am J Surg 154:687, 1987

54. Tyler DC, Redding G, Hall D, Lynn A: Increased intracranial pressure: An indication to decompress a tension pneumomediastinum. Crit Care Med 12:467, 1984

37 *Pericardial Tubes*

Mary Ann Fletcher
Martin Raymond Eichelberger

A. INDICATIONS

1. Pneumopericardium with tamponade[1-5]
   a. Decreased or distant heart sounds, bradycardia
   b. Decreased blood pressure
   c. Pulsus paradoxus[6]
   d. Decreased EKG voltage
   e. Cardiac halo on transillumination or radiograph
2. Pericardial effusion with tamponade
3. Aspiration of pericardial fluid for diagnosis

B. CONTRAINDICATION

Asymptomatic pericardial collections

C. EQUIPMENT

1. Transillumination device with sterile, transparent bag to cover tip (for pneumopericardium)
2. Antiseptic solution
3. Sterile swabs or gauze pads
4. Surgical aperture drapes
5. Surgical gloves
6. No. 11 surgical blade
7. Drainage cannula
   a. Preassembled closed drainage system as for Emergency Evacuation of Air Leaks, Thoracostomy Tubes (Fig. 36-24), or
   b. 18- to 20-gauge intravenous cannula with inner needle
      (1) Short IV extension tubing
      (2) Three-way stopcock
8. 10- or 20-ml syringe
9. ½-inch adhesive tape
10. 4-0 nonabsorbable suture on small cutting needle with needle holder (optional)
11. Connecting tubing and underwater seal device for indwelling tube

D. PRECAUTIONS AND COMPLICATIONS

The problems encountered in evacuating material from the pericardium are the same as those encountered in thoracostomy tubes. Because of the site of insertion, there is particular risk of puncturing the liver or heart (see Fig. 36-19).

E. TECHNIQUE

See Figure 37-1.

Emery illustrates the surgical placement of a permanent pericardial tube by incising the linea alba and dissecting away the diaphragmatic fibers to allow direct incision of the pericardial sac.[7] See below. While this technique is relatively rapid in experienced hands, the indirect puncture described in this section is faster when there is life-threatening tamponade.

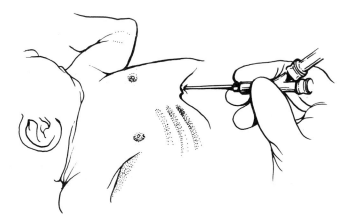

FIG. 37-1
Insertion of pericardial tube in the xiphisternal space with the direction toward the tip of the left scapula. This location is also satisfactory for drainage of large, tension pneumomediastinum.

1. Transilluminate chest over precordium to outline area of air accumulation.[8]

   A significant air collection appears with borders more rounded than seen in an intrapleural collection and extends as a complete halo around the heart. The cardiac pulsations should be evident within the area of transillumination. While fluid will not transilluminate, it is prudent to keep the transillumination equipment available in case of a complicating air leak during pericardiocentesis.

2. Cleanse skin over xiphoid, precordium, and upper abdomen with antiseptic. Blot to remove excess.
3. Cover tip of transillumination device with sterile glove to allow continued use within sterile field.
4. Apply drapes, leaving precordium and xiphoid exposed.
5. Put three-way stopcock on syringe and attach it open to cannula, or use preassembled device.
6. Make small stab wound in left xiphisternal angle.
7. Insert cannula at 30- to 45-degree angle from the skin and direct it toward tip of left scapula. Use transillumination as guide to area of accumulation.
8. While advancing cannula, apply constant suction on syringe. Advance until air is obtained and then remove stylet. Center cannula in area of maximal transillumination. Evacuate as much as possible, remembering that accumulation may recur.
9. If air reaccumulates as detected either by transillumination or clinically, secure cannula in place and attach to continuous suction via underwater seal, 5 to 10 cm H_2O. Evacuate manually any time there is a reaccumulation not cleared by continuous suction.

   Continuous drainage using a small gauge cannula is often ineffective because tubing resistance may be too great for low suction pressures. If there is reaccumulation, a permanent tube inserted by cutdown is indicated.

10. Confirm position of indwelling catheter with radiograph (Fig. 37-2).

A   B

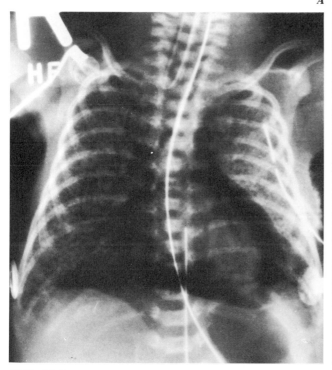 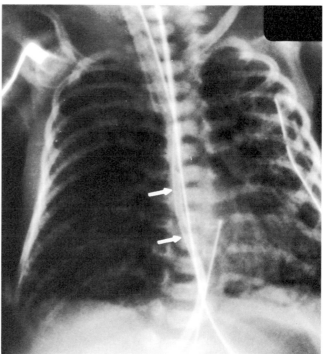

FIG. 37-2
(*A*) Pneumopericardium sufficient to cause tamponade. (*B*) Successful drainage with an indwelling tube (*arrows*).

Insertion of Pericardial Tube by Cutdown

A. EQUIPMENT

1. Same as for emergency percutaneous cannulation, 1–7 above.
2. Slightly curved hemostatic forceps
3. Fine scissors, sharp/sharp
4. Chest tube, 8 or 10 Fr
5. Local anesthetic as required
6. Connecting adaptor, tubing, and underwater seal device

B. TECHNIQUE

1. Follow steps 1–4 above.
2. Instill 0.25 to 0.5 ml local anesthetic in skin 1 to 2 cm below sternum.
3. In the midline at the tip of the xiphoid process, make a horizontal incision through the skin just slightly wider than the diameter of the tube to be placed.
4. Dissect with slightly curved hemostatic forceps along the linea alba in a cephalad direction through the diaphragmatic fibers until the pericardium is reached.
5. Grasp the pericardium with forceps and open the sac in a small incision with fine scissors.

   > Because the pericardium is under tension, it bulges into view. As soon as pericardial sac is entered, there is a rush of air or fluid with relief of the tamponade. The rest of the procedure can be completed less urgently.

6. Thread chest tube through pericardium above the heart until side holes are within sac. Keep tube open during insertion.
7. Secure chest tube at skin insertion and connect to underwater drainage system.
8. Confirm position and efficacy of drainage by transillumination and radiograph.

References

1. POMERANCE JJ, WELLER MH, RICHARDSON CJ, ET AL: Pneumopericardium complicating respiratory distress syndrome: Role of conservative management. J Pediatr 84:883, 1974
2. BRANS YW, PITTS M, CASSADY G: Neonatal pneumopericardium. Am J Dis Child 130:393, 1976
3. REPPERT SM, MENT LR, TODRES ID: Treatment of pneumopericardium in the newborn infant. J Pediatr 90:115, 1977
4. HIGGINS CB, BRODERICK TW, EDWARDS DK, SHUMAKER A: The hemodynamic significance of massive pneumopericardium in preterm infants with respiratory distress syndrome. Clinical and experimental observations. Radiology 133:363, 1979
5. LAWSON EE, GOULD JB, TAEUSCH HW JR: Neonatal pneumopericardium: Current management. J Pediatr Surg 15:181, 1980
6. BERG RA: Pulsus paradoxus in the diagnosis and management of pneumopericardium in an infant. Crit Care Med 18:340, 1990
7. EMERY RW, LINDSAY WG, NICOLOFF DM: Placement of pericardial drainage tube for the treatment of pneumopericardium in the neonate. Ann Thorac Surg 26:84, 1978
8. CABATU EE, BROWN EG: Thoracic transillumination: Aid in the diagnosis and treatment of pneumopericardium. Pediatrics 64:958, 1979

38 Gastric and Transpyloric Tubes

Mary Ann Fletcher

Oral or Nasal Gastric Tubes

A. INDICATIONS[1,2]

1. To provide a route for enteric feedings
   a. Abnormal gag reflex
      (1) Immaturity
      (2) Neurologic disease
   b. Insufficient oral intake
   c. Respiratory symptoms sufficiently severe to interdict oral intake
2. To administer medications
3. To sample gastric contents for analysis
4. To decompress and empty stomach

B. CONTRAINDICATION

Recent esophageal repair or perforation

C. EQUIPMENT

1. Suction equipment
2. Cardiac monitor
3. 5 or 8 Fr infant feeding tube
4. 1/2-inch adhesive tape
5. Sterile water or saline
6. 5- and 20-ml syringes
7. Stethoscope
8. Gloves

D. PRECAUTIONS

1. Measure and note appropriate length for insertion.
2. Have suction apparatus readily available in case there is any regurgitation.
3. Do not push against any resistance. Perforation occurs even with very little force or sensation of resistance.

4. Do not instill any material if position of tube is unclear.
5. Evaluate for possible esophageal perforation after insertion[3,4] if there is
   a. Bloody aspirate
   b. Increased oral secretion
   c. Acute respiratory symptoms
   d. Pneumothorax
   e. Failure to obtain acid gastric contents and air with tube at calculated depth
6. Ensure that open tube drains below level of infant's stomach.

E. TECHNIQUE

1. Put on gloves.
2. Clear nose and oropharynx by gentle suctioning as necessary.
3. Monitor infant's heart rate and observe for arrhythmia or respiratory distress throughout procedure.
4. Position infant on back with head of bed elevated.
5. Measure length for insertion by estimating distance from nose to ear to xiphisternum. Mark length on feeding tube with a loop of tape.
6. Moisten end of tube with sterile water or saline.
7. Oral insertion

   Slightly depressing the tongue seems to ease oral pharyngeal passage and should decrease the risk of pharyngoesophageal perforation in small infants.

   a. Depress anterior portion of tongue with forefinger, and stabilize head with free fingers.
   b. Insert tube along finger to oropharynx.
8. Nasal insertion[5] (Avoid this route if there is critical airway compromise.)
   a. Stabilize head. Elevate tip of nose to widen nostril.

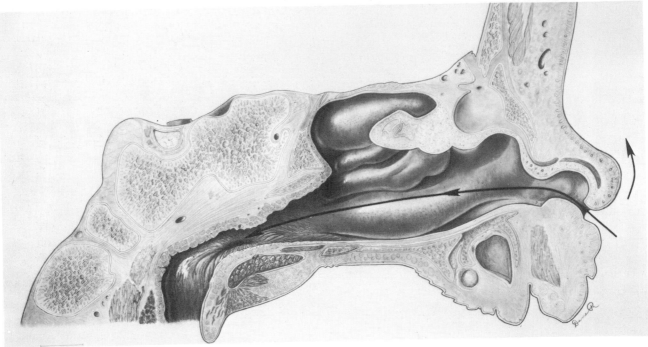

FIG. 38-1
Anatomical view of the neonatal nasopharynx. The natural direction in tube insertion is toward the nasal turbinates where it might stop and give an impression of obstruction. By pushing the nostril up, one can direct a tube toward the occiput with less trauma.

b. Insert tip of tube, directing it toward occiput rather than toward vertex (Fig. 38-1).

c. Advance tube gently to oropharynx.

d. Observe for bradycardia.

9. If possible, use pacifier to encourage sucking and swallowing.

10. Tilt head forward slightly.

11. Advance tube to predetermined depth.

   a. Do not push against any resistance.

   b. Stop procedure if there is onset of any respiratory distress, cough, or struggling.

12. Determine location of tip.

   Injecting air to verify position is a standard practice, but a rush of air also occurs when the tip is positioned within the distal esophagus; therefore, the method is unreliable.[6]

   a. Aspirate any contents; describe and measure; determine acidity by pH tape.

   b. Observe and palpate abdomen gently for tip of tube.

c. Suspect perforation or misplacement if there is no air or fluid returned, or if there is onset of respiratory distress.

13. Secure indwelling tube to face with ½-inch tape.

   a. For feedings, attach to syringe.

   b. For gravity drainage, attach specimen trap and position below level of stomach.

   c. For decompression, connect to intermittent pressure.

14. Pinch or close gastric tube during removal to prevent emptying contents into pharynx.

F. COMPLICATIONS

1. Apnea or bradycardia
2. Hypoxia[7]
3. Obstruction of obligatory nasal airway[5]
4. Irritation and necrosis of nasal mucosa
   a. Epistaxis
   b. Ulceration

A   B

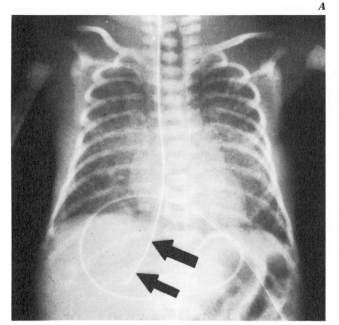 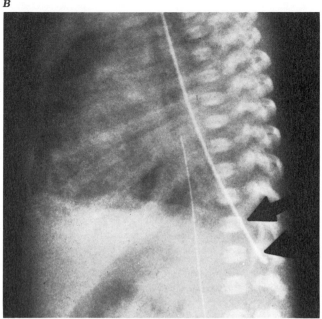

FIG. 38-2
Two radiographic views demonstrating a typical nasopharyngeal perforation with extra pleural malposition of a nasogastric tube at the right lung base (*arrows*). Either a traumatic endobronchial intubation or primary trauma from the nasogastric tube accounts for the perforation.

5. Perforation[8–11] (Figs. 38-2, 38-3)
   a. Posterior pharynx, particularly at level of cricopharynx
   b. Esophagus
      (1) Submucosal and remaining within mediastinum
      (2) Complete into thorax
   c. Stomach
   d. Duodenum
6. Misplacement on insertion [12]
   a. Coiled in oropharynx (Fig. 38-4A)
   b. Trachea (Fig. 38-4B)
   c. Esophagus (Figs. 38-4C–E)
7. Displacement after insertion due to inappropriate length or fixation
   a. Pulling back into esophagus
   b. Prolapsing into duodenum (see Fig. 36-21)

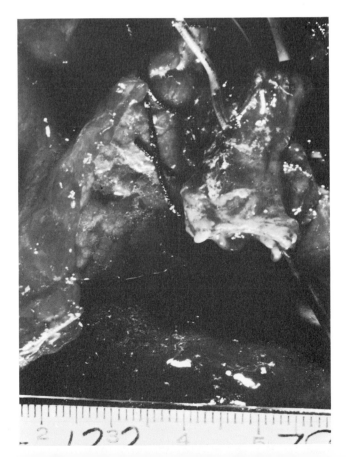

FIG. 38-3
Posterior perforation of the esophagus demonstrated in postmortem examination of 26-week gestational age infant. Upper probe is through perforation. Barium from a premortem study spilled through the perforation, causing pleuritis. Perforation may have occurred as a result of endotracheal intubation, suctioning, or passage of a gastric tube and is more common is smaller, premature infants.

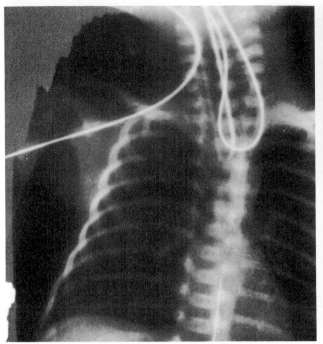
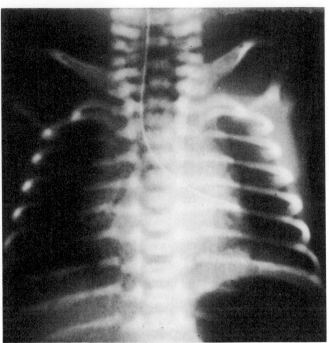

A B
C D

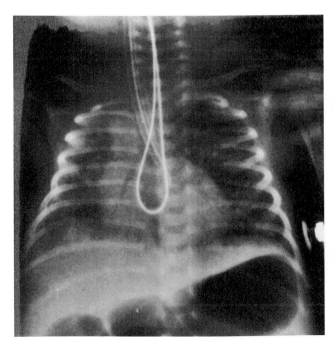
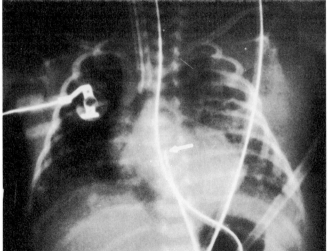

FIG. 38-4
Radiographic examples of misplaced feeding tubes. (*A*) Tube coiled in the oropharynx and upper esophagus, simulating an esophageal atresia. (*B*) Tube into the left mainstem bronchus. (*C*) Tube coiled in the lower esophagus. (*D*) Tube doubled on itself in the stomach with its distal end in the esophagus (*arrow*). (*E*) Tube only into the esophagus. A rush may be heard on auscultation over the stomach when air is injected through a tube lying in this position, making that an unreliable sign of gastric location.

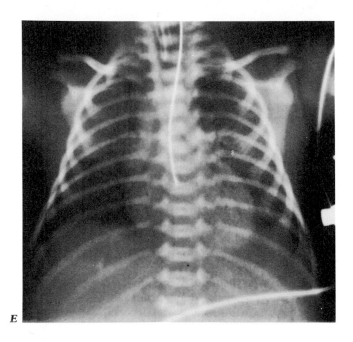

E

FIG. 38-4
(*continued*)

8. Coiling and knotting[13]
9. Obstruction of tube[14]
10. Staphylococcal enterocolitis after nasal colonization, particularly with indwelling tubes[15]
11. Interference with development of normal palate by indwelling tube[16]

Transpyloric Feeding Tube

A. INDICATIONS[17]

1. Clinical condition dictating transpyloric feeding
2. Sampling of duodenal–jejunal contents

B. CONTRAINDICATIONS[1,2]

1. Clinical condition allowing feeding into prepyloric region
2. Clinical condition compromising duodenojejunal integrity: necrotizing enterocolitis, fulminant sepsis, shock, patent ductus arteriosus

C. EQUIPMENT

1. Feeding tube
   a. 3.5 or 5 Fr, 36-inch
   b. Nontoxic, nonstiffening polyurethane

2. 20-ml syringe
3. ½-inch tape
4. pH tape
5. Continuous infusion pump and connecting tubing

D. PRECAUTIONS

1. Use oral route whenever possible to avoid compromise of nasal airways.[5]
2. Avoid pushing against any obstruction or resistance.
3. Replace tubes as per manufacturer's recommendations. If the tube is stiff on removal, replace next tube sooner.

   Polyvinyl chloride tubes require replacement every 4 days because the plasticizers are leached, stiffening the tube. "Nonstiffening" tubes lose some of their compliance when left in place, but stay softer for longer periods.

4. If a tube has become partially dislodged, replace it rather than pushing it in further.
5. When using feedings that tend to coagulate in tubing, it may be necessary to flush periodically with air or water.
6. Use reliable infusion pumps that control rate and detect obstructions.
7. Limit infusion of hypertonic solutions beyond pylorus.

8. Consider the effect of continuous feedings on medication absorption.[18]

E. TECHNIQUE[19]

1. Insert orogastric tube as per gastric tubes, above. Aspirate gastric contents.
2. Measure distance from glabella to heels, or 10 cm longer than distance for gastric tube. Mark point with tape on transpyloric tube.
3. Turn patient onto right side.
4. Inject air through orogastric tube to distend stomach. Close orogastric tube.
   a. 10 ml for babies less than 1 kg
   b. 15 to 20 ml for babies more than 1 kg
5. Pass transpyloric tube to predetermined depth.
6. After approximately 10 minutes with infant remaining on right side, gently aspirate through transpyloric tube. Tube may be in position within duodenum if aspirate is
   a. Without air
   b. Alkaline
   c. Bilious
7. If not beyond pylorus, leave long tube open and orogastric tube closed for up to 4 hours or until bilious secretions return, keeping infant on right side.
8. When passage across pylorus is suspected, confirm position by x-ray film. Tip of catheter should be just beyond second portion of duodenum (Fig. 38-5).
9. If, after 4 hours, there are no bilious secretions, remove tube and repeat procedure.
10. Avoid pushing to advance tube after initial placement. If tube is not in far enough, retape to give external slack and to allow peristalsis to carry tip to new position.

> Most often if the tube does not cross the pylorus within the first ½ hours after passage, it is unlikely to pass in the next few hours, and it may be better to restart the procedure.

11. When positioned, close transpyloric tube or start continuous infusion. Open gastric tube with syringe-barrel chimney or specimen trap to decompress stomach and to detect any transpyloric regurgitation.

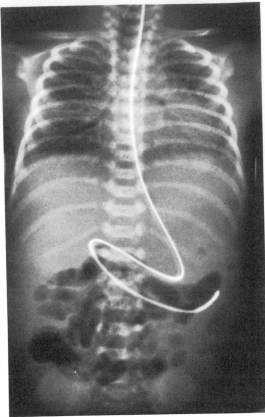

FIG. 38-5
Radiographic demonstration of a transpyloric feeding tube that has passed the ligament of Treitz, well below the more appropriate level and increasing the risk of perforation or nutritional dumping.

F. COMPLICATIONS

See also Gastric Tubes.

1. Misplacement into tracheobronchial tree, esophagus, or stomach, or incorrect position within proximal duodenum[12,20] (see Figs. 38-4A–E)
   a. Aspiration
   b. Pneumonia[21]
2. Kinking or knotting of tube
3. Hardening of PVC tube with leaching of bioavailable plasticizers
4. Obstruction of tube[14]
5. Perforation of esophagus, stomach, duodenum[8,9,11,22-26]
6. Perforation of kidney[24]
7. Sepsis

8. Local infection (nasal colonization with staphylococci)[15]
9. Enterocolitis
   a. Staphylococcus[15]
   b. Necrotizing enterocolitis[27]
10. Development of pyloric stenosis[28]
11. Formation of enterocutaneous fistula[29]
12. Interference with absorption of medications[18]
13. Malabsorption
    a. If fats enter bowel too distally[30]
    b. If hypertonic medications or feedings instilled too rapidly[30]

References

1. CAILLIE MV, POWELL GK: Nasoduodenal versus nasogastric feeding in the very low birthweight infant. Pediatrics 56:1065, 1975
2. PEREIRA G, LEMONS J: Controlled study of transpyloric and intermittent gavage feeding in the small preterm infant. Pediatrics 67:68, 1981
3. BLAIR GK, FILLER RM, THEODORESCU D: Neonatal pharyngoesophageal perforation mimicking esophageal atresia: Clues to diagnosis. J Pediatr Surg 22(8):770, 1987
4. KRASNA IH, ROSENFELD D, BENJAMIN BG, ET AL: Esophageal perforation in the neonate: An emerging problem in the newborn nursery. J Pediatr Surg 22(8):784 1987
5. VAN SOMEREN V, LINNETT SJ, STOTHERS JK, SULLIVAN PG: An investigation into the benefits of resiting nasoenteric feeding tubes. Pediatrics 74:379, 1984
6. METHENY N: Measures to test placement of nasogastric and nasointestinal feeding tubes: A review. Nurs Res 37(6):324, 1988
7. HERRILL N, MARTIN RJ, FANAROFF A: Arterial oxygen tension during nasogastric feeding in the preterm infant. J Pediatr 96:914, 1980
8. FOGLE RS, SMITH WL, GRESHAM EL: Perforation of feeding tube into right renal pelvis. J Pediatr 93:122, 1978
9. NAGARAJ HS, MULLEN P, GROFF DB, ET AL: Iatrogenic perforation of the esophagus in premature infants. Surgery 86:583, 1979
10. FLEMING PJ, VENUGOPAL S, LEWINS MJ, ET AL: Esophageal perforation into the right pleural cavity in a neonate. J Pediatr Surg 15:335, 1980
11. MCALISTER WH, SIEGEL MJ, SHACKELFORD GD, ET AL: Intestinal perforations by tube feedings in small infants: Clinical and experimental studies. AJR 145:687, 1985
12. MCWEY RE, CURRY NS, SCHABEL SI, REINES HD: Complications of nasoenteric feeding tubes. Am J Surg 155:253, 1988
13. ARMSTRONG MAM, MINTZ AA: Method for removing a knotted nasogastric feeding tube in an infant. J Pediatr 85:732, 1974
14. MOYER L, CHAN G: Clotted transpyloric feeding tube using a premature formula. Pediatr Res 15 (Part 2):542, 1981
15. GUTMAN L, IDRISS Z, GEHLBACH S, BLACKMON L: Neonatal staphylococcal enterocolitis: Association with indwelling feeding catheters and *S. aureus* colonization. J Pediatr 88:836, 1976
16. NEAL P, BULL MJ, JANSEN RD, ET AL: Palatal grooves secondary to oral feeding tubes. J Perinatol 5:41, 1986
17. PRICE E, GYOTOKU S: Using the nasojejunal feeding technique in a neonatal intensive care unit. American Journal of Maternal Child Nursing 3:361, 1978
18. SNEED RC, MORGAN WT: Interference of oral phenytoin absorption by enteral tube feedings. Arch Phys Med Rehabil 69:682, 1988
19. SCHAFF-BLASS ES, KUHNS LR, WYMAN ML: Gastric air insufflation as an aid to placement of oro-duodenal tubes. J Pediatr 89:954, 1976
20. RHEA JW, GHAZZAWI O, WEIDMAN W: Nasojejunal feeding: An improved device and intubation technique. J Pediatr 82:951, 1973
21. HENDRY PJ, AKYUREKLI Y, MCINTYRE R, ET AL: Bronchopleural complications of nasogastric feeding tubes. Crit Care Med 14:892, 1986
22. BOROS SJ, REYNOLDS JW: Duodenal perforation: A complication of neonatal nasojejunal feeding. J Pediatr 85:109, 1974
23. CHEN JW, WONG BWK: Intestinal complications of nasojejunal feeding in low birth-weight infants. J Pediatr 85:109, 1974
24. PEREZ-RODRIGUES J, QUERO J, FRIAS, ET AL: Duodenal perforation by silicone rubber tube. J Pediatr 92:113, 1978
25. SIEGLE RL, RABINOWITZ JG, SARASOHN C: Intestinal perforation secondary to nasojejunal feeding tubes. AJR 126:1229, 1976
26. SUN SC, SAMUELS LJ: Duodenal perforation: A rare complication of neonatal nasojejunal tube feeding. Pediatrics 55:371, 1975
27. DRYBURGH E: Transpyloric feeding in 49 infants undergoing intensive care. Arch Dis Child 55:879, 1980
28. LATCHAW LA, JACIR NN, HARRIS BH: The development of pyloric stenosis during transpyloric feedings. J Pediatr Surg 24:823, 1989
29. PATRICK CH, GOODIN J, FOGARTY J: Complication of prolonged transpyloric feeding: Formation of an enterocutaneous fistula. J Pediatr Surg 23:1023, 1988
30. CURET-SCOTT M, SHERMETA A: A comparison of intragastric and intrajejunal feedings in neonatal piglets. J Pediatr Surg 21:552, 1986

39 Gastrostomy

Mary Ann Fletcher
Martin Raymond Eichelberger

A. INDICATIONS[1-3]

1. Inability to swallow
   a. Neurologic or neuromuscular deficit
   b. Complex congenital malformations including esophageal atresia not undergoing early correction
2. Administration of supplemental feedings despite normal deglutition but with grossly inadequate oral intake
   a. Chronic disease states
   b. Requirement for nonpalatable diet
3. Presence of complex bowel disorders for long-term continuous delivery of gastric nutrients
4. Gastrointestinal decompression particularly when respiratory compromise makes prolonged presence of nasogastric tube undesirable
   a. Chronic gastrointestinal decompression: gastroschisis, duodenal atresia, gastric volvulus
   b. Emergency gastric decompression during respiratory failure with diaphragm compressed by inflated stomach: TE fistula with esophageal atresia and need for artificial ventilation

B. CONTRAINDICATIONS

The presence of remediable conditions that unduly increase operative risks

C. EQUIPMENT

Operative Insertion

1. Sterile pediatric instruments appropriate for laparotomy
2. 12 to 14 Fr mushroom (de Pezzer or Malecot) single-lumen latex catheter

Maintenance Care After Insertion

1. Fixation device
   a. Modified, soft, feeding nipple, or
   b. Firm latex catheter bridge
2. Stomahesive (Squibb, Princeton, NJ)
3. 1% hydrogen peroxide
4. Cotton-tipped applicators
5. 2 × 2 gauze sponges

D. TECHNIQUES FOR INSERTION

Placement of gastrostomy tubes in neonates most often requires general anesthesia and frequently occurs as an adjunct to other abdominal surgery. The technique varies according to the individual preferences of the surgeon, but the Stamm procedure described in 1894 is still the most frequently used.[4] The gastrostomy should lie in the center of a triangle formed by the costal margin, umbilicus, and xiphoid.

> There is some suggestion that gastrostomy on the lesser curvature may reduce the incidence of new onset, postoperative gastroesophageal reflux.[5,6]

1. After insertion of nasogastric tube and aseptic preparation of skin, enter abdomen in left upper quadrant through a transverse incision (Fig. 39-1). Expose stomach and pull it into wound.
2. Place two concentric purse-string sutures 0.5 to 1-cm apart on the anterior surface of the stomach toward its greater curvature and halfway between the esophagus and pylorus. Avoid the gastroepiploic vessels (Fig. 39-2).
   a. Inner pursestring for hemostasis
   b. Outer pursestring for inverting and fixing site to abdominal wall
3. Make stab wound through stomach wall in the center of purse-string sutures. With stylet inside catheter, flatten mushroom catheter head and introduce

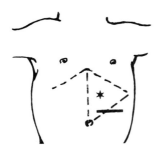

FIG. 39-1
Landmarks for gastrostomy. The primary horizontal incision is left supraumbilical. The gastrostomy tube will pass through the abdomen at a separate site in the center of a triangle formed by the xiphoid, umbilicus, and left costal margin.

catheter through gastric opening. Verify its intragastric placement.

4. Tie sutures sequentially. First suture secures stomach around catheter, providing hemostasis. Second suture inverts first (Stamm method).[4]

5. At center of triangle formed by umbilicus, left costal margin, and xiphoid, make stab wound through abdominal wall, smaller than diameter of catheter (see Fig. 39-1). Insert curved hemostat through stab wound and expose undersurface of abdominal wall through transverse incision. To secure the stomach to the abdominal wall, place, but do not tie, three or four equidistant sutures through seromuscular layers of stomach near gastrostomy and of anterior abdominal wall near hemostat (Fig. 39-3).

6. With hemostat, pull gastrostomy tube through stab incision until stomach is snug against abdominal wall. Tie the previously placed sutures, while placing gentle traction on gastrostomy tube (Fig. 39-3).

   A 4-0 nylon suture in skin helps secure gastrostomy tube and prevent inadvertent removal.

7. Close abdominal incision in layers.

8. Document length of gastrostomy tube outside abdomen.

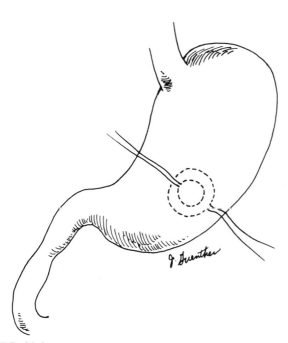

FIG. 39-2
Site for concentric rings for Stamm procedure. Entrance into stomach is on greater curvature midway between esophagus and pylorus.

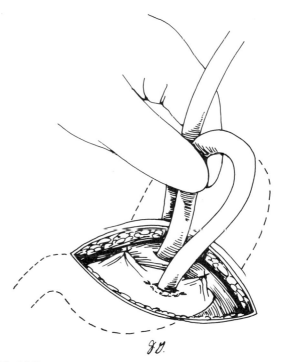

FIG. 39-3
After the tube is secured inside the stomach and passed through a stab wound in the abdominal wall, the anterior wall of the stomach is sutured to the inner wall of the abdomen.

E. FIXATION OF TUBE AFTER SURGICAL PLACEMENT

Attention to fixation of the gastrostomy tube on the anterior abdominal wall is critical to encourage proper gastrocutaneous tract formation and helps prevent many of the most common complications. The gastrostomy tube should exit the abdominal wall at a 90-degree angle to maintain the smallest possible orifice and to minimize leakage. A dressing that supports the tube in an immobile, perpendicular position for 5 to 7 days postoperatively is important. Once the dressing is removed and the wound healed, the gastrostomy tube is secured to the anterior abdominal wall with porous tape to avoid maceration of the skin.

> Feedings may begin as soon as 24 hours postoperatively and increase gradually as clinically indicated. Never clamp a gastrostomy tube for more than a few seconds. Use gravity suspension to prevent loss of gastric contents while preserving the pressure release possible through the tube.

Fixation Materials: Select One Type

1. Latex bridge (Fig. 39-4) (Put on catheter prior to its insertion or replacement.)
   a. Cut large, firm latex catheter at its wider end to length of 3 to 4 cm.
   b. Cut opposing holes at midpoint of latex bridge just wide enough to admit but not constrict gastrostomy tube.

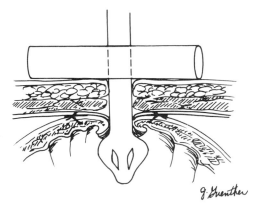

FIG. 39-4
Latex bridge at gastrostomy exit stabilizes tube perpendicular to skin, keeping stoma narrow to avoid leakage. Rotating the bridge around the tube allows change in contact points with the skin. Note how the flared end of the mushroom catheter is pulled to keep the stomach apposed to the abdominal wall.

   c. Pull gastrostomy tube through holes to create tight seal on catheter but without constricting lumen of tube.
   d. Insert distal end of catheter into gastrostomy site as described above. If using a Foley catheter, inject 2 to 4 ml of saline into balloon.
   e. Push latex bridge snug against skin of abdominal wall.
      (1) Pulls balloon of Foley catheter or flange of mushroom catheter against interface between peritoneum and stomach
      (2) Provides support of catheter, exiting abdomen at 90 degrees
   f. For skin care
      (1) Periodically, rotate catheter around gastrostomy tube to vary area of catheter contacting skin.
      (2) Prevent excoriation of skin.
         (a) Apply light coat of antifungal powder.
         (b) Place Stomahesive between skin and bridge.
         (c) Change Stomahesive only every 3 to 4 days, as long as seal around stoma is maintained.
2. Gauze stint
   a. Fold 4 × 4 gauze pad 2 to 4 cm in height and place next to gastrostomy tube at abdominal exit.
   b. Loop gastrostomy catheter over gauze stint.
   c. Secure gauze and tube to abdominal wall with tape.
   d. Apply Stomahesive and antifungal powder.
   e. Keep gastrostomy catheter exiting abdomen at 90 degrees, and stoma exposed for continuous examination.
3. Modified, soft, feeding nipple (Fig. 39-5)[7]

   > Because it is critical to keep site as dry as possible, there must be modification of nipple for good circulation of air.

   a. Excise an elliptical window in flared base of nipple in circumferential direction (1–1.5 cm in length).
   b. Make 1-cm crosscut in tip of nipple.
   c. Coat undersurface of nipple flange with Stomahesive as well as skin area around gastrostomy.
   d. Slide nipple over gastrostomy tube until there is contact with anterior abdominal wall.

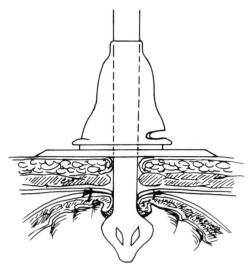

FIG. 39-5
Modified feeding nipple. The elliptical hole at the base allows air circulation and regular cleaning of the skin as important factors in avoiding maceration of the site. (Kappell DA, Leape LL: A method of gastrostomy fixation. J Pediatr Surg 10:523, 1975. Modified by permission.)

e. Adjust tension on tube to pull flange or balloon of catheter against internal wall of stomach.
f. Tape nipple flange to skin, without covering elliptical hole to allow air circulation and visualization of site.
  (1) Dislodgement
  (2) Necrosis of underlying skin
g. Clean skin around gastrostomy site with cotton applicators inserted through elliptical window.
  (1) Moisture under nipple leads to maceration. Keep area under nipple dry to avoid skin maceration.
  (2) Replace Stomahesive around gastrostomy site as needed.

F. MAINTENANCE CARE OF GASTROSTOMY

1. Maintain apposition of anterior gastric wall to peritoneum.
  a. Prevent gastric distention.
  b. Keep flared end of tube pulled snugly against stomach wall, but avoid pressure necrosis of abdominal wall (see Figs. 39-4, 39-5).

2. Keep tube immobile at insertion site to maintain stoma as small as possible.
  a. Use careful fixation to maintain perpendicular position
  b. Keep some slack in tube when it is suspended.
3. Prevent migration of tube through pylorus or esophagus by
  a. Proper fixation
  b. Comparing length of external tube with postoperative length
  c. Observing for signs of obstruction, for example,
    (1) Gastric distention
    (2) Increased drainage from oral gastric or gastrostomy tubes
    (3) Bilious drainage
    (4) Gastroesophageal reflux, new or increased
4. Minimize leak from gastrostomy site in long-term gastrostomies.
  a. Maintain tight fit of tube in stoma.
  b. Avoid local infection.
  c. Treat leaking gastrostomy early.
    (1) Remove tube for 24 hours to allow partial closure.
    (2) Replace mushroom catheter with Foley catheter, and pull balloon (inflated with 2–ml H_2O) against abdominal wall to seal leak. Use latex bridge to secure tube.
    (3) Apply Stomahesive around catheter to decrease excoriation and to encourage epithelialization. Change Stomahesive only every 3 to 4 days, as long as seal remains.
    (4) Maintain perpendicular position of gastrostomy tube.
    (5) Keep tube unclamped.
    (6) Maintain skin and stoma hygiene.
      (a) Cleanse daily with 1% hydrogen peroxide.
      (b) Keep area dry. Change dressing after cleansing skin and whenever wet.

G. REPLACING GASTROSTOMY TUBE

1. During first week after gastrostomy, reoperation for replacement is usually necessary.
2. After formation of fistulous tract, nonoperative placement is possible.
  a. To avoid stoma closure, replace within 4 to 6 hours.

b. Use deflated Foley catheter for replacement prior to formation of epithelialized tract.
  (1) Probe stoma with hemostat or thin dilator to establish course of tract, which is usually medial toward vertebral column at 45-degree angle.
  (2) Lubricate catheter generously with water-soluble lubricant, and insert gently. Use hemostat to guide tube if it does not pass alone.
  (3) Inflate balloon with 2 to 4 ml of water, and pull against stomach wall.
  (4) Secure with fixation device.
  (5) Mark outside length of catheter to help detect internal or external migration of balloon.

c. Use mushroom catheter replacement in well-established tract.
  (1) Carefully determine direction of tract.
  (2) Lubricate catheter.
  (3) Stretch tip of mushroom catheter with thin, metal dilator or cotton-tipped applicator to decrease angle of flange.
  (4) Apply gentle pressure to insert catheter.

Avoid force, which may lead to traumatic separation of stomach from abdominal wall.

d. Confirm intragastric position by one of following methods.
  (1) For recent gastrostomy
    (a) Instill 30 ml of air, clamp, and obtain decubitus radiograph for evidence of pneumoperitoneum.
    (b) Instill 15 to 30 ml of $^{1}/_{4}$-strength Gastrografin and obtain decubitus radiograph. Remove Gastrografin.
  (2) For well-established gastrostomy, aspirate and determine acidity.

H. DISCONTINUATION OF GASTROSTOMY TUBE[8]

General
1. Remove tube, and apply gauze dressing.
2. Allow spontaneous closure, usually 4 to 7 days, or
3. Approximate skin edge with skin closure tape.

Persistent Gastrocutaneous Fistula
1. Cause: granulation and epithelialization of gastrocutaneous tract
2. Remove tube.
3. Cauterize granulation tissue or epithelium within stoma with silver nitrate sticks.
4. Seal orifice with Stomahesive.
5. Approximate edges with surgical tape.
6. Persistent gastrocutaneous fistula of 4 to 6 weeks: surgical closure required.

I. EMERGENCY PERCUTANEOUS CELIOTOMY

The use of percutaneous gastrostomy placement has gained favor in certain conditions, particularly in older patients where general anesthesia can be avoided. There are several techniques well described in the literature that are performed either with or without endoscopy.

a. Percutaneous endoscopic gastrostomy (PEG)
  (1) "Pull" technique[9]
  (2) "Push" technique[10]
  (3) "Poke" technique[11]
b. Nonendoscopic[12]

Percutaneous gastrostomy has limited indications for use in neonates because many of the advantages offered to older patients do not transfer to neonates.

The original method of PEG described by Gauderer in 1980 involves four basic elements.
  (1) Gastroscopic insufflation to appose stomach to abdominal wall
  (2) Percutaneous introduction of tapered cannula under direct endoscopic guidance
  (3) Introduction of a long suture through cannula with one end withdrawn through patient's mouth
  (4) Tying to the oral end of the suture a modified mushroom catheter and pulling it through the stomach and abdominal wall. The catheter is modified with a tapered end where it is pulled through the abdominal wall and with a latex bridge at its mushroom end to keep it from pulling out of the stomach.[3]

We describe an emergency percutaneous celiotomy that may be used as a life-saving measure when there is either respiratory failure or a high probability of gastric rupture in the presence of extreme gastric distention and when surgical gastrostomy is not immediately available.

> The primary indication for this type of procedure is in infants with esophageal atresia and fistula who have critical diaphragmatic constriction from gastric distention prior to interhospital transport.

1. Prepare skin in upper left abdomen with antiseptic solution. Blot excess.
2. If possible, transilluminate abdomen to verify position of distended stomach away from liver.
3. Using 20-gauge catheter with needle stylet, puncture abdominal wall at the junction of the left anterior rib cage and the lateral border of the rectus abdominis muscle. Advance needle through wall into stomach.
4. Remove needle while advancing cannula to a depth of several centimeters, depending on infant size. Attach short IV extension tubing, three-way stopcock, and syringe. Aspirate only enough air to relieve tamponade effect and improve ventilation. Avoid completely emptying stomach.
5. Secure cannula and keep in place until surgical evaluation is possible.

J. COMPLICATIONS[1–3,13,14]

1. Separation of stomach from anterior abdominal wall: peritonitis
2. Wound separation, dehiscence, ventral hernia
3. Intraperitoneal spillage
4. Hemorrhage
5. Injury to posterior wall of stomach on initial insertion or reinsertion
6. Perforation of or injury to other organs
   a. Diaphragm
   b. Esophagus[15]
   c. Liver, spleen
   d. Colon
7. Pneumoperitoneum (after PEG)
8. Prolonged ileus, gastric atony, failure to accept feedings
9. Gastric torsion around catheter
10. Adhesive bowel obstruction
11. Dislodgement
    a. Inadvertent removal
    b. Intraperitoneal, extragastric placement
    c. Internal or external migration[16]
12. Catheter deterioration
    a. Fractured catheter
    b. Rupture of balloon
13. Tube occlusion
14. Persistent leak
    a. Wound breakdown
       (1) Granulation tissue and skin irritation
       (2) Infection, particularly moniliasis
       (3) Dislodgement because of loosening
    b. Electrolyte imbalance
    c. Malnutrition
15. Prolapse of gastric mucosa
    a. Bleeding
    b. Excessive leakage
16. Gastroesophageal reflux: new onset or exacerbation[17]
17. Gastrocutaneous fistula[8,18]

References

1. GALLAGHER MW, TYSON KRT, ASCHCRAFT KW: Gastrostomy in pediatric patients: An analysis of complications and techniques. Surgery 536:74, 1973
2. CYWES S: Stomas in children. S African Med J 50:815, 1976
3. GAUDERER MWL, STELLATO TA: Gastrostomies: Evolution, techniques, indications and complications. Curr Probl Surg 23:661, 1986
4. STAMM M: Gastrostomy by a new method. Med News (NY) 65:324, 1894
5. STRINGEL G: Gastrostomy with antireflux properties. J Pediatr Surg 25:1019, 1990
6. SEEKRI IK, RESCORIA FJ, CANAL DF, ET AL: Lesser curvature gastrostomy reduces the incidence of postoperative gastroesophageal reflux. J Pediatr Surg 26:982, 1991
7. KAPPEL DA, LEAPE LL: A method of gastrostomy fixation. J Pediatr Surg 10:523, 1975
8. DUCHARME JC, YOUSEFF S, TILKIN F: Gastrostomy closure: A quick, easy and safe method. J Pediatr Surg 12:729, 1977
9. GAUDERER MWL, PONSKY JL, IZANT RJ JR: Gastrostomy without laparotomy: A percutaneous endoscopic technique. J Pediatr Surg 15:872, 1980
10. SACHS BA, VINE HS, PALESTRANT AM, ET AL: A nonoperative technique for establishment of a gastrostomy in the dog. Invest Radiol 18:485, 1983

11. Russell TR, Brotman M, Norris F: Percutaneous gastrostomy. A new simplified and cost-effective technique. Am J Surg 148:132, 1984

12. Cory DA, Fitzgerald JF, Cohen MD: Percutaneous nonendoscopic gastrostomy in children. AJR 151:995, 1988

13. Campbell JR, Sasaki TM: Gastrostomy in infants and children: An analysis of complications and techniques. Am Surg 40:505, 1974

14. Gauderer MWL: Percutaneous endoscopic gastrostomy: A 10-year experience with 220 children. J Pediatr Surg 26:288, 1991

15. Kenigsberg K, Levenbrown J: Esophageal perforation secondary to gastrostomy tube replacement. J Pediatr Surg 21:946, 1986

16. Currarino G, Votteler T: Prolapse of the gastrostomy catheter in children. American Journal of Roentgenology, Radium Therapy and Nuclear Medicine 123:737, 1975

17. Jolley SG, Tunnel WB, Hoelzer DJ, et al: Lower esophageal pressure changes with tube gastrostomy: A causative factor of gastroesophageal reflux in children? J Pediatr Surg 21:624, 1986

18. Aronian JM, Redo SF: Gastrocutaneous fistula after tube gastrostomy. Incidence in infants and children. NY State J Med 74:2364, 1974

Part 8
Transfusions

40 Transfusion of Blood and Blood Products

Naomi L.C. Luban

Red Blood Cell Transfusions

A. INDICATIONS[1-9]

1. Replace acute blood loss.
2. Correct anemia that is
   a. Compromising cardiovascular status
   b. Compromising oxygen-carrying capacity
3. Correct iatrogenic blood loss when 2.a. or 2.b. are anticipated.

B. CONTRAINDICATIONS

1. None absolute
2. Exert caution in patient with
   a. Volume overload
   b. Congestive heart failure

C. EQUIPMENT

1. Blood product (Appendix C)
2. Cardiorespiratory monitor
3. Blood filter: all blood, blood products, must be filtered prior to transfusion.[10]
   a. Standard administration set filter
      (1) 120 to 170 μ particle size
      (2) Appropriate for red cells, plasma, and platelets
   b. Microaggregate filter[11]
      (1) 20 to 40 μ particle size
      (2) Must follow manufacturer's instructions
      (3) Some only function if product dripped
      (4) Not advisable for syringe administration
   c. Third generation leukocyte removal filters
      (1) "Ultrafiltration" capability removes 99.9% of WBC or 3 log leukodepletion
      (2) Must follow manufacturer's instructions
      (3) May be useful for attenuation/abrogation of CMV and other viruses harbored in WBC
      (4) Most are not suitable as bedside filters in neonatal ICU as yet[12]
4. Sterile syringes
5. Blood administration set (includes standard filter)
6. Automated syringe pump with appropriate tubing to patient[11,13]

   Least hemolysis occurs with straight syringe pumps (e.g., Harvard; Auto-syringe).[14,15]

7. Vascular access through 23 or larger gauge needle, cannula, or catheter.

   The amount of hemolysis that results from infusion of RBCs is directly proportionate to length of storage of blood and rate of transfusion, and inversely to needle size. Hyperkalemia, hemoglobinuria, and renal dysfunction may result if hemolyzed blood is transfused.[16]

8. Normal saline flush (1–3 ml) to clear IV solution
9. Specialized blood warmer and appropriate tubing (optional)

   Warming blood is only necessary when large volumes of blood are being used for whole and/or partial exchange transfusions. Inappropriate warming by exposure of blood to heat lamps or phototherapy lights may produce hemolysis.[17]

D. PRECAUTIONS

1. Limit use of transfusions to true indications.[2]
2. Select blood product appropriate for infant's condition.
3. Carefully confirm that blood product received is correct one for patient, prior to transfusion.
4. Avoid excessive transfusion volume or rate unless acute blood loss or shock dictates faster transfusion.

a. 10 ml/kg red cells in single transfusion at 2 to 5 ml/kg/hr

b. 20 ml/kg whole blood in single transfusion at 5 to 10 ml/kg/hr

5. Store blood and blood products appropriately.

a. Use blood bank refrigerator for storage of RBC, whole blood, thawed FFP, and thawed cryoprecipitate.

(1) Temperature controlled at $4 \pm 2°C$ with constant temperature monitors and alarm systems

(2) Refrigerator is quality-controlled at least daily.

(3) Designated for blood products only

b. Limit time blood is at room temperature as much as possible. Should never exceed 4 hours to minimize

(1) Bacterial contamination

(2) Red blood cell hemolysis

c. Platelets should never be refrigerator-stored[10] and never transfused through a blood warmer. Syringe storage at 20 to 22°C and electromechanical infusion do not harm platelets.[18]

6. Heat only in quality-controlled blood warmer.

7. Stop transfusion or slow rate if baby manifests any adverse side-effects.

a. Tachycardia, bradycardia, or arrhythmia

b. Tachypnea

c. Systolic blood pressure increases of more than 15 mm Hg, unless this is the desired effect

d. Temperature above 38°C

e. Hyperglycemia or hypoglycemia

f. Cyanosis

g. Skin rash, hives, or flushing

h. Hematuria

8. Use cautiously in incipient or existing cardiac failure

a. Monitor heart rate, blood pressure, and peripheral perfusion.

b. Transfuse packed red blood cells, or

c. Consider partial exchange transfusion

(1) With hemoglobin level less than 5 to 7 g/dl

(2) With cord hemoglobin less than 10 g/dl

9. Prevent hypoglycemia.

a. In infants less than 1200 gm or in other unstable infants

(1) Establish separate IV for blood administration.

(2) Continue parenteral glucose administration.

b. Expect rebound hypoglycemia when transfused blood has elevated glucose concentration.

E. TECHNIQUE

1. Determine total amount of blood needed.

a. Calculate volume of blood for transfusion.

b. Include volume of blood needed for deadspace of tubing, filter, pump mechanism. (Varies from system to system; may be as much as 30 ml.)

2. Obtain blood product

a. Verify whether crossmatched or uncrossmatched product necessary.[19–21]

b. Confirm that restrictions have been adhered to on blood product and transfusion tag.

(1) CMV—tested/untested[22–24]

(2) Irradiated—yes/no[25–27]

(3) Directed donation—yes/no[19]

(4) RBC antigen negative—yes/no[10]

(5) Sickledex negative—yes/no[28]

(6) Other restrictions specified—yes/no

3. Verify blood identification by comparing blood-bank slip and patient identification.

a. Hospital number or other designated number of blood unit

b. Patient hospital number

c. Patient identification by armband or footband

d. Blood group and type of both donor and recipient

e. Expiration date and time

4. Adhere to sterile technique throughout procedure.

5. Warm blood as indicated.[29,30]

a. Smaller-volume transfusions, over a 1-hour duration: allow blood to remain at room temperature for 20 minutes before starting infusion.

b. Large-volume transfusions, primarily exchange transfusions: use controlled blood warmer.

6. Attach filter and tubing as indicated by manufacturer's instructions for selected automated pump, warmer, and infusion route.

7. If desired, prepare for use of more than one aliquot from a single bag (i.e., small volumes to be removed from single blood unit over time).

a. Use multi-injection site coupler following sterile technique.

(1) Use large bore needle (18 g or >).

(2) Remove ml needed into syringe (Fig. 40-1).

Use in-line filter to prepare filtered syringe ready to mount into infusion device. Filter should be placed between bag and syringe or syringe and infusion line.

(3) Primary bag outdates 24 hours from entry with coupler.

b. Use sterile connecting device to splice single or multiple satellite bags onto primary bag. (Fig. 40-2 A to F)

(1) Handle each satellite bag as a primary bag with lesser volume.

(2) Satellite bags outdate at same time as primary bag.

8. Clear syringe and tubing of bubbles.

9. Verify patency of vascular access.

10. Clear line into patient with normal saline.

11. Record and monitor vital signs.

12. Determine spot glucose test (Dextrostix). Repeat hourly.

13. Begin transfusion at controlled rate.

14. Gently invert container of blood every 15 to 30 minutes to minimize sedimentation.

15. Stop transfusion when any adverse change in condition occurs.

16. At end of infusion, clear blood from line with saline prior to reinitiating glucose solutions.

17. Check recipient hemoglobin and hematocrit at least 2 hours post-transfusion.

18. If post-transfusion hematocrit/hemoglobin is not up to expected level, check following.

a. Inappropriate calculation of transfusion requirement

b. Ongoing blood loss

c. Transfusion reaction

d. Hemolysis due to ABO or other RBC incompatibility[19,31]

(1) Infant has circulating anti-A, anti-B, and anti-AB which is bound to A or B antigens on transfused RBCs.

(2) Direct antiglobulin (Coombs) test negative initially, now positive

(3) Unexpected increase in bilirubin

(4) Infant has RBC antibody other than ABO.

e. Hemolysis from extrinsic damage to RBCs[17,30]

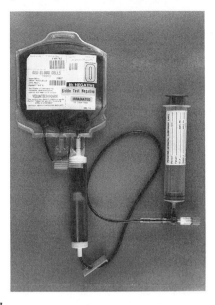

FIG. 40-1
Drawing up red blood cells via in-line filter. RBCs or washed RBCs can be pre-filtered in the blood bank using a standard blood transfusion filter, three-way stopcock, and labelled syringe. Aliquots can be drawn off as needed. Because the blood is pre-filtered, only a minimal extra volume is required to fill the short tubing. Expiration time of the blood is reduced to 24 hours. The same system may be used for FFP and platelets.

F. COMPLICATIONS

1. Transmission of infectious diseases

a. Bacterial organisms[32]

b. Cytomegalovirus[12,23,33,34]

c. Epstein-Barr virus[22]

d. Hepatitis A, B and C, non-A, non-B[35–38]

e. Human immunodeficiency virus I and human T-lymphotrophic virus I/II[39–41]

f. Malaria

g. Syphilis

h. Toxoplasmosis

2. Circulatory overload with/without intravascular hemorrhage[42]

3. Transfusion reaction[28]

a. Hemolytic

(1) Immunologic

(2) Overheating of blood[17,30]

(3) Improper freezing of blood

(4) Exposure to hypertonic or hypotonic solutions

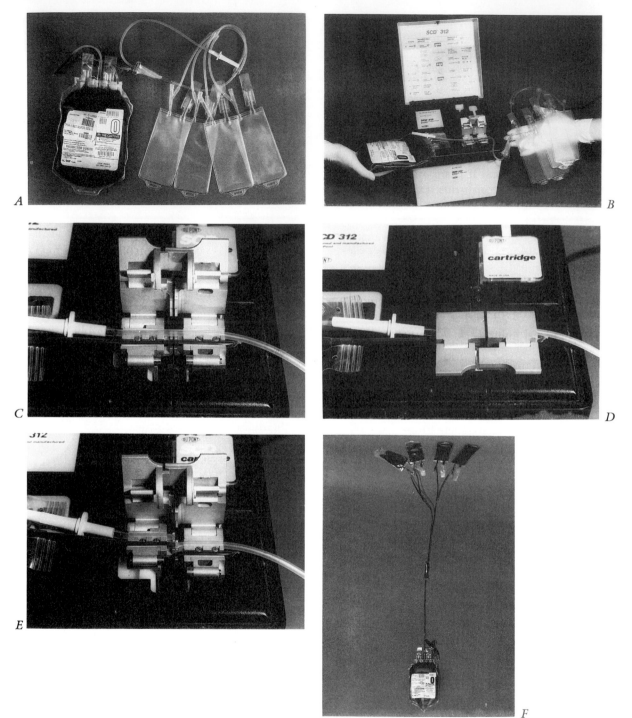

FIG. 40-2
Use of a sterile connecting device. (*A*) An adult RBC unit is shown along with a set of pediatric transfer bags. (*B*) The transfer bags can be attached by spiking the unit, causing it to expire in 24 hours; or alternately, the transfer bags can be connected using a sterile connection device. (*C*) The separate tubings are loaded into the tubing holders of the device. (*D*) The covers are closed. (*E*) A welding wafer heated to about 500°F melts through the tubing. The tubing holders realign and the welding wafer retracts allowing the tubing ends to fuse together. (*F*) The unit can now be aliquoted as needed. Because a functionally closed system has been maintained, the expiration date of the blood has not changed.

(5) Trauma to cells
   (a) Small needle size
   (b) Excessive handling in preparation
  b. Febrile, nonhemolytic
  c. Allergic, anaphylactic[19,26,43]
  d. Graft versus host
4. Intravenous sickling
5. Metabolic[44]
  a. Hyperkalemia[45,46]
  b. Hypoglycemia or hyperglycemia
  c. Hypocalcemia
  d. Acidosis from acid pH of blood
  e. Post-transfusion alkalosis from citrate metabolism
6. Retrolental fibroplasia (may be a contributing factor among several others)[47]
7. Technical problems relating to route of administration
  a. Catheter-related or IV-related (see Part V, Vascular Access)
  b. Air embolism[5,30]
  c. Inadvertant heating
8. T-cell activation, especially in infants with necrotising enterocolitis[48]

Autologous Fetal Blood (AFB) Transfusions

A. INDICATIONS

Emergency transfusion at birth of infant with unexpected hypovolemic shock

B. CONTRAINDICATIONS[49,50]

1. Maternal infection
  a. Chorioamnionitis
  b. Sepsis
  c. Hepatitis
2. Prolonged rupture of membranes > 24 hours
3. Rapid availability of properly collected O-negative packed cells

C. EQUIPMENT

Keep all equipment sterile.

1. Antiseptic solution (e.g., iodophor)

2. Swab or gauze sponge for antiseptic
3. Saline in 5- to 10-ml syringe (for cord rinse)
4. Three 18-gauge needles
5. 50-ml syringe for blood collection
6. Three-way stopcock
7. Saline for dilution of heparin
8. Heparin (prepare proper dilution)
  a. 1:1000 diluted to 1:3300 for syringe prime, or
  b. 1:100 for direct addition to blood
9. 20 to 40 μ microaggregate blood filter
10. Laboratory tubes
  a. Platelet count, hemoglobin, hematocrit
  b. Prothrombin, partial thromboplastin times
  c. Thrombin time or reptilase time
  d. Anaerobic and aerobic culture medium

D. PRECAUTIONS

1. Use strict asepsis throughout procedure and transfusion.
2. Use only correctly diluted heparin in priming syringe for anticoagulation.
3. Use blood within 15 to 30 minutes of collection.
  a. Better protection against bacterial growth
  b. Better anticoagulation
  c. More physiologic preparation
4. Filter blood at time of transfusion.
5. Follow coagulation profile in recipient.

E. TECHNIQUE

1. Calculate amount of blood needed.
  a. For studies (10 ml–15 ml)
  b. For transfusion (10ml/kg)
2. Heparinize (requires 2 units–3 units per ml of AFB drawn).
  a. 0.5 ml of 1:3300 heparin in 50-ml syringe
   (1) 1 ml heparin (1:1000), plus
   (2) 2 ml saline
   (3) Prime in syringe, and then expel, or
  b. 1:100 heparin in tuberculin syringe
   (1) Add by way of three-way stopcock as blood is drawn.
   (2) 0.2 ml for each 10 ml of AFB
3. Prepare umbilical cord or placenta for sterile venipuncture.
  a. Umbilical cord: after vaginal delivery of infant, but prior to delivery of placenta

(1) Using antiseptic, clean umbilical cord 1 to 3 inches above cord clamp. Keep cleansed area away from perineum.

(2) Rinse venipuncture site on umbilical cord with sterile saline.

(3) Using prepared syringe, perform venipuncture, and aspirate with free flow of blood without bubbles.

  b. Placenta

(1) After delivery of placenta, clean area on fetal surface near insertion of cord with antiseptic.

(2) Rinse with sterile saline.

(3) Select superficial prominent vessel close to cord, and perform venipuncture with primed syringe.

(4) Aspirate with free flow of blood without bubbles.

4. Periodically, invert syringe carefully until transfusion is complete to mix heparin.

5. Transfer blood for laboratory studies.

> Do laboratory studies before attaching filter, because forcing blood through microaggregate filter may prolong activated prothrombin time (PT) and partial thromboplastin time (PTT).

  a. Do coagulation studies first.
  b. Change needle before adding blood to culture media.

6. Remove needle, and attach microaggregate filter to blood syringe.

7. Transfuse blood as per Blood Transfusions.

8. Obtain laboratory samples from infant post-transfusion.
  a. Coagulation profile
  b. Aerobic and anaerobic blood cultures
  c. Hemoglobin and hematocrit

F. COMPLICATIONS

1. Excess heparinization, causing prolonged coagulation profile or clinical bleeding in infant

2. Inadequate heparinization, causing clotting before administration, or thromboemboli if not removed by filter

3. Bacterial sepsis from contaminated collection

Platelet Transfusions

A. INDICATIONS[2]

Severe thrombocytopenia or thrombocytopathy with symptomatic bleeding; moderate thrombocytopenia in association with intraventricular hemorrhage[51–55]

B. CONTRAINDICATIONS

Because the half-life of platelets is so limited in conditions of rapid consumption or immune destruction, platelet transfusions are rarely helpful. Additionally, platelet transfusions may in some instances worsen the pathologic process. Their use in these conditions is reserved for life-threatening situations in which other therapy is ineffective.

1. Immune thrombocytopenia
2. Consumptive coagulopathy with marked coagulation defects

C. EQUIPMENT

1. Platelets[56]
  a. Random donor, platelet concentrate (5.5×10^{10} platelets/bag)
    (1) Separated from whole blood by centrifugation within 8 hours of blood draw
    (2) Resuspended in plasma
    (3) May be maternal if indicated for isoimmune thrombocytopenia of newborn
  b. Plateletpheresis (3×10^{11} platelets/bag)
    (1) Removes only platelets, returns RBC and plasma to donor
    (2) Permits repeated donations from same donor every 48 hours under select circumstances
    (3) High yield of platelets
    (4) More costly product
    (5) May be HLA typed or PLA1 typed
    (6) Rarely indicated in newborn. Feasible if sterile connecting device is used to permit multiple sterile aliquots to be removed over 5-day dating period

In alloimmune neonatal thrombocytopenia, when infant is platelet antigen PLA1 negative and has circulating anti-PLA1, use maternal PLA1 negative platelets washed and resuspended in group compatible ABO plasma.[57]

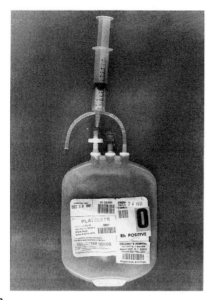

FIG. 40-3
Platelet unit. Platelet aliquots in small volume may be required for neonatal use. They may be drawn up in a syringe for administration, but must be filtered prior to infusion. An alternate method of providing platelets in a syringe is to prefilter them as shown in Fig. 40-1.

2. Platelet or blood administration set with 120 to 170 μ in-line filter.

> If using a leukodepletion filter, only use filters approved for use with platelet concentrates.

3. Sterile syringe for automated pump infusion (Fig. 40-3)

> Use of syringe technique will increase handling of platelets. Administer by drip if clinically feasible

4. Automated syringe pump
5. Connecting IV tubing
6. IV access, preferably through 23-gauge or larger needle or through umbilical venous catheter
7. Normal saline flush solution

D. PRECAUTIONS

1. Use type-specific platelets when potential for sensitization is present (i.e., in Rh-negative female).

> Although platelets do not have Rh antigens, there is usually some degree of red blood cell

TABLE 40-1
Choice of Platelets

Baby	Donor
O	O
A	A, AB
B	B, AB
AB	AB

contamination in platelet preparations that may cause Rh sensitization.[51]

2. Use platelets from donor with ABO-compatible plasma (Table 40-1).

> Isohemagglutinins in ABO-incompatible plasma may result in hemolysis, a positive direct Coombs' test, and poorer in vivo platelet survival than anticipated.

3. Transfuse platelets as soon after preparation as possible.
4. If fluid overload is a significant concern, two possible options are
   a. Remove aliquot of 15 ml/kg from random donor platelet concentrate.[51]
   b. Concentrate random donor platelets by reducing volume from 45–75 ml to 25 ml by centrifugation[10]

> The increased handling of platelets in concentrating them may decrease their number and viability.

   (1) Centrifuge at 22°C, with lateral plasma packs at 1500 rpm (580 g) for 20 minutes.
   (2) Express all but 15 to 20 ml of platelet-poor plasma.
   (3) Allow to stand at 20 to 24°C for 15 minutes.
   (4) Resuspend by rocking action.
   (5) Transfuse immediately.

E. TECHNIQUE OF PLATELET ADMINISTRATION BY AUTOMATED SYRINGE

1. Estimate by weight the volume of platelets in single bag to determine fluid load to infant. Deter-

mine what volume will be tolerated, plus volume needed for deadspace of tubing.

One unit of platelets should increase the count by 50,000 per mm³ per 5 kg of body weight, with a decrement of 10% per day in the absence of abnormal consumption.

2. Confirm correct platelet product.
   a. Infant and unit identification
   b. Infant and donor blood group, and Rh type
   c. That restrictions (i.e., CMV negative,[23] irradiated[60] other) have been honored.
3. Attach, aseptically, in sequence.
   a. Platelet pack
   b. Platelet administration set, including filter
   c. Three-way stopcock
   d. Transfusion syringe
4. Draw into syringe volume of platelets for transfusion and tubing deadspace. Clear air bubbles.
5. Remove syringe from three-way stopcock and attach to connecting tubing.
6. Establish IV access. If infant is at risk for hypoglycemia, with interruption of continuous glucose source, start new IV or monitor closely throughout infusion.
7. Clear IV of glucose solution with 1 to 3 ml of saline.
8. Attach connecting tubing and syringe to IV.
9. Monitor vital signs of patient.
10. Infuse platelets over 1- to 2-hour period

    Faster if tolerated by infant

11. After infusion is complete, flush IV with 1 to 3 ml of normal saline before restarting glucose solution.
12. Determine survival time of transfused platelets by obtaining counts at 1, 2, or 24 hours.

F. COMPLICATIONS

See list of complications for all blood products (Blood Transfusion, F).

1. Accentuated hemolysis in sensitized but Coombs-negative ABO setup
2. Rh sensitization in Rh-negative recipient
3. Volume overload
4. Decreased platelet adhesion because of donor ingestion of aspirin
5. Sepsis

Fresh Frozen Plasma and Cryoprecipitate

A. INDICATIONS[2]

Complex factor deficiency unresponsive to Vitamin K, isolated congenital factor deficiency or congenital or acquired dys or hypofibrinogenemia.

B. CONTRAINDICATIONS

1. None absolute.
2. Exert caution when possibility of volume overload.
3. Do not use for volume expansion or provision of trace minerals.[2]
4. Necrotizing enterocolitis (NEC)—use with extreme caution.[48] May aggravate hemolysis in child with NEC and T activation.

C. EQUIPMENT AND TECHNIQUE SEE PLATELET TRANSFUSION

References

1. ALVERSON DC, ISKEU VH, COHEN RSA: Effect of booster blood transfusions on oxygen utilization in infants with bronchopulmonary dysplasia. J Pediatr 113:722, 1988
2. BLANCHETTE VS, HUME HL, LEVEY GL, ET AL: Guidelines for auditing pediatric blood transfusion practices. Am J Dis Child 145:787, 1991
3. BROWN MS, BERMAN ER, LUCKEY D: Prediction of the need for transfusion during anemia of prematurity. J Pediatr 116:773, 1990
4. HUDSON I, COOKE A, HOLLAND B, ET AL: Red cell volume and cardiac output in anaemic preterm infants. Arch Dis Child 65:672, 1990
5. JONES JG, HOLLAND BM, HUDSON IR, ET AL: Total circulating red cells versus hematocrit as the primary descriptor of oxygen delivery. Br J Haematol 76:228, 1990
6. JOSHI A, GERHARDT T, SHANDLOFF P, ET AL: Blood transfusion effect on the respiratory pattern of preterm infants. Pediatrics 80:79, 1987
7. KEYES WG, DONOHUE PK, SPIVAK JL, ET AL: Assessing the need for transfusion of premature infants and role of hematocrit, clinical signs and erythropoietin level. Pediatrics 84:412, 1989
8. LENES BA, SACHER RA: Blood component therapy in neonatal medicine. Clin Lab Med 1:285, 1981

9. Ross MP, Christensen RD, Rothstein G, et al: A randomized trial to develop criteria for administering erythrocyte transfusions to anemic preterm infants 1 to 3 months of age. J Perinatol 9:246, 1989

10. Standards for Blood Banks and Transfusion Services, 14th Ed. Arlington, VA, American Association of Blood Banks, 1991

11. Ciavarella D, Synder E: Clinical use of blood transfusion devices. Transfus Med Rev 2:95, 1988

12. Gilbert GL, Hayes K, Hudson IL, James J: Prevention of transfusion-acquired cytomegalovirus infection in infants by blood filtration to remove leukocytes. Lancet II:1288, 1989

13. Gurdak RG, Anderson G, Mintz G. Evaluation of IVAC variable pressure volumetric pump Model 560 for the delivery of red blood cells, adenine-saline added. Am J Clin Pathol 91:199, 1989

14. Veerman MW, Leff RD, Roberts RJ: Influence of two piston-type infusion pumps on hemolysis of infused red blood cells. Am J Hosp Pharm 42:626, 1985

15. Wilcox GJ, Barnes A, Modanlou H: Does transfusion using a syringe infusion pump and small-gauge needle cause hemolysis? Transfusion 21:750, 1981

16. Herrera A, Corless J: Blood transfusions: Effect of speed of infusion and of needle gauge on hemolysis. J Pediatr 99:757, 1981

17. Opitz JC, Baldauf MC, Kessler DL, Meyer JA: Hemolysis of blood in intravenous tubing caused by heat. J Pediatr 112:111, 1988

18. Pisciotto PT, Snyder EL, Napychank PA, Hopfer SM: In vitro characteristics of volume-reduced platelet concentrate stored in syringes. Transfusion 31:404, 1991

19. Elbert C, Strauss RG, Barrett F, et al: Biological mothers may be dangerous blood donors for their neonates. Acta Haematol 85:189, 1991

20. Floss AM, Strauss RG, Goeken N, Knox L: Multiple transfusions fail to provoke antibodies against blood cell antigens in human infants. Transfusion 26:419, 1986

21. Ludvigsen CW, Swanson JL, Thompson TR, McCullough J: The failure of neonates to form red blood cell alloantibodies in response to multiple transfusions. Am J Clin Pathol 87:250, 1987

22. Luban NLC: Transfusion-associated infection. In Donowitz LC (ed): Hospital Acquired Infection in the Pediatric Patient. Baltimore, Williams and Wilkins, 1988, p 109

23. Yeager AS, Grumet FC, Hafleigh EB, et al: Prevention of transfusion acquired cytomegalovirus infection in newborn infants. J Pediatr 98:281, 1981

24. Tegtmeier GE: The use of cytomegalovirus-screened blood in neonates [Editorial]. Transfusion 28:201, 1988

25. Funkhouser AW, Vogelsang G, Zehnbauer B, et al: Graft versus host disease after blood transfusions in a premature infant. Pediatrics 87:247, 1991

26. Holland PV: Prevention of transfusion-associated graft-versus-host disease. Arch Pathol Lab Med 113:285, 1989

27. Thaler M, Shamiss A, Orgad S, et al: The role of blood from HLA-homozygous donors in fatal transfusion-associated graft-versus-host disease after open heart surgery. N Engl J Med 321:25, 1989

28. Luban NLC: Adverse reactions to blood and blood products. In Kasprisin DO, Luban NLC (eds): Pediatric Transfusion Medicine. Boca Raton, FL, CRC Press, 1987, p 127

29. Luban NLC, Mikesell J, Sacher RA: Techniques for warming red blood cells packaged in different containers for neonatal use. Clin Pediatr 24:642, 1985

30. Strauss RG, Bell EF, Snyder EL, et al: Effect of environmental warming on blood components dispensed in syringes for neonatal transfusions. J Pediatr 109:109, 1986

31. Falterman CG, Richardson CJ: Transfusion reaction due to unrecognized ABO hemolytic disease of the newborn infant. J Pediatr 97:812, 1980

32. Tipple MA, Bland LA, Murphy JJ, et al: Sepsis associated with transfusion of red cells contaminated with yersinia enterocolitica. Transfusion 30: 207, 1990

33. Adler SP: Data that suggest that FFP does not transmit CMV [letter]. Transfusion 28:604, 1988

34. Yeager AS: Transfusion-acquired cytomegalovirus in newborn infants. J Pediatr 98:281, 1981

35. Alter HJ, Purcell RH, Shih JW, et al: Detection of antibody to hepatitis C virus in prospectively followed transfusion recipients with acute and chronic non-A and non-B hepatitis. N Engl J Med 321:1494, 1989

36. Esteban JI, Gonzales A, Hernandez JM, et al: Evolution of antibodies of hepatitis C virus in a study of transfusion-associated hepatitis. N Engl J Med 323:1107, 1990

37. Hoofnagle JH: Post-transfusion hepatitis B. Transfusion 30:384, 1990

38. Polesky HF, Hanson MR: Transfusion-associated hepatitis C virus (non-A, non-B) infection. Arch Pathol Lab Med 113:232, 1989

39. Alter HJ, Epstein JS, Swenson SG, et al: Prevalence of human immunodeficiency virus type 1 p24 antigen in US blood donors: An assessment of the efficacy of testing in donor screening. N Engl J Med 323:1312, 1990

40. Cummings PD, Wallace EL, Schorr JB, Dodd RY: Exposure of patients to human immunodeficiency virus through transfusion of blood components that test antibody negative. N Engl J Med 321:941, 1989

41. Dodd RY: The risk of transfusion—transmitted infection. N Engl J Med 327:419, 1992

42. Phillips H, Holland BM, Wardrop CAJ, et al: Determination of red cell mass in assessment and management of anemia in babies needing blood transfusion. Lancet i:882, 1986

43. Sanders MR, Graeber JE: Post-transfusion graft-versus-host disease in infancy. J Pediatr 117:159, 1990

44. LUBAN NLC, STRAUSS RG, HUME HA: Commentary on the safety of red blood cells preserved in extended storage media for neonatal transfusions. Transfusion 31:229, 1991

45. BROWN KA, BISSONNETTE B, MACDONALD M, POON AO: Hyperkalemia during massive blood transfusion in pediatric craniofacial surgery. Can J Anaesth 37:401, 1990

46. SCANLON JW, KRAKAUR R: Hyperkalemia following exchange transfusion. J Pediatr 96:108, 1980

47. SACHS L, SCHAFFER DB, ANDAY EK, ET AL: Retrolental fibroplasia and blood transfusion in very low birth weight infants. Pediatrics 68:770, 1981

48. WILLIAMS RA, BROWN EF, HURST D, FRANKLIN LC: Transfusion of infants with activation of erythrocyte T antigen.J Pediatr 115:949, 1989

49. GOLDEN SM, O'BRIEN WF, LISSNER C, ET AL: Hematologic and bacteriologic assessment of autologous cord blood for neonatal transfusions. J Pediatr 97:810, 1980

50. PAXON CL JR: Collection and use of autologous fetal blood. Am J Obstet Gynecol 134:708, 1979

51. ANDREW M, CASTLE V, SAIGAL S, ET AL: Clinical impact of neonatal thrombocytopenia. J Pediatr 110:457, 1987

52. BADA HS, KORONES SB, PERRY EH, ET AL: Frequent handling in the neonatal intensive care unit and intraventricular hemorrhage. J Pediatr 117:126, 1990

53. BALLIN A, KOREN G, KOHELET D, ET AL: Reduction of platelet counts induced by mechanical ventilation in newborn infants. J Pediatr 111:445, 1987

54. CASTLE V, ANDREW M, KELTON J, ET AL: Frequency and mechanism of neonatal thrombocytopenia. J Pediatr 108:749, 1986

55. SETZER ES, WEBB IB, WASSENAAR JW, ET AL: Platelet dysfunction and coagulopathy in intraventricular hemorrhage in the premature infant. J Pediatr 100:599, 1982

56. SILLS RH, STUART MJ: Platelet transfusion in the newborn. In Sherwood WC, Cohen A (eds): Transfusion Therapy: The Fetus, Infant, and Child. New York: Masson Publishing, 1980, p 95

57. PEARSON HA, SHULMAN NR, MARDER VJ, ET AL: Isoimmune neonatal thrombocytopenic purpura: Clinical and therapeutic considerations. Blood 23:154, 1964

58. LEE EJ, SCHIFFER CA: ABO compatibility can influence the results of platelet transfusion: Results of a randomized trial. Transfusion 29:384, 1989

59. PIERCE RN, REICH LM, AND MAYER K: Hemolysis following platelet transfusion from ABO incompatible donors. Transfusion 25:60, 1985

60. READ EJ, KODIS C, CARTER CS, LEITMAN SF: Viability of platelets following storage in the irradiated state. Transfusion 28:446, 1988

41 Exchange Transfusions

Maureen C. Edwards
Mary Ann Fletcher

The frequency with which postnatal exchange transfusions are performed appears to be decreasing.[1,2] This decrement relates to newer approaches to prenatal management of hemolytic disease and more aggressive management of jaundice in the newborn, as well as changing levels of concern regarding bilirubin encephalopathy and risks associated with exchange transfusions.[3,4]

A. INDICATIONS

1. To regulate antibody–antigen levels[5]
   a. Removal in isoimmune disease (e.g., Rh, ABO disease)[6]
   b. Removal in maternal autoimmune disease[7–9]
   c. Augmentation in sepsis[10]
2. To remove toxins significantly concentrated in the blood and not otherwise removable (e.g., by forced diuresis, dialysis, or chelation)
   a. Metabolic products
      (1) Bilirubin[11]
      (2) Ammonia[12]
      (3) Amino acids
   b. Drugs[13–15]
   c. Bacterial toxins[10]
3. To correct life-threatening electrolyte and fluid imbalance[16]
4. To regulate the level and type of hemoglobin (Hbg)

   Partial exchange transfusion is usually indicated for these conditions.

   a. Severe anemia in face of normal or excess blood volume[17,18]
   b. Clinical polycythemia[19]
5. To treat coagulation defects not remedied by single-component replacement[7]

B. CONTRAINDICATIONS

1. When alternatives such as simple transfusion or phototherapy would be just as effective with less risk
2. When a contraindication to placement of necessary lines outweighs indication for exchange transfusion
3. When patient is unstable and not likely to benefit from procedure

   Partial exchange transfusion, particularly to correct severe anemia in the face of cardiac failure or hypervolemia, can be used to stabilize the patient's condition. A complete exchange can then be performed when the patient and equipment are optimally prepared.

C. EQUIPMENT

1. Infant care center (see Chap. 2, Maintenance of Homeostasis)
   a. Automatic and manually controlled heat source
   b. Temperature monitor
   c. Cardiorespiratory monitor
   d. Transcutaneous oxygen monitor
2. Resuscitation equipment and medication (immediately available)
3. Infant restraints
4. Orogastric tube
5. Suctioning equipment
6. Equipment for line insertion (see Part V, Vascular Access)
7. Blood warmer and appropriate coils (see precautions)
8. Sterile exchange transfusion equipment
   a. Preassembled disposable set with special stopcock (Pharmaseal*) or
   b. Nonassembled
      (1) 20-ml syringe
      (2) Two 3-way stopcocks with locking connections
      (3) Waste receptacle (empty IV bottle or bag)
      (4) IV connecting tubing

*American Pharmaseal Company, Valencia, CA

Use a smaller syringe if aliquot per pass is smaller.

9. Appropriate blood product
10. Syringes and tubes for pre- and post-exchange blood tests

D. PRECAUTIONS

1. Stabilize infant before initiating exchange procedure.
2. Check potassium of donor blood if patient has hyperkalemia or renal compromise.[20]
3. Monitor infant closely during and after procedure.
4. Do not rush procedure.
    a. May necessitate repeat if efficacy is decreased by haste.
    b. Stop or slow if patient becomes unstable.
5. Use blood product appropriate to clinical indication. Use freshest blood available, preferably less than 5 to 7 days.[6,21]
6. Use only thermostatically controlled blood-warming device that has passed quality control for temperature and alarms. Do not overheat blood, i.e., beyond 38°C.[22]

    Be sure to review operating and safety procedures for specific blood warmer.

7. Do not start exchange procedure until personnel are available for monitoring and as backup for other emergencies or fatigue.
8. Do not apply excessive suction if it becomes difficult to draw blood from line. Reposition line or replace syringes, stopcocks, and any adapters connected to line.
9. Leave anticoagulated, banked blood in line or clear line with heparinized saline if the procedure is interrupted.
10. Clear line with heparinized saline if administering calcium.
11. Follow pertinent precautions listed in Part V, Vascular Access.

E. PREPARATION FOR TOTAL OR PARTIAL EXCHANGE TRANSFUSION

1. Determine type of blood product needed. Whole blood or packed red cells reconstituted with plasma may be used as indicated and available.[21,22] Notify blood bank of indication for exchange to aid in preparation of proper product (see Table 40-1, Blood Products).

    In a healthy term infant, small volume partial exchange transfusion for polycythemia may be performed with isotonic saline replacement rather than a blood-bank product.

    a. Hematocrit (Hct) may be adjusted within the range of 45 to 60%, depending on desired end result.
    b. In face of renal compromise or abnormal serum electrolytes, consider determination of electrolyte content of donor blood.
    c. Blood should be as fresh as possible.[6]
    d. Standard blood-bank screening is particularly important, including sickle cell preparation, HIV, Hepatitis B, and CMV. Irradiated blood may limit complications in at-risk patients.[23]

    In presence of isoimmunization, e.g., Rh, ABO, special attention to compatibility is necessary. Donor blood should be compatible with both mother and infant's serum.

    (1) For ABO incompatibility, use O cells reconstituted with AB plasma.[5]
    (2) For Rh incompatibility, use Rh-negative blood, whole or reconstituted.
2. Determine volumes of donor and infant blood required.
    a. Quantity needed for total procedure
        (1) Blood volume of infant (70–90 ml/kg for term and 85–110 ml/kg for preterm infant) times factor determined by exchange indication (Fig. 41-1).[24] Use no more than equivalent of one whole unit of blood for each procedure, to decrease donor exposure.
            (a) Double volume for removal of plasma-bound substance (e.g., bilirubin, antibodies: 2×80–100 ml/kg).
            (b) Single volume for correction of coagulopathies or anemia
            (c) Partial volume to change hemoglobin level

    These formulas are approximation, because mixing of patient and donor blood somewhat reduces the efficiency of exchange transfusion.

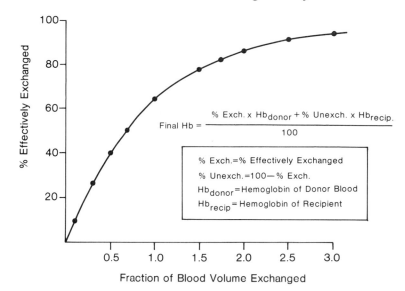

$$\text{Final Hb} = \frac{\%\ \text{Exch.} \times \text{Hb}_{donor} + \%\ \text{Unexch.} \times \text{Hb}_{recip.}}{100}$$

% Exch. = % Effectively Exchanged
% Unexch. = 100 − % Exch.
Hb_{donor} = Hemoglobin of Donor Blood
Hb_{recip} = Hemoglobin of Recipient

FIG. 41-1
Graph depicting the effectiveness of exchange transfusion against the fraction of blood volume exchanged. The formula permits the calculation of the final hemoglobin.

1) Polycythemia

Volume replaced (ml) =
$$\frac{\text{Blood volume} \times (\text{Hct observed} - \text{Hct desired})}{\text{Hct observed}}$$

2) Anemia

Volume exchanged (ml) =
$$\frac{\text{Blood volume} \times (\text{Hbg desired} - \text{Hbg initial})}{(\text{Hbg PRBCs}^* - \text{Hbg initial})}$$

*Hbg PRBC $\cong$ 22 g/100 ml; PRBC = packed red blood cells

   (2) Tubing dead space including blood warmer requires at least 25 to 30 ml.
 b. Aliquot for each pass in push–pull technique
   (1) 5% of estimated blood volume, plus dead space in catheter and stopcocks
   (2) Minimum of 5 ml per pass
   (3) Maximum of 20 ml per pass
 c. Infant blood for laboratory tests pre- and postexchange as indicated. Consider
   (1) Pre-exchange diagnostic studies. Note that diagnostic serological test on the infant, such as antiviral antibody titers or studies to evaluate unexplained hemolysis, should be drawn prior to the exchange transfusion.

   (2) Hemoglobin, hematocrit, platelets
   (3) Electrolytes, calcium, blood gas
   (4) Glucose
   (5) Bilirubin
   (6) Coagulation profile
   (7) Drug levels
   (8) Postexchange crossmatch and Coombs' test
3. Determine rate of exchange procedure
 a. Rate for maximum benefit
 b. Tolerance of infant to abrupt changes
   (1) Hemodynamics, particularly in push–pull techniques

Aortic blood pressure changes occur with each pass. When following too rapidly, there may be a progressive fall in aortic pressure and narrowing of pulse pressures.[25] Additionally, withdrawal from the umbilical vein induces a negative pressure that may be transmitted to the mesenteric veins and contribute to the high incidence of ischemic bowel complications.[26]

   (2) Acid load of anticoagulant
   (3) Oxygen saturation and content
   (4) Electrolyte, calcium, glucose
 c. Mechanical limitations: blood warmer, filters
 d. Average time per pass for push–pull technique is approximately 3 to 5 minutes.

(1) Total duration of 90 to 120 minutes for double-volume exchange

(2) Total duration of 45 to 60 minutes for iso-volumetric or single-volume exchange in stable infant

4. Prepare infant as per Chapters 2 and 3.

   a. Place infant on warmer with total accessibility and controlled environment.

   b. Connect physiologic monitors, and establish baseline values. (temperature, respiratory and heart rates, oxygenation)

   c. Empty infant's stomach.

     (1) Do not feed for 4 hours prior to procedure, if possible.

     (2) Place orogastric tube, and remove gastric contents.

   d. Apply urine collector to infant.

   e. Start IV for glucose and medication infusion.

     (1) If exchange procedure interrupts previous essential infusion rate, or

     (2) If prolonged lack of oral or parenteral glucose will lead to hypoglycemia

5. Whenever possible, treat any remediable conditions that contribute to patient's instability prior to starting exchange procedure; e.g., give packed-cell transfusion when severe hypovolemia and anemia are present, or modify ventilator or ambient oxygen when there is respiratory decompensation.

6. Determine if albumin infusion is indicated before or during exchange for hyperbilirubinemia.

   a. Increases circulating volume. Increase must not jeopardize infant.

   b. Provides benefit probably only in infants with low reserve albumin-binding capacity for bilirubin, notably, small, sick, premature infants.

7. Prepare blood

   a. Verify identification of blood product (see Chap. 40).

     (1) Type and crossmatch data

     (2) Expiration date

     (3) Donor and recipient identities

   b. Attach blood administration set to blood-warmer tubing and to blood bag.

   c. Allow blood to run through blood warmer.

8. Identify person who will record the exchange on flow sheet and monitor infant's condition throughout.

F. TECHNIQUE

Exchange Transfusion by Push–Pull Technique Through Special Stopcock with Pre-assembled Tray

1. Read instructions provided by manufacturer carefully.

2. Scrub as for major procedure. Wear gloves and gown.

3. Open preassembled equipment tray, using techniques of asepsis.

4. Identify positions on special stopcock in clockwise rotation (Fig. 41-2). The direction that the handle is pointing indicates the port that is open to syringe.

> The special stopcock allows clockwise rotation in the order used: (1) withdraw from patient, (2) clear to waste bag, (3) draw new blood, (4) inject

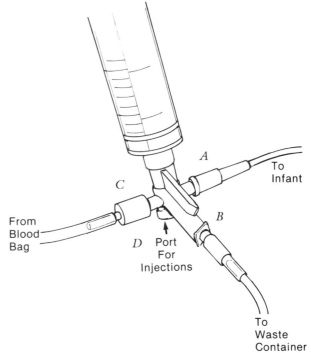

FIG. 41-2
Special four-way stopcock. (*A*) Male adapter to infant line; (*B*) female adapter to waste container; (*C*) attachment to blood tubing; (*D*) "off" position (180 degrees from adapter to waste container) allowing injection through rubber stoppered port "below" syringe. The stopcock is used in clockwise rotation when correctly assembled.

into patient. Always rotate in clockwise direction to follow proper sequence, and keep connections tight.

   a. Male adapter to umbilical or peripheral line
   b. Female adapter to the extension tubing to which waste bag will be attached.
   c. Pre-attached to tubing for attachment to blood-warmer coil
   d. Neutral "off" position in which additives may be administered through rubber stopper. (180 degrees from waste receptacle port)

5. Follow steps as illustrated by manufacturer to make all connections to blood and waste bags.

6. With stopcock open to blood source, clear all air into syringe. Turn in clockwise direction 270 degrees and evacuate into waste.

7. Turn stopcock to "off," and replace onto sterile field.

8. Insert umbilical venous catheter, as described in Chapter 40, Umbilical Vein Catheterization.
   a. Use side-hole catheter
   b. Consider CVP measurement, using pressure transducer, in unstable baby.
   c. Place catheter in IVC and verify position by radiograph. The venous catheter on commercial exchange tray is not radiopaque.
      or
      Place in umbilical vein and use cautiously for exchange in an emergent situation (see Chap. 26, Umbilical Vein Catheterization).
      Alternatively
      Use pre-existing umbilical line.
   a. Cleanse line and connectors with antiseptic.
   b. Stop IV pump.
   c. Minimize deadspace by removing stopcocks and connectors already in place.
   d. Attach special stopcock.

9. Have an assistant document all vital signs, volumes, and other data, on the exchange record.

10. Draw blood for diagnostic studies (see E2c).

11. If infant is hypovolemic or has low CVP, start exchange with transfusion of aliquot into catheter. If infant is hypervolemic or has high CVP, start by withdrawing precalculated aliquot.

12. Gently agitate the blood bag every 10 to 15 minutes to prevent red cell sedimentation.[27]

13. Check peripheral glucose estimation every 30 min-

utes. Follow continuous oxygen assessment. Determine blood gases as often as indicated by pre-existing clinical condition and stability.

14. Remeasure CVP if indicated.
   a. Expect rise as plasma oncotic pressure increases, if CVP low at start.
   b. Monitor the effect of each push-pull on the blood volume, and vary aliquots accordingly.

15. Consider giving calcium supplement.

   Modern blood-banking technique has reduced the requirement to administer calcium during exchange transfusion. It is rarely necessary or advantageous to give calcium during an exchange if the infant is normocalcemic. When administered, the effect may last only a few minutes.[28] Calcium will reverse the effect of the anticoagulant in the donor blood and may cause clotting of the line. Prior to administration, clear the line of donor blood with 0.9% NaCl.

   a. When hypocalcemia is documented
   b. With symptoms or signs of hypocalcemia
      (1) Change in Q-Tc interval
      (2) Agitation and tachycardia: these symptoms are not reliably correlated with ionized calcium levels.
   c. Give 1 ml of 10% calcium gluconate per kg body weight.
   d. Administer slowly, with careful observation of heart rate and rhythm.

16. Perform calculated number of passes, until desired volume has been exchanged.

17. Be sure there is adequate volume of donor blood remaining to infuse after last withdrawal, if a positive intravascular balance is desired.

18. Clear umbilical line of banked blood and withdraw amount of infant's blood needed for laboratory testing, including recrossmatching.

19. Document procedure in patient's hospital record.

Exchange Transfusion by Isovolumetric Technique (Central or Peripheral Lines)[29-31]

1. Scrub as for major procedure.
2. Select two sites for line placement, and insert as per Part V, Vascular Access.
   a. Venous for infusion
      (1) Umbilical venous catheter
      (2) Peripheral IV that is at least 23 gauge

b. Arterial for removal
   (1) Umbilical artery catheter
   (2) Peripheral, usually radial if infant's size permits
3. Connect arterial line to three-way stopcock.
   a. Use short, connecting IV tubing to extend peripheral line.
   b. Attach additional connecting tubing to stopcock and place into sterile waste container.
   c. Attach empty 3- to 10-ml syringe to stopcock, for withdrawal of blood.

   > An additional stopcock may also be placed on this port so that a syringe of heparinized saline (5 U/ml) may be attached for use as needed. Be cautious about total volume infused.

4. Connect venous line to single, three-way stopcock, which in turn connects to empty 5- to 10-ml syringe and to blood-warming coil.
5. Start exchange-transfusion record.
6. Withdraw and discard blood from arterial side at rate of 2 to 3 ml/kg/min, and infuse at same rate into venous side. Keep flow as steady as possible, and volumetrically equal for infusion and removal.
7. Intermittently, flush arterial line with heparinized saline to clear.

   > The heparin solution remaining in tubing will be removed with next withdrawal, thus reducing significantly the total heparin dose actually received by the patient.

8. Follow steps as for push–pull technique until exchange is complete.

Exchange Transfusion Using a Single Umbilical Line and Two Three-Way Stopcocks in Tandem

The principles and techniques for using either the special stopcock or two three-way stopcocks in tandem are the same. It is important to ensure that all junctions are tight to produce a closed, sterile system. It is also essential to understand the working positions of the stopcocks before starting the exchange.

1. Scrub as for major procedure. Wear gown and gloves.
2. Attach stopcock and tubing in sequence (Fig. 41-3).
   a. Proximal stopcock
      (1) Umbilical catheter
      (2) IV extension tubing to sterile waste container
   b. Distal stopcock
      (1) Tubing from blood-warming coil
      (2) 10- or 20-ml syringe
3. Clear lines of air bubbles.
4. Start exchange record.
5. Follow steps of push–pull technique until exchange is completed.

G. POSTEXCHANGE FOR ALL TECHNIQUES

1. Continue to monitor vital signs closely for at least 4 hours.
2. Rewrite orders: adjust any drug dosages as needed to compensate for removal by exchange (Table 41-1).[32–34]

TABLE 41-1

Hypothetical Drug Loss by Exchange Transfusion Calculated by First Order Elimination from a Single Compartment $(1 - e^{-V/Vd})*$

	Percent Loss	
Drug	One Volume	Two Volume
Amikacin	7.1	13.8
Ampicillin	7.7	14.7
Carbamazepine	3.7	7.2
Carbenicillin	5.6	10.9
Colistin	18.7	33.9
Diazepam	2.3	4.5
Digoxin†	1.2	2.4
Furosemide	4.9	9.5
Gentamicin	5.2	10.1
Kanamycin	5.6	10.9
Methicillin	10.1	19.1
Oxacillin	19.6	35.4
Penicillin G (crystalline)	6.0	11.6
Penicillin G (procaine)	2.4	4.8
Phenobarbital	6.4	12.3
Phenytoin	3.1	6.2
Theophylline†	17.8	32.4
Tobramycin	10.3	19.6
Vancomycin	5.7	11.0

*V = plasma volume exchanged in liters; Vd = apparent volume of distribution

†Whole blood volume used in calculation

(Lackner TE: J Pediatr 100:813, 1982. Copyright © 1982 by C. V. Mosby)

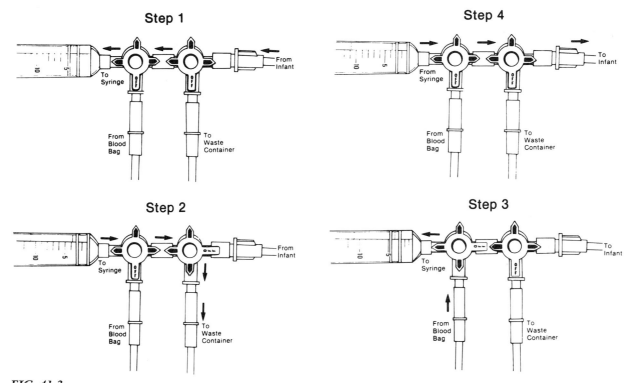

FIG. 41-3
Three-way stopcocks in tandem. Step 1: stopcocks positioned for withdrawing blood from infant; Step 2: stopcocks positioned for emptying withdrawn blood to waste container; Step 3: stopcocks positioned for filling syringe from blood bag; Step 4: stopcocks positioned for injecting blood into infant line.

3. Keep infant NPO for at least 4 hours.
4. Follow glucose levels until normal and infant is re-stabilized on pre-exchange glucose intake.
5. Repeat blood gases as often as clinically indicated.
6. Repeat hemoglobin, hematocrit, and bilirubin measurements approximately 4 hours after exchange.

H. COMPLICATIONS

The following long list of reported complications emphasizes the hazards of this procedure and the need to follow all precautions.

Related Primarily to Blood Product

1. Potentially, all complications of simple transfusions (see Chap. 40)

   Because of larger volumes used for exchange and increased handling of blood, there is enhanced risk of complications.

2. Transmission of infectious agents
   a. Transient bacteremia[35]
   b. HIV
   c. Cytomegalovirus[36]
   d. Hepatitis[37]
   e. Malaria[38]
   f. Syphilis[39]
   g. Endocarditis[40]
   h. Septic arthritis and osteomyelitis[41]
3. Hemolysis of transfused blood
   a. Sickle hemoglobin[42]
   b. G-6-PD deficiency[43]
   c. Blood mismatching
   d. Traumatic handling
      (1) Overheating[44]
      (2) Excessive agitation
      (3) Injection rate too rapid for catheter or IV diameter

4. Hematologic/immunologic aberrations
  a. Inappropriate final hemoglobin level (anemia or polycythemia)
     (1) Donor hematocrit inappropriate
     (2) Inadequate mixing during transfusion
     (3) Inappropriate volume surplus or deficit in recipient
  b. Coagulopathy
     (1) Alteration of coagulation factors[45]
     (2) Disseminated intravascular coagulation[44]
     (3) Excessive heparinization
     (4) Thromboembolization
  c. Thrombocytopenia[46]
  d. White blood cell deficiency
     (1) Neutropenia[47]
     (2) Alteration of granulocyte function[48]
  e. Suppressed production of autologous IgG and IgA with provoked IgM synthesis[49]
  f. Graft versus host reaction[23]
5. Metabolic changes
  a. Hyperkalemia/hypokalemia[50]
  b. Hypernatremia[51]
  c. Hyperglycemia from excessive glucose load[52]
  d. Hypoglycemia during or after exchange[53]
  e. Hypocalcemia during or after exchange[54]
  f. Hypercalcemia from overdose[54]
  g. Acidosis during exchange[55]
  h. Alkalosis after exchange, resulting from citrate metabolism[65]
6. Cardiovascular reactions
  a. Arrhythmia or arrest[57]
     (1) Due to hyperkalemia, hypocalcemia, or hypomagnesemia
     (2) Temperature stress
  b. Volume overload[58]
     (1) Due to change in central vascular oncotic pressure mobilizing peripheral fluids (hydrops)
     (2) Due to excessive transfusion
  c. Myocardial infarction[59]
  d. Aggravation of pulmonary hypertension[60]
7. Other
  a. Temperature instability[61]
     (1) Hypothermia
     (2) Hyperthermia
  b. Splenic rupture[62]

Related Primarily to Exchange Technique and Catheterization

1. Potentially, all complications of placement and use of umbilical and peripheral lines
2. Gastrointestinal

   Most of the reported gastrointestinal complications are related to exchanges through umbilical vein catheters.

   a. Emesis with aspiration
   b. Ischemic bowel[63]
      (1) Necrotizing enterocolitis
      (2) Isolated bowel perforations
      (3) Stenosis
   c. Portal vein thrombosis[64]
   d. Portal hypertension[65]
   e. Portal venous gas[66]
   f. Hepatic necrosis
3. Other
   a. Air embolism
   b. Change in intracranial pressure[67]
   c. Omphalitis
   d. Hemoperitoneum[68]
   e. Hydrothorax[69]

References

1. HOVI L, SIIMES MA: Exchange transfusion with fresh heparinized blood is a safe procedure. Acta Pediatr Scand 74:360, 1985
2. KALPOYIANNIS N, ANDROULAKIS N, HADJIGEORGIOU E, ET AL: Efficacy of phototherapy and/or exchange transfusion in neonatal jaundice. Clin Pediatr 21:602, 1982
3. KEENAN WJ, NOVAK KK, SUTHERLAND JM, ET AL: Morbidity and mortality associated with exchange transfusion. Pediatrics 75 (Suppl):471, 1985
4. WATCHKO JF, OSKI FA: Bilirubin 20 mg/dL = vigintiphobia. Pediatrics 71:660, 1983
5. COHEN A, SHERWOOD WC, BUSCH S: Transfusion therapy in hemolytic disease of the newborn. In Sherwood WC, Cohen A (eds): Transfusion Therapy: Fetus, Infant and Child. New York, Masson Publishing, 1980, p 113
6. DEPALMA L, LUBAN NC: Blood component theory in the perinatal period: Guidelines and recommendations. Sem Perinatol 14:403, 1990
7. GREENBERG J, SACHER RA: Exchange transfusion in the newborn. In Luban, NC, Keating LJ (eds): Hemo-

therapy of the Infant and Premature. Arlington, VA, American Association of Blood Banks, 1983, p 76

8. MOREL E, EYMARD B, VERNET-DER GARABEDIAN B, ET AL: Neonatal myasthenia gravis: A new clinical and immunologic appraisal of 30 cases. Neurology 38:138, 1988

9. WIT JM, GERARDS LH, VERMEULEN-MEINERS C, BRUINSE HW: Neonatal thyrotoxicosis treated with exchange transfusion and Lugol's iodine. Eur J Pediatr 143:317, 1985

10. HALL RT: Exchange transfusion in neonatal sepsis. In Blood Component Therapy of Neonatal Disease. Mead Johnson Symposium on Perinatal and Developmental Medicine, No. 28. Vail CO, 1986

11. HARPER RG, SIA CG, KIERNEY CMP: Kernicterus 1980: Problems and practices viewed from the perspective of the practicing clinician. Clin Perinatal 7:75, 1980

12. WIEGAND C, THOMPSON T, BOCK GH, ET AL: The management of life-threatening hyperammonemia: A comparison of several therapeutic modalities. J Pediatr 96:142, 1980

13. KESSLER DL JR, SMITH AL, WOODRUM DE: Chloramphenicol toxicity in a neonate treated with exchange transfusion. J Pediatr 96:140, 1980

14. THEARLE MJ: Exchange transfusion for diazepam intoxication at birth followed by jejunal stenosis. Proceedings of the Royal Society of Medicine 66:349, 1973

15. PERRIN C, DEBRUYNE D, LACOTTE J, ET AL: Treatment of caffeine intoxication by exchange transfusion in a newborn. Acta Paediatr Scand 76:679, 1987

16. SETZER ES, AHMED F, GOLDBERG RN, ET AL: Exchange transfusion using washed red blood cells reconstituted with fresh-frozen plasma for treatment of severe hyperkalemia in the neonate. J Pediatr 104:443, 1984

17. BIANCHI DW, BEYER EC, STARK AR, ET AL: Normal long-term survival with alpha-thalassemia. J Pediatr 108:716, 1986

18. NIEBURG PI, STOCKMAN JA: Rapid correction of anemia with partial exchange transfusion. Am J Dis Child 131:60, 1977

19. HEIN HA, LATHROP SS: Partial exchange transfusion in term polycythemic neonates: Absence of association with severe gastrointestinal injury. Pediatrics 80:75, 1987

20. BLANCHETTE VS, GRAY E, HARDIE MJ, ET AL: Hyperkalemia after neonatal exchange transfusion: Risk eliminated by washing red cell concentrates. J Pediatr 105:321, 1984

21. BARNARD DR, CHAPMAN RG: Blood for use in exchange transfusion in the newborn. Transfusion 20:401, 1980

22. American Association of Blood Banks, Standards Committee: Standards for blood banks and transfusion services, 13th Ed., 1989

23. SANDER MR, GRAEBER JE: Posttransfusion graft-versus-host disease in infancy. J Pediatr 117:159, 1990

24. AMATO M, BLUMBERG A, HERMANN U, ZURBRUGG R: Effectiveness of single versus double volume exchange transfusion in newborn infants with ABO hemolytic disease. Helv Paediatr Acta 43:177, 1988

25. ARANDA JV, SWEET AY: Alterations in blood pressure during exchange transfusion. Arch Dis Child 52:545, 1977

26. MINTZ AA, VALLBONA C: A hazard of exchange transfusion in newborn infants—negative pressure in the umbilical vein. Pediatrics 26:661, 1960

27. SCHUERGER G, ROBERTSON A: Effects of agitation of donor blood on neonatal exchange transfusions. Clin Pediatr 9:715, 1970

28. WEILAND P, DUC G, BINSWANGER U, FISCHER JA: Parathyroid hormone response in newborn infants during exchange transfusion with blood supplemented with citrate and phosphate: Effect of IV calcium. Pediatr Res 123:963, 1979

29. FOK TF, SO LY, LEUNG KW, ET AL: Use of peripheral vessels for exchange transfusion. Arch Dis Child 65:676, 1990

30. MARTIN JR: A double catheter technique for exchange transfusion in the newborn infant. NZ Med J 77:167, 1973

31. SCARCELLA A, GAMBARDELLA P: Partial exchange transfusion using peripheral vessels. Eur J Pediatr 144:545, 1986

32. ASSAEL, BM, CACCAMO ML, GERNA M: Effect of exchange transfusion in the elimination of theophylline in premature infants. J Pediatr 91:331, 1977

33. ENGLUND JA, FLETCHER CV, JOHNSON D, ET AL: Effect of blood exchange on acyclovir clearance in an infant with neonatal herpes. J Pediatr 110:151, 1987

34. LACKNER TE: Drug replacement following exchange transfusion. J Pediatr 100:811, 1982

35. NELSON JD: The significance of bacteremia with exchange transfusion. J Pediatr 66:291, 1965

36. KUMAR A, NANKERVIS GA, COOPER AR, ET AL: Acquisition of cytomegalovirus infection in infants following exchange transfusion, a prospective study. Transfusion 20:327, 1980

37. PAXSON CL, MORRISS FH, ADCOCK EW: Neonatal exchange transfusion with blood containing hepatitis B antigen. J Pediatr 88:357, 1976

38. SHULMAN IA, SAXENA S, NELSON JM, FURMANSKI M: Neonatal exchange transfusions complicated by transfusion-induced malaria. Pediatrics 73:330, 1984

39. RISSEEUW-APPEL IM, KOTHE FC: Transfusion syphilis: A case report. Sex Transm Dis 10:200, 1983

40. SYMCHYCH PS, KRAUSS AN, WINCHESTER P: Endocarditis following intracardiac placement of umbilical venous catheters in neonates. J Pediatr 90:287, 1977

41. JURESHI ME: Osteomyelitis after exchange transfusion. Br Med J 2:28, 1971

42. MURPHY RJC, MALHOTRA C, SWEET AY: Death follow-

ing an exchange transfusion with hemoglobin SC blood. J Pediatr 96:110, 1980

43. GULATI S, SINGH S, NARANG, A, BHAKOO ON: Exchange transfusion with G-6-PD deficient donor blood causes exaggeration of neonatal hyperbilirubinemia. Indian Pediatr 26:499, 1989

44. SESHADRI RS, BLAKE GP: Disseminated intravascular coagulation due to an exchange transfusion with overheated blood. Aust Paediatr J 15:33,1979

45. NIELSON NC: The influence of exchange transfusion upon coagulation and fibrinolysis in newborn infants with erythroblastoses. Acta Obstet Gynecol Scand 49:71, 1970

46. PODOLSAK B: Thrombopoiesis in newborn infants after exchange blood transfusion. Zeitschrift fur Kinderheilkunde 114:13, 1973

47. PHIBBS RH: Response of newborn infants to leukocyte depletion during exchange transfusion. Biol Neonate 15:112, 1970

48. PELET B: Exchange transfusion in newborn infants: Effects on granulocyte function. Arch Dis Child 54:687, 1979

49. MANTALENKI-ASFI K, MORPHIS L, NICOLOPOULOS D, MATSANIATIS N: Influence of exchange transfusion on the development of serum immunoglobulin. J Pediatr 87:396, 1975

50. SCANLON JW. KRAKAUR R: Hyperkalemia following exchange transfusion. J Pediatr 96:108, 1980

51. STEELE AM, BROWN DL, LIPSITZ PJ: Relationship of exchange transfusion to hypernatremia. J Pediatr 94:168, 1979

52. FERNANDEZ A, SUBRAMANIAM S, CHAWLA C, GAIKWAD P: Changes in biochemical parameters following exchange transfusion. Indian Pediatr 23:429, 1986

53. BECA JP, FILIPPA R, ROMAN C: Hypoglycemia and exchange transfusion. Rev Chil Pediatr 47:388, 1976

54. NELSON N, FINNSTROM O: Blood exchange transfusions in newborns, the effect on serum ionized calcium. Early Hum Dev 18:157, 1988

55. GANDY G, PARTRIDGE JW: Control of acidosis during exchange transfusion with citrated blood. Arch Dis Child 43:147, 1968

56. RATZMAN VGW, ZOLLNER H, BEYERSDORFF E, JAHRIG K: Magnesium- kalzium- and phosphat-veranderungen im serum von neugeborenen bei austauschtransfusionen. Kinderarztl Praxis 53:119, 1985

57. SINGH M, SINGHI S: Cardiac arrest during exchange transfusions. Indian J Pediatr 46:131, 1979

58. MacLAURIN JC, COULTER JB, HOBY AM: Changes in blood volume associated with exchange transfusion. Arch Dis Child 50:404, 1975

59. VANDER HAUWAERT LG, LOOS MC: Myocardial infarction during exchange transfusion in a newborn infant. J. Pediatr 70:745, 1967

60. GRIFFITH R: Effect of transfusion of RBC in pulmonary hypertension. J Pediatr 99:670, 1981

61. HEY EN, KOHLINSKY S, O'CONNELL B: Heat-losses from babies during exchange transfusion. Lancet i 1:335, 1969

62. SIMMONS MA, BURRINGTON JD, WAYNE ER, HATHAWAY WE: Splenic rupture in neonates with erythroblastosis fetalis. Am J Dis Child 126:679, 1973

63. TOULOUKIAN RJ, KADAR A, SPENCER RP: The gastrointestinal complications of neonatal umbilical venous exchange transfusion: A clinical and experimental study. Pediatrics 51:36, 1973

64. THOMPSON EN, SHERLOCK S: The etiology of portal vein thrombosis with particular reference to the role of infection and exchange transfusion. Q J Med 33:421, 1964

65. OSKI A: Portal hypertension-a complication of umbilical vein catheterization. Pediatrics 31:297, 1963

66. SCHMIDT AG: Portal vein gas due to administration of fluids via the umbilical vein. Radiology 88:293, 1967

67. BADA HS, CHUA C, SALMON JH, HAJJAR W: Changes in intracranial pressure during exchange transfusion. J Pediatr 94:129, 1979

68. HILLARD J, SCHREINER RL, PRIEST J: Hemoperitoneum associated with exchange transfusion through an umbilical arterial catheter. Dis Child 133:216, 1979

69. KULKARNI PB, DORANO RD: Hydrothorax: A complication of intracardiac placement of umbilical venous catheter. J Pediatr 94:813, 1979

Part 9

Miscellaneous Procedures

42 Extra Digits and Skin Tags

Mary Ann Fletcher

A. INDICATIONS

Removal of Nonfunctional Extra Digit

1. Prevention of accidental avulsion or torsion around narrow base
2. Cosmetic correction at parental request

B. CONTRAINDICATIONS

1. Presence of illness in infant

   This is an elective procedure that is painful when the clamp is applied. To prevent accidental avulsion of appendage if extra digit on a narrow base were to become entangled, apply a soft dressing or adhesive bandage until infant is stable enough for removal.

2. Presence of any other hand anomaly when further surgical correction may be necessary[1]
3. Base of extra digit greater than 5 to 6 mm in width
4. Bone crossing the isthmus between extra digit and hand

C. EQUIPMENT

1. Iodophor antiseptic solution and swabs
2. Straight mosquito hemostat
3. Surgical silk suture, 3-0 or 4-0
4. Fine or delicate scissors
5. Adhesive bandage

D. PRECAUTIONS

1. Perform procedure only on stable, healthy infant.
2. Consider surgical evaluation for any questionable digit.
   a. When base is more than 5 to 6 mm in width
   b. When extra digit is on radial side of hand
   c. When clamping will not crush base to a thin, translucent layer indicative of hemostasis after excision
   d. When there appears to be a joint at the base
3. Apply hemostat to base of extra digit prior to placing ligature.
   a. Allows closer amputation without residual bump
   b. Allows faster autoamputation or removal of most of digit within a few hours

E. TECHNIQUE

1. Cleanse digit and the surrounding skin with iodophor antiseptic. Allow to dry.
2. Clamp hemostat as close to the base of extra digit as possible but without drawing up extra skin (Fig. 42-1A).
3. Tightly tie suture around digit between hemostat and hand.
4. Keep clamp in place until digit turns white for at least 5 minutes.
5. Using as a cutting guide the edge of the hemostat further from the hand, excise the digit (Fig. 42-1B).
6. Remove hemostat and observe for hemostasis, leaving ligature in place. If there is any bleeding, reapply hemostat and ligature.
7. Cover with an adhesive bandage until residual stump autoamputates.

Removal of Skin Tags (Fig. 42-2)

The removal of small skin tags follows essentially the same technique as for extra digits: Clamp close to base of lesion to achieve hemostasis and apply ligature between hemostat and normal area. If the lesions are large or in critical areas, removal is best delayed beyond the neonatal period. Consider other diagnoses associated with skin tags.[2]

375

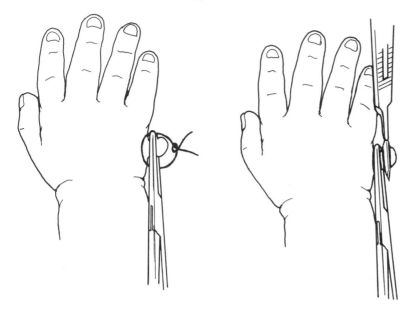

FIG. 42-1
(*A*) Place fine hemostat as close to base of extra digit as possible and firmly secure ligature between clamp and hand. (*B*) After finger turns white, excise digit tag outside hemostat, leaving ligature in place for autoamputation of residual stump.

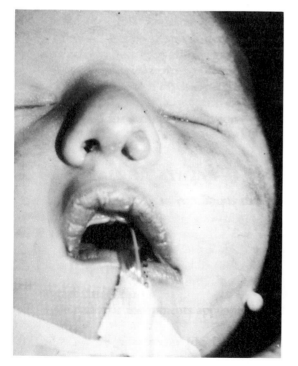

FIG. 42-2
Skin tags of naris and cheek. Removal of tags this large requires surgical excision rather than ligation for best result and may be associated with other malformations.

G. COMPLICATIONS

1. Hemorrhage
   a. Failure to achieve complete hemostasis prior to excision
   b. Loosening of ligature before blood supply is retracted
2. Infection
3. Inappropriate removal of digit in presence of related anomalies

References

1. NAKAMURA J, KANAHARA K, ENDO Y, HIRASE Y: Effective use of portions of the supernumerary digit to correct polydactyly of the thumb. Ann Plast Surg 15:7 1985
2. Syndromes associated with preauricular tags. In Jones KL(ed): Smith's Recognizable Patterns of Human Malformations, 4th Ed. Philadelphia, WB Saunders, 1988, p 733.

43 Circumcision

Mhairi G. MacDonald

A. INDICATIONS

Non-ritual newborn circumcision is a controversial procedure.[1] Many physicians and layman consider circumcision routine, but complications, although rare, can be severe. Therefore, despite the simplicity of procedure, meticulous attention to anatomic landmarks, wound care, and followup are necessary. The occurrence of severe complications of circumcision must be weighed against increasing evidence that noncircumcised boys are at greater risk for ascending infections of the urinary tract than are circumcised boys.[2]

B. CONTRAINDICATIONS

1. Age less than 1 day (i.e., before complete physical adaptation to extrauterine life has occurred)
2. Any current illness
3. Prematurity (< 36 weeks' gestation)
4. Bleeding diathesis or family history of bleeding disorder
5. Abnormality of urethra or penile shaft (Foreskin may be essential for later reconstruction [e.g., hypospadias, chordee, very small penis].)[3]
6. Local infection

C. EQUIPMENT

Necessary for All Methods
Sterile

a. Gown and gloves
b. Cup with antiseptic
c. 4 × 4 gauze pads
d. Small, flexible, blunt probe
e. Two straight mosquito hemostats
f. Large, straight hemostat
g. Tissue scissors

Unsterile
Materials for restraint

Optional Equipment

a. Local anesthetic: 1% lidocaine hydrochloride *without* epinephrine in a tuberculin syringe with a 1.2 cm × 27-gauge needle

Circumcision of neonates has frequently been used as a model to study the response of the newborn to pain (see Chap. 5). However, until recently neonatal circumcision has been performed without anesthesia. Since the initial report by Kirya and Werthman in 1978,[4] there have been reports of several controlled studies that have concluded that the use of dorsal penile nerve block is both effective and safe.[5–7]

b. Sterile fine-tipped marking pen
c. Sterile gauze impregnated with petroleum jelly (e.g., Vaseline)

Additional Equipment for Use with Gomco Clam
All equipment is sterile.

a. Gomco circumcision clamp*[8,9] size 1 to 2 cm for average newborn glans (size range: 1–3.5 cm).

Be sure to use the size that is large enough to protect the glans.

b. No. 11 scalpel blade and holder
c. A small safety pin

Additional Equipment for Use with Plastibell
All equipment is sterile.

a. Plastibell plastic cone.† Available in presterilized packs; size range based on size of glans penis: 1.1 cm, 1.3 cm, and 1.5 cm. A linen suture is included in pack (Fig. 43-1).

When selecting size make sure that it is not so large that it allows proximal migration of the bell

---

*Gomco Surgical Manufacturing Corp., Buffalo, NY 14211
†Hollister, Inc., Chicago, IL

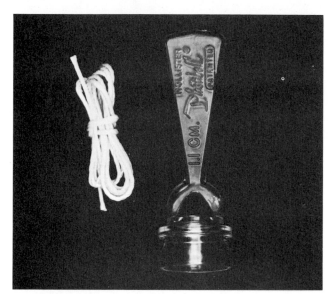

FIG. 43-1
Plastibell with linen suture.

and excessive loss of penile skin, nor so small that it could impair penile circulation.

b. Scissors capable of cutting through plastic.

D. PRECAUTIONS

1. Obtain informed consent.
   a. Explain expected course of circumcision to parents. When Plastibell is used they should be told to call their physician if ring has not fallen off within 10 days.[10]
   b. Be aware of laws surrounding ritual circumcision (e.g., Jewish "Brit Milah").[11,12]
   　(1) Should be performed on 8th day of life, unless infant is ill.
   　(2) Should be performed (or at least attended) by a qualified mohel.
2. Never circumcise at time of delivery. Circumcise long enough before discharge to allow adequate wound observation.
3. Do not use local anesthetic containing epinephrine.
4. Specifically locate coronal sulcus and urethral meatus.
5. Make sure that inner epithelium is completely separated from glans penis and that prepuce can be retracted to visualize entire circumference of coronal sulcus.

6. *Never use electrocautery.*
7. Do not use circumferential dressing.
8. Recheck wound prior to discharging patient and 1 to 2 weeks post-circumcision. Residual skin should retract completely and *entire* coronal sulcus must be visible to avoid post-circumcision adhesions, the most common complication.

E. TECHNIQUE

A complete description of formal surgical excision has been excluded from this edition because of the requirement to use sutures and the associated increased risk of bleeding compared with methods that involve crushing of tissue.

Ritual circumcisions are most commonly performed using a Mogen clamp. The method involves no dorsal incision or sutures,[13] however, because the glans is not visible at the time of excision of the prepuce, there is potential for damage to the glans and urethra.

1. Immobilize infant in supine position.
2. Put on cap and mask.
3. Scrub as for major procedure (see Chap. 4).
4. Put on gown and gloves.
5. Prepare skin with antiseptic, and drape.
6. Perform penile dorsal nerve block if desired.[4,14–15]

   Use of topical lidocaine and local anaesthesia at the level of the glans has also been described in the neonate.[16,17]

   a. Be familiar with anatomy of dorsal nerves of penis (Fig. 43-2).[4]

   Although only the two dorsal penile nerves are targeted by the injection of lidocaine, the ventral penile nerve is also blocked by infiltration through the subcutaneous tissue.

   b. Identify dorsal nerve roots at 10 o'clock and 2 o'clock positions.
   c. Identify by palpation the symphysis pubis and corpora cavernosa at the penile base.
   d. Estimate depth of pubic bone from penile base to indicate necessary depth of injection (should not exceed 0.5 cm).

   Although the ideal area for infiltration corresponds to the 2 and 10 o'clock position, 1 cm distal to the penile base, if the base is buried in pubic fat the injection must be done at the junction of pubic and pelvic skin.

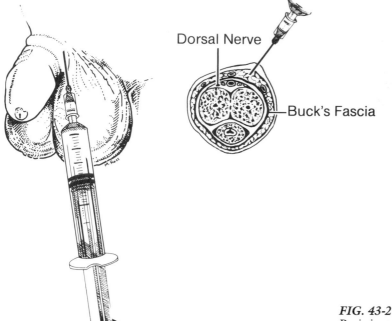

Dorsal Nerve

Buck's Fascia

FIG. 43-2
Penis is stabilized at angle of 20 to 25 degrees from midline. The formation of a lidocaine ring is shown (see text).

e. Stabilize organ, with gentle traction, at angle of 20 to 25 degrees from midline.

f. Pierce skin over one of dorsal nerves at penile root, and advance carefully posteromedially (0.25–0.5 cm) (Fig. 43-2) into subcutaneous tissue to avoid lodging in the erectile tissue.

After entering skin, needle should not meet resistance and tip should remain freely movable. If the tip of the needle is not freely mobile, it is probably embedded in the corpora cavernosum beneath the dorsal nerve, and should be withdrawn slightly.

g. Aspirate to rule out intravascular position.

h. Slowly infiltrate area with 0.2 to 0.4 ml lidocaine (never infiltrate as needle is advanced or withdrawn).

Arnett et al have reported good results using 0.2 ml lidocaine.[18]

i. Repeat procedure at other dorsolateral position.

After infiltration a small lidocaine ring forms (see Fig. 43-2). The swelling is minimal and does not interfere with the circumcision procedure.

j. Wait 3 to 5 minutes for analgesia.

Analgesia is usually obtained after 3 minutes, and typically disappears within 20 to 30 minutes. However, there is individual variation, and testing of the prepuce with a hemostat is suggested prior to dissection.

7. Locate coronal sulcus (Fig. 43-3A). Marking the position of the sulcus with ink on the skin of the penile shaft, prior to the procedure, is helpful in demarcating this vital landmark.

8. Use mosquito hemostat to dilate prepucial ring (Fig. 43-3B).

9. Use blunt probe to separate inner epithelium of prepuce from glans penis (Fig. 43-3C).

Failure to do this completely may result in concealed penis (see Complications).

10. Perform dorsal slit if desired.

This step is not mandatory as long as there is adequate separation of the glans from the prepuce.

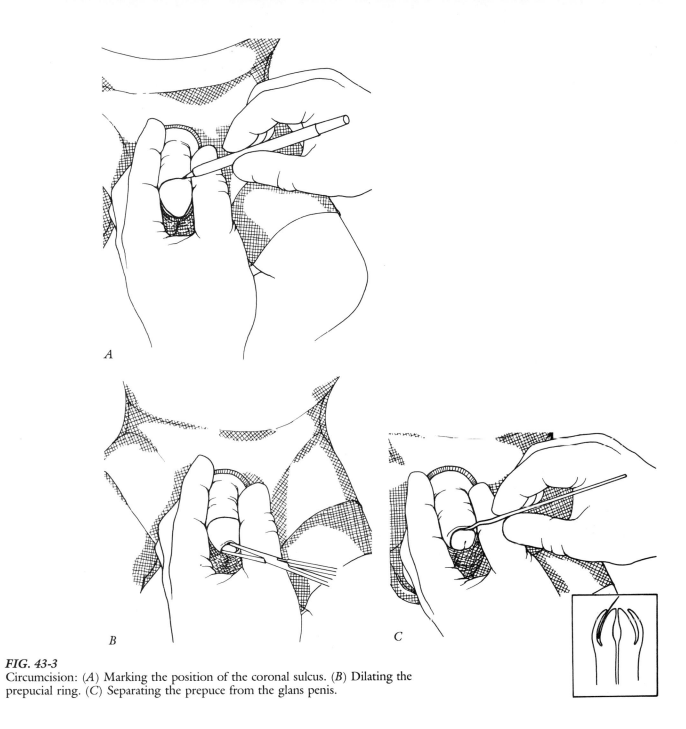

FIG. 43-3
Circumcision: (*A*) Marking the position of the coronal sulcus. (*B*) Dilating the prepucial ring. (*C*) Separating the prepuce from the glans penis.

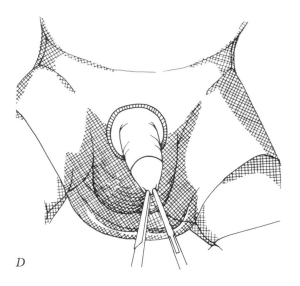

D

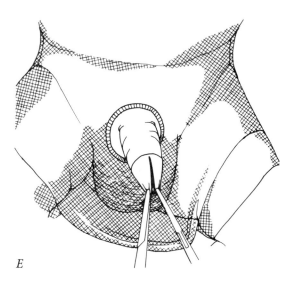

E

FIG. 43-3 (*continued*)
(*D*) Grasping the prepuce with mosquito hemostats in preparation for the dorsal-slit procedure. (*E*) Dorsal slit.

a. Grasp rim of prepuce on dorsal aspect with mosquito hemostats, approximately 2 to 4 mm apart (Fig. 43-3D).
b. Visualize urethra.
c. Place lower blade of large, straight hemostat between prepuce and glans to within 3 to 4 mm of corona, making sure to avoid urethra.
d. Close hemostat for 5 to 10 seconds to crush foreskin in dorsal midline.
e. Use tissue scissors to cut prepuce along crush line (Fig. 43-3E).
f. Check that prepuce is freed from entire surface of glans. Complete separation if necessary.
11. Complete circumcision using method of choice.

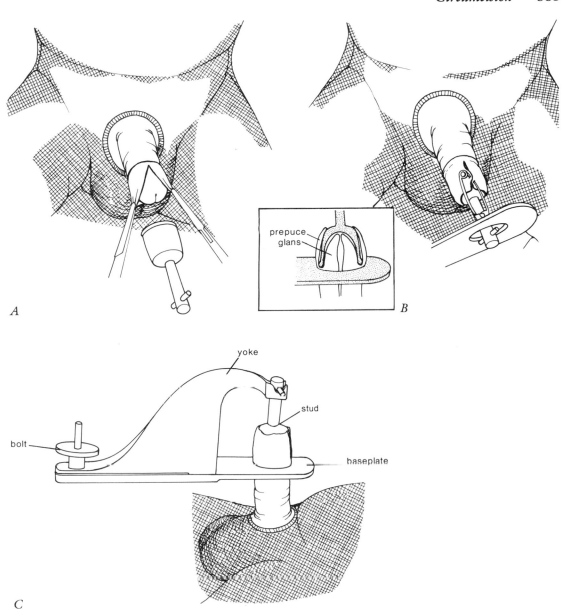

FIG. 43-4
Circumcision with a Gomco clamp. (*A*) Placing the stud over the glans. (*B*) Placing the base-plate of the clamp over the stud until the stud engages with the baseplate (*inset*). (*C*) Gomco clamp in position for circumcision.

a. Use of Circumcision Clamp

(1) Check clamp to ensure that all parts are present, fit well, and are in good working order.

(2) Assemble clamp, ensuring that yolk (arm) articulates correctly with baseplate.

(3) Draw prepuce backward gently to expose entire glans penis.

(4) Break down all residual adhesions and observe position of meatus. If meatus abnormal, cease at this point.

(5) Sponge glans dry with gauze swabs.

(6) Select stud (bell) of adequate size (see equipment), and place over glans (Fig. 43-4A).

(7) Pull prepuce over stud.

  (a) Approximate edge of dorsal slit. (A sterile safety pin may be used.)

  (b) Observe amount of skin remaining under baseplate for accuracy.

Proper placement of prepuce over stud is essential. Pulling too taut may lead to removal of excessive penile skin. Insufficient tension may lead to incomplete circumcision.

(8) Place baseplate of clamp over stud (with pin perpendicular to shaft of penis) so that prepuce is sandwiched between them (Fig. 43-4B).

(9) Continue to pull upward on stud until entire prepuce is drawn through baseplate and stud engages with baseplate.

(10) Hook yoke (arm) of clamp under side arms on shaft of stud and bolt firmly to baseplate, after checking position of prepuce between stud and baseplate (Fig. 43-4C).

(11) Remove safety pin.

(12) Wait 10 minutes.

Hemostasis is produced by pressure between baseplate and rim of stud. If the clamp is removed before 10 minutes have elapsed, wound edge hemostasis may be inadequate. If significant bleeding occurs during the procedure, remove the device and search for bleeding vessel—avoid blindly placing sutures.

(13) Remove prepuce with scalpel held parallel to and flush with upper surface of baseplate. *Never use electrocautery.*

(14) Loosen bolt on clamp and remove.

(15) Optional: Dress with loose, non-circumferential sterile gauze impregnated with vaseline.

Gough et al have shown that the addition of tincture of benzoin to the dressing adversely affected wound healing and the addition of Soframycin did not produce better results than those achieved with ordinary paraffin gauze.[19]

(16) Apply tight diaper for 1 hour.

(17) For 24 hours after circumcision, check (or instruct parents to check) for bleeding, excessive swelling, and difficulty voiding.

(18) Until circumcised area is completely healed, do not immerse; give sponge bath.

b. Use of Plastibell

(1) Follow steps (3) to (5) under Use of Circumcision Clamp.

(2) Select bell of correct size (see equipment).

  (a) Cone should fit snugly without pressure on glans.

  (b) Grooved rim of bell should be just distal to apex of dorsal slit.

(3) If necessary, cut small segment out of cone so that it clears frenulum.

(4) Hold prepuce firmly in place over cone (Fig. 43-5A)

(5) Tie suture tightly around rim of bell so that prepuce is firmly compressed into groove.

(6) Trim prepuce distal to ligature with tissue scissors. Use outer rim of cone as guide.

(7) Break off cone handle. Tissue beneath ligature will atrophy and separate with bell in 5 to 8 days (max. 10–12 days) (Fig. 43-5B).

(8) Observe and care for circumcision as in steps (17) and (18) for Gomco clamp.

F. MANAGEMENT OF POSTOPERATIVE BLEEDING

Postoperative bleeding usually stems from inadequate hemostasis or hereditary clotting disorders. Rarely, anomalous vessels are responsible.

Continuous Ooze

1. Apply manual pressure for 5 to 10 minutes.

Check that the string on the Plastibell is in place and is sufficiently tight.

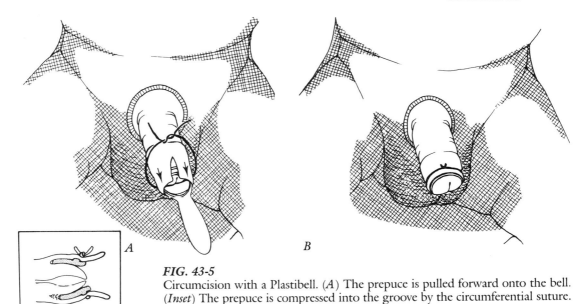

FIG. 43-5
Circumcision with a Plastibell. (*A*) The prepuce is pulled forward onto the bell. (*Inset*) The prepuce is compressed into the groove by the circumferential suture. (*B*) Appearance of the completed circumcision.

2. Assess bleeding site. If continued oozing:
   a. Apply topical thrombin (Thrombostat) on absorbable gelatin sponge (Gelfoam) *or* oxidized cellulose (Oxycel, Surgicel); do not use circumpherential dressing.
   b. Silver nitrate and epinephrine have also been used topically to control bleeding. To avoid local ischemia or systemic effects, do not exceed a 1:100,000 concentration of epinephrine.

Active Hemorrhage or Uncontrolled Ooze

1. Surgical assessment—ligation of bleeding vessel.
2. Consider underlying coagulopathy.

G. COMPLICATIONS

The overall incidence of complications associated with circumcision ranges from approximately 0.2 to 7%.[20,21]

1. Hemorrhage[3,22,23]
2. Infection[9]

   More common with the Plastibell. Most are mild and respond to wet to dry dressings and Sitz baths, but fatalities have been reported.[9]

   a. Local[4,24,25]
   b. Systemic[22,26,27]
   c. Necrotizing fasciitis[28]
3. Incomplete circumcision (most common complication)[3,29,30]

   a. Phimosis[3]
   b. Skin bridge between penile shaft and glans (commonly due to inadequate skin removal and failure to visualize the corona on followup examination)[3,31]
   c. Concealed penis (see 13a)[3,22,26,32,33]
4. Trauma
   a. Urethral laceration during dorsal-slit procedure (avoided by keeping urethra in view at all times during the procedure)
   b. Loss of penis (most commonly due to injuries related to cautery)[34,35]
   c. Hypospadias/epispadias[36]
   d. Cyanosis/necrosis of glans penis caused by overly tight Plastibell, misplaced sutures, or overtight circumpherential bandage[3,22,37]
   e. Urethrocutaneous fistula associated with use of

Gomco clamp or Plastibell (most commonly caused by using a Plastibell or clamp of incorrect size or failure to recognize congenital megaloureter).[26,38–41]

5. Urinary retention
   a. Tight (or occlusive) dressing or Plastibell[3,24,41-43]
   b. Meatal stenosis resulting from urethral meatitis[3,4]
6. Inflammation/ulceration of meatus[4,38,44–47]
7. Circumcision of hypospadias[3,22]
8. Chordee[3] (most commonly is the result of dense ventral scarring from inflammation; may be due to removal of excess skin from shaft or secondary to a skin bridge)
9. Inclusion cyst of prepuce[41]
10. Lymphedema[3,41]
11. Displacement with lodging of Plastibell around penile shaft or glans penis[10,48–50]
12. Death
    a. Anesthetic[45,50,51]
    b. Infection[52]
13. Wound separation/removal of excess skin (Fig. 43-6)[22,41,51,53]

Buried penis is usually the result of inappropriate circumcision in a chubby baby with a small or concealed penis. Excessive removal of skin should be treated with application of antiseptic (Betadine) daily and not with grafting or burying the penis in scrotum. The skin will grow back.

Circumcision by a Mohel, belonging to some Orthodox Jewish sects (Hassidim), involves removal of some skin from the shaft of the penis. This is covered by an oil-soaked bandage ("Haluk"). Only men may remove the dressing.

14. Recurrence of pneumothorax[54]
15. Reaction to epinephrine, used to control bleeding[55]
    a. Tachycardia
    b. Local vasospasm (may lead to necrosis of the glans)
16. Complications due to local anesthetic
    a. Methemoglobinemia has been reported following exposure to prilocaine, procaine, benzocaine, and lidocaine[56]
    b. Hematoma[15] (Those reported in neonates have resolved spontaneously.)
17. Mechanical problems with Gomco clamp[57]
    a. Loss of a part
    b. Warping of the plate after multiple use
    c. Breakage of arm during tightening
    d. Grooves and nicks in bell at junction of bell and plate

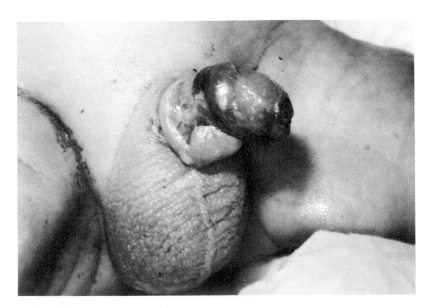

FIG. 43-6
Complication of circumcision: removal of excessive skin from the penile shaft.

References

1. POLAND RL: The question of routine circumcision. New Engl J Med 322:1312, 1990

2. WISWELL TE, ENZENAUER RW, HOLTON ME, ET AL: Declining frequency of circumcision: Implications for changes in the absolute incidence and male to female sex ratio of urinary tract infections in early infancy. Pediatrics 79:338, 1987

3. KAPLAN GW: Circumcision—an overview. Curr Probl Pediatr VII(5):3, 1977

4. KIRYA C, WERTHMANN MW JR: Neonatal circumcision and penile dorsal nerve block—a painless procedure. J Pediatr 92:998, 1978

5. PELOSI AP, APUZZIO J: Making circumcision a painless event. Contemporary Pediatrics (Jan):85, 1985

6. MAXWELL LG, YASTER M, WETZEL RC, ET AL: Penile nerve block for newborn circumcision. Obstet Gynecol 70:415, 1987

7. SFEZ M, LEMAPIHAN Y, MAZOIT X, DREUX-BOUCARD H: Local anesthetic concentrations after penile nerve block in children. Anesth Analg 71:423, 1990

8. YELLEN HS: Bloodless circumcision of the newborn. Am J Obstet Gynecol 30:146, 1935

9. GEARHART JP, CALLAN NA: Complications of circumcision. Contemporary Ob/Gyn 27:57, 1986

10. RUBENSTEIN MM, BASEN WM: Complication of circumcision done with a plastic bell clamp. Am J Dis Child 116:381, 1968

11. GOTTLIEB N: A Jewish child is born. New York, Block Publishing, 1960

12. SHECHET J: The layman's guide to the covenant of circumcision. Los Angeles, California (tel. 213-656-3938)

13. DUBRISIN R, ZAPRUDSKY P: Circumcising neonates with the Mogen clamp. Contemporary OB/Gyn 36:79, 1991

14. WILLIAMSON PS, WILLIAMSON ML: Physiologic stress reduction by local anesthetic during newborn circumcision. Pediatrics 71:36, 1983

15. FONTAINE P, TOFFLER WL: Dorsal nerve block for newborn circumcision. Am Fam Practitioner 43:1327, 1991

16. MUDGE D, YOUNGER JB: The effects of topical lidocaine on infant response to circumcision. J Nurse Midwifery 34:335, 1989

17. MASCIELLO AL: Anaesthesia for neonatal circumcision: Local anaesthesia is better than dorsal penile nerve block. Obstet Gynecol 75:834, 1990

18. ARNETT RM, JONES JS, HORGER EO: Effectiveness of 1% lidocaine dorsal penile nerve block in infant circumcision. Am J Obstet Gynecol 163:1074, 1990

19. GOUGH DCS, LAWTON N: Circumcision—which dressing? Brit J Urol 65:418, 1990

20. WISWELL TE, GESCHKE DW: Risks from circumcision during the first month of life compared with those for uncircumcised boys. Pediatrics 83:1011, 1989

21. MORENO CA, REALINI JP: Infant circumcision in an outpatient setting: Texas Medicine 85:37, 1989

22. GEE WF, ANSELL JS: Neonatal circumcision: A ten year overview with comparison of the Gomco clamp and the Plastibell device. Pediatrics 58:824, 1976

23. PATEL H: The problem of routine circumcision. Can Med Assoc J 95:576, 1966

24. FRAND M, BERANT N, BRAND N, ROTEM Y: Complications of ritual circumcision in Israel. Pediatrics 54:521, 1974

25. ROSENSTEIN JL: Wound diphtheria in the newborn infant following circumcision. J Pediatr 18:657, 1941

26. BYARS LT, TRIERS WC: Some complications of circumcision and their surgical repair. Arch Surg 76:477, 1958

27. KIRKPATRICK BV, EITZMAN DV: Neonatal septicemia after circumcision. Clin Pediatr 13:767, 1974

28. WOODSIDE JR: Necrotizing fasciitis after neonatal circumcision. Am J Dis Child 134:301, 1980

29. LEITCH IOW: Circumcision—a continuing enigma. Aust Pediatr J 6:59, 1970

30. WYNDER EL, LICKLIDER SD: The question of circumcision. Cancer 13:442, 1960

31. KLAUBER GT: Circumcision and phallic fallacies, or the case against routine circumcision. Conn Med 37:445, 1973

32. TALARICO RD, JASAITIS JE: Concealed penis: A complication of neonatal circumcision. J Urol 110:732, 1973

33. TRIER WC, DRACH GW: Concealed penis—another complication of circumcision. Am J Dis Child 125:276, 1973

34. IZZIDIEN AY: Successful reimplantation of a traumatically amputated penis in a neonate. J Pediatr Surg 16:202, 1981

35. MONEY J: Ablatio penis: Normal male infant sex-reassignment as a girl. Arch Sex Behav 4:65, 1975

36. MCGOWAN AJ JR: Letter to the Editor: A complication of circumcision. JAMA 207:2104, 1969

37. ROSEFSKY JB: Glans necrosis as a complication of circumcision. Pediatrics 39:774, 1967

38. LACKEY JT, MANNION RA, KERR JE: Urethral fistula following circumcision. JAMA 206:2318, 1968

39. LIMAYE RD, HANCOCK RA: Penile urethral fistula as a complication of circumcision. J Pediatr 72:105, 1968

40. SHIRAKI IW: Congenital megalourethra with urethro cutaneous fistula following circumcision: A case report. J Urol 109:723, 1973

41. SHULMAN J, BEN-HUR N, NEUMAN Z: Surgical complications of circumcision. Am J Dis Child 107:149, 1965

42. BERMAN W: Urinary retention due to ritual circumcision. Pediatrics 56:621, 1975

43. HOROWITZ J, SUSSHEIM A, SCALETTAR HE: Abdominal distention following ritual circumcision. Pediatrics 57:579, 1976

44. DALEY MC: Circumcision. JAMA 214:2195, 1970

45. GAIRDNER D: The fate of the foreskin—a study of circumcision. Br Med J 2:1433, 1949

46. GALLAGHER AGP: Complications of circumcision. Br J Urol 44:720, 1972

47. MACKENZIE AR: Meatal ulceration following neonatal circumcision. Obstet Gynecol 28:221, 1966

48. JOHNSONBAUGH RE, MEYER BP, CATALANO JD: Complication of a circumcision performed by a plastic bell clamp. Am J Dis Child 118:781, 1969

49. MALO T, BONFORTE RJ: Hazards of plastic bell circumcision. Obstet Gynecol 33:869, 1969

50. WRIGHT JE: Non-therapeutic circumcision. Med J Aust 1:1083, 1967

51. MAL HERBE WOF: Injuries to the skin of the male genitalia in South Africa. South Afr Med J 49:147, 1975

52. GROSSMAN E, POSNER NA: Surgical circumcision of neonates: A history of its development. Obstet Gynecol 58:241, 1981

53. VAN DUYN J, WARR WS: Excessive penile skin loss from circumcision. J Med Assoc Ga 51:394, 1962

54. AUERBACH MR, SCANLON JW: Recurrence of pneumothorax as a possible complication of elective circumcision. Am J Obstet Gynecol 132:583, 1978

55. DENTON J, SCHRIENER RL, PEARSON J: Circumcision complication: Reaction to treatment of local hemorrhage with topical epinephrine in high concentration. Clin Pediatr 17:285, 1978

56. MANDEL S: Methemoglobinemia following circumcision (Letter) JAMA 261:702, 1989

57. FEINBERG AN, BLAZEK MA: Mechanical complications of circumcision with a Gomco clamp. Am J Dis Child 142:813, 1988

44 Drainage of Superficial Abscesses

Marilea Kay Miller

A. INDICATIONS

1. To identify pathogens[1]
2. To differentiate infectious from noninfectious lesions[2-5]
3. To establish free drainage of contents from a superficial abscess, which is a localized collection of pus causing fluctuant soft tissue swelling and which may have associated erythema and induration[6-11]

B. CONTRAINDICATIONS

1. Carefully identify and avoid
   a. Cephalohematoma
   b. Hemangioma
   c. Cystic hygroma
   d. Encephalocele

C. EQUIPMENT

Sterile

1. Gloves and gown
2. Antiseptic swabs or cup containing antiseptic solution
3. 1-ml syringe
4. Nonbacteriostatic, isotonic saline without preservative
5. 23-gauge needle
6. 2 × 2 gauze squares
7. Scalpel with No. 11 blade
8. Cotton-tipped culture swab
9. Mosquito hemostat
10. 1/2-inch, fine-mesh, plain gauze

Unsterile

1. Ethyl chloride spray as topical anesthetic
2. Mask and cap
3. Adhesive tape

D. PRECAUTIONS

1. Use appropriate isolation techniques to safeguard other infants.
2. Obtain blood cultures after drainage.
3. Do not suture abscess cavity following incision and drainage.
4. Debride all tissue undergoing putrefaction and digestion thoroughly.[7,12]

E. TECHNIQUE[1,4,7,8]

1. Prepare as for major procedure if abscess is to be drained, or for minor procedure if needle aspiration alone is to be performed (see Chap. 4).
2. Put on mask and cap.
3. Spray roof of abscess with ethyl chloride until skin becomes white.
4. Scrub and put on gown and gloves.
5. Prepare local area with antiseptic (e.g. iodophor)
6. Aspiration
   a. Attach sterile needle to syringe.
   b. Insert needle into pustule, abscess cavity, or advancing border of cellulitis.
   c. Aspirate the material deep within the lesion.
   d. If no material is aspirated, inject 0.1 to 0.2 ml of nonbacteriostatic saline and withdraw immediately.
   e. Process aspirated material immediately. Gram stain and culture for anaerobic and aerobic organisms. Giemsma stain for suspected herpes. Perform other special stains as warranted.
7. Drainage
   a. Insert scalpel blade and incise at point of maximum fluctuance (Fig. 44-1). The size of the incision should be as small as possible, yet allow for continued adequate drainage.

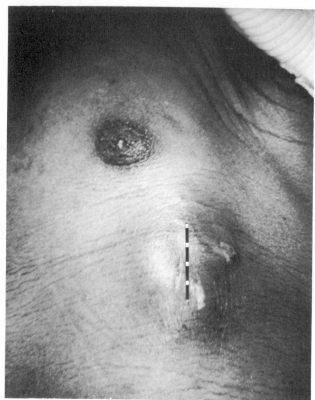

FIG. 44-1
Superficial abscess in the site of an electrode placed in the left anterior axillary line for cardiorespiratory monitoring. The site for incision is indicated.

11. Remove half of gauze packing in 24 hours and remainder within 48 hours.
12. Check abscess wound, and apply sterile warm soaks for 20 to 30 minutes, three times a day, until healing has commenced as indicated by
    a. Cessation of drainage
    b. Formation of granulation tissue
    c. Resolution of local tissue inflammation

D. COMPLICATIONS

1. Introduction of infection into sterile abscess or hematoma
2. Local bleeding
3. Injury to blood vessels, nerves, or tendons (deep to abscess cavity)[6]
4. Incomplete drainage with recurrent abscess formation[7,8]
5. Systemic infection[13]
6. Scar formation at drainage site, requiring skin graft[14]

   b. Obtain specimen for culture with cotton-tipped applicator, if not obtained by prior aspiration with syringe and needle.
   c. Evacuate exudate from abscess with gentle finger pressure to surrounding area.
   d. If necessary, insert mosquito hemostat into abscess cavity, and spread blades to break septa and to release remaining collections of pus (Fig. 44-2A). Recognize that this may cause discomfort and should be done rapidly.
8. Lavage area with sterile saline to remove residual pus (optional).
9. If indicated, insert plain, ½-inch gauze into abscess cavity to stop bleeding and/or to serve as a wick to promote drainage (Fig. 44-2B).
10. Apply dry, sterile dressing.

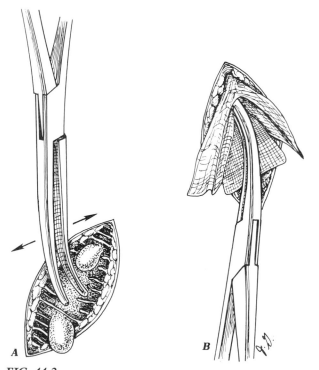

FIG. 44-2
Drainage of a superficial abscess. (*A*) Breaking the septa with a clamp. (*B*) Packing the wound.

7. Reduction of breast size following incomplete drainage of breast abscess[9]

References

1. GOETZ J, TAFARI N, BOXERBAUM B: Needle aspiration in *Haemophilus influenzae* type B cellulitis. Pediatrics 54:504, 1974
2. JARRATT M, RAMSDELL W: Infantile acropustulosis. Arch Derm 115:834, 1979
3. KAHN G, RYWLIN A: Acropustulosis of infancy. Arch Derm 115:831, 1979
4. RUDOY R, NAKASHIMA G: Diagnostic value of needle aspiration in *Haemophilus influenzae* type B cellulitis. J Pediatr 94:924, 1979
5. ZELMAN S: Abscesses from parenteral injection. JAMA 240:23, 1978
6. ALBOM M: Surgical gems: Surgical management of a superficial cutaneous abscess. J Dermatol Surg Oncol 2:120, 1976
7. MACFIE J, HARVEY J: The treatment of acute superficial abscesses: A prospective clinical trial. Br J. Surg 64:264, 1977
8. MEISLIN HN, LERNER SA, GRAVES MH, ET AL: Cutaneous abscesses: Anaerobic and aerobic bacteriology and outpatient management. Ann Intern Med 87:145, 1977
9. RUDOY R, NELSON J: Breast abscess during the neonatal period. Am J Dis Child 129:1031, 1975
10. TURBEY W, BUNTAIN W, DUDGEON D: The surgical management of pediatric breast masses. Pediatrics 56:736, 1975
11. WINKEL CA, SNYDER DL, SCHLAERTE JB: Scalp abscess: A complication of the spiral fetal electrode. Am J Obstet Gynecol 126:720, 1976
12. RAMAMURTHY R, SRINIVASAN G, JACOBS N: Necrotizing fasciitis and necrotizing cellulitis due to group B Streptococcus. Am J Dis Child 131:1169, 1977
13. GORMLEY D: Neonatal anaerobic (clostridial) cellulitis and omphalitis. Arch Dermatol 113:683, 1977
14. FEDER H, McLEAN WC, MOXON R: Scalp abscess secondary to fetal scalp electrode. J Pediatr 89:808, 1976

45 Phototherapy

Dorothy S. Hsiao

Phototherapy is a mechanism for reducing bilirubin levels and the risk of bilirubin toxicity. Detoxification begins immediately by producing configurational and structural photoisomers of bilirubin in the skin and precedes the fall in serum bilirubin. Increasing irradiance improves excretion of bilirubin, presumably via increased production of the structural photoisomer lumirubin.[1,2] Phototherapy is effective,[3] easy to use, and without any major short- or long-term side-effects.[4]

A. INDICATIONS

Clinically significant indirect hyperbilirubinemia

A convenient guideline is to use phototherapy when bilirubin levels are 86 μM/L (5 mg/dL) less than the level at which an exchange transfusion would be performed.[5] Phototherapy is minimally efficacious at bilirubin levels of 86 μM/L.[6] Indications vary with gestational age, birth weight, day of life, serum albumin, factors indicating acuity of illness, and institutional and physician practices (Table 45-1). Indications established for Rh isoimmunization[7] do not directly apply to other etiologies for hyperbilirubinemia, for example, ABO incompatibility[8] or breast milk jaundice.[9]

B. RELATIVE CONTRAINDICATIONS

1. As an isolated therapy when exchange transfusion is directly indicated for removal of antibodies in the presence of rapidly rising bilirubin
2. In the presence of direct hyperbilirubinemia

Bronze baby syndrome occurs when phototherapy is used in the presence of hepatic dysfunction and cholestasis leading to high serum porphyrins and copper. Bilirubin photoproducts sensitize copper porphyrins to form brown photoproducts that bronze the skin.[10,11] Phototherapy with a direct bilirubin, >34 μm/L (2 mg/dL) or > 20% of the total serum bilirubin level indicates cholestasis[12] and may result in bronzing in susceptible infants.

3. Porphyria[13]
4. Concurrent therapy with tin protoporphyrin[14]

C. EQUIPMENT

1. Phototherapy unit
   a. Free standing
   b. Attached to radiant warmer
   c. Wall mounted or suspended from ceiling
2. Bulbs (Fig. 45-1)
   a. Fluorescent tubes: High Intensity (Special®) Blue, blue, green, daylight, cool white, or gold

   High intensity blue fluorescent bulbs are most effective in reducing bilirubin levels.[15] Green light penetrates the skin more deeply but provides no advantage over blue light.[16] Daylight

---

TABLE 45-1

Serum Bilirubin Concentrations Commonly Used as Guidelines for Initiating Phototherapy*

Birth Weight	Bilirubin†
<1500 gm	8–10 mg/dL
1501–2500 gm	10–12 mg/dL
>2500 gm	15–18 mg/dL

Adapted with permission from Neonatal Hyperbilirubinemia. American Board of Pediatrics Program for Renewal of Certification in Pediatrics. Supplement to Pediatrics in Review.

*These guidelines represent the current practice of many practitioners but they have not been validated by clinical studies.

†In the presence of hemolysis or risk factors such as hypoxia, acidosis, hypoalbuminemia, or sepsis, these values should be reduced by 2 mg/dL. The smaller and younger the infant is within the weight group, the more liberal the use of phototherapy. These values do not pertain to healthy infants whose jaundice is believed to be due to breast feeding.

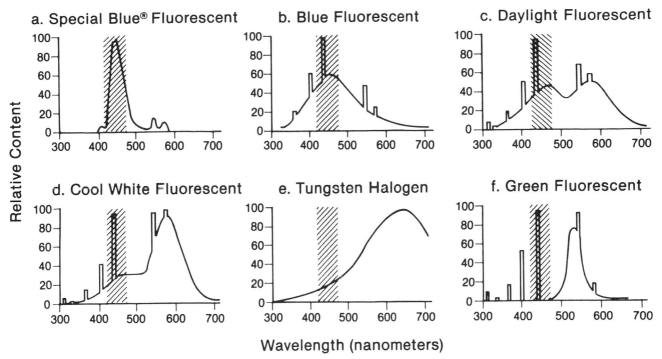

FIG. 45-1
Relative spectral content of phototherapy bulbs. Shaded area indicates wavelength effective for phototherapy. Absolute spectral irradiance (μW/cm²/nm) depends not only on relative power across wavelength of bilirubin absorption, but also on total wattage and distance from infant. While all bulbs provide effective phototherapy for the same wattage, Special® Blue and blue fluorescent bulbs provide the most amount of power in the bilirubin wavelength. (Based on data from Olympic Medical [*a–d*]. Warshaw JB, et al: A comparison of fluorescent and nonfluorescent light sources for phototherapy. Pediatrics 65:796, 1980 [*e*]. Farr PM: Arch Dis Child 63:461, 1988 [*f*])

bulbs have a greater relative power than cool white in the bilirubin wavelength. Gold light decreases some of the side-effects when special blue light bulbs are used but are themselves not effective in reducing bilirubin.

b. Nonfluorescent lamps: quartz-halogen or tungsten-halogen

Halogen lamps produce a more intense light over a smaller surface area. They are effective[17] but more expensive than fluorescent bulbs.

3. Eye patches
a. Opaque
b. Soft, nonshredding
c. Stable in place

Masks adhering directly to velcro tabs on the temples are preferable to circumferential head bands.

4. Photoradiometer with fixed bandwidth at 425 to 275 nm
5. Optional: yellow or amber-tinted transparent plastic curtain (4 × 4) fastened as a skirt around phototherapy unit

When high intensity blue fluorescent bulbs are in use, the staff may suffer nausea, eye strain, and headache. There are fewer symptoms if a curtain filters the blue light. Alternatively, one of the blue lamps may be replaced with a gold or white fluorescent bulb, although the saturation of the blue light will be diluted.

D. PRECAUTIONS

Infant
1. Protect eyes from phototherapy light and irritation.
2. Monitor temperature to avoid hypothermia and

hyperthermia, especially in infants in incubators (greenhouse effect).

3. Prevent dehydration secondary to increased insensible water loss.

4. Avoid fully occlusive dressings, bandages, topical skin ointments, and plastic in direct in contact with infant's skin (diapers or plastic wrap) to prevent burns.

5. Remove plastic heat shields and plastic wrap that decrease irradiance delivered to the skin.[18]

> Heat shields constructed with plastic wrap tightly stretched over a frame insignificantly affects irradiance, while those with wrinkled plastic wrap or thick and scratched walls decrease it.

6. Recognize that clinical assessment of skin color for cyanosis or jaundice and transcutaneous bilirubinometry are not as accurate once phototherapy is started.
   a. Use oxygen saturation monitor as needed but shield the monitor probe from the phototherapy light.[19]
   b. Monitor serum bilirubin levels.

7. Turn off unit during phlebotomy for bilirubin levels.

Phototherapy Unit

1. Maintain intact Plexiglass shield over phototherapy light bulbs.
   a. Block ultraviolet radiation.
   b. Protect infant from accidental bulb breakage.

2. Maximize bulb life.
   a. Provide good air ventilation to the phototherapy unit to prevent overheating light bulbs.
   b. Protect unit from jarring by staff or other equipment.

3. Maintain cleanliness and electrical safety.

4. Keep photoradiometer calibrated. Follow manufacturer's instructions for proper use.

E. TECHNIQUE

1. Monitor infant's temperature, weight, intake, and output. Supplement fluids as clinically indicated: Increase by 10 to 60 ml/kg/day.

2. Shield eyes with patches or mask.

3. Clean eyes regularly and check for discharge.

4. Maximize skin exposure to phototherapy source.
   a. Change infant's position regularly.
   b. Cover gonads only as clinically necessary.

   > DNA damage as demonstrated in human tissue culture exposed directly to ultraviolet and visible light is a theoretical risk.[20,21] High intensity blue lights minimize ultraviolet light exposure.

   c. Keep diapers, blanket rolls, or bandages from blocking light.

5. Select type of light bulb (Fig. 45-1)

6. Position phototherapy unit over infant to obtain desired irradiance (10–40 $\mu W/cm^2/nm$).

   > Increasing irradiance increases efficacy.[6] Maximal amount of irradiance achieved by standard technique is 30–50 $\mu W/cm^2/nm$.

7. Check and document irradiance daily. If increased irradiance is desired
   a. Shorten distance between infant and phototherapy unit. Make certain closer position does not overheat infant.
   b. Add additional phototherapy units.
      (1) Fluorescent panel perpendicular to incubator
      (2) Fiberoptic halogen pad underneath infant
   c. Line incubator with white cloth without blocking light.
   d. Change light bulbs.

8. Encourage family visitation.

9. Discontinue phototherapy when bilirubin is low enough not to suggest rebound to levels requiring therapy.

F. ALTERNATIVE TECHNIQUES

1. Home phototherapy

   > Home phototherapy decreases costs of hospitalization and eliminates separation of mother and infant. It is a safe and effective therapy for selected infants.[22] Equipment has not been standardized for home use so precautions listed earlier apply. The following guidelines are based on recommendations by the American Academy of Pediatrics.[23]

a. Limit use to
  (1) Term infants, otherwise healthy and older than 48 hours
  (2) Serum bilirubin >239 μm/L (14 mg/dL) but <308 μm/L (18 mg/dL)
  (3) No elevation of direct bilirubin
  (4) Diagnostic evaluation negative
      (a) Physical exam
      (b) CBC, differential, smear and reticulocyte count
      (c) Fractionated bilirubin
      (d) Blood type and Coombs reaction on both mother and infant
      (e) Urinalysis
      (f) Urine reducing substances
b. Estimate current rate of rise of serum bilirubin not to exceed 17 μm/L (1mg/dL) every 3 to 4 hours.
c. Judge caretakers as to capacity to follow instructions.
d. Hospitalize infant if signs of illness develop.
e. Obtain informed consent from caregivers.
f. Use only a reliable equipment vendor who maintains safe and effective equipment for home use and who will provide full time support as needed.
g. Have infant seen daily for exam and bilirubin level.
  (1) Visiting nurse or
  (2) Office visit

2. Fiberoptic halogen pad

The fiberoptic halogen pad is available for home and hospital use and is safe and effective.[24] It minimizes infant/parent separation; theoretically has less risk for hypothermia, hyperthermia, and insensible water loss; eliminates the need for occlusive eye patches; and is less cumbersome.[25,26]

a. Equipment
  (1) Illuminator unit
  (2) Fiberoptic panel and cable
  (3) Disposable covers
  (4) Replacement bulbs
b. Precautions
  (1) Ensure stability and adequate ventilation of illuminator unit.
      (a) Place on secure surface.
      (b) Place outside incubator, warmer, or bassinet.
  (2) Keep fiberoptic panel and illuminator clean and dry, according to manufacturer's instructions.
  (3) Turn off and unplug illuminator when servicing or when panel is not on unit. Allow lamp to cool for 10 to 20 minutes before moving illuminator.
  (4) Verify that line voltage matches the level specified for the unit.
  (5) Do not place sharp or heavy objects on panel or cable.
  (6) Avoid carrying infant wrapped in panel.
  (7) Avoid constriction and skin irritation under infant's arms.
      (a) Place panel properly.
      (b) Do not wrap too tightly.
      (c) Verify that proper side of disposable cover touches the skin.
  (8) Use disposable cover on only one infant and discard if soiled.
  (9) Use eye patches if any direct exposure to lights in panel or if used with conventional phototherapy for double-sided effect.
c. Technique
  (1) Place illuminator on hard surface less than 4 feet from infant.
  (2) Insert panel into disposable cover so it is flat and directed toward infant.
  (3) Place covered panel around infant's back or chest and secure in position but not tight.
      (a) Ensure proper ventilation under panel.
      (b) Maximize skin exposure.
  (4) Connect fiberoptic panel to illuminator.
  (5) Swaddle infant in blanket or dress in sleeper.
  (6) Turn illuminator on at the highest irradiance levels.
  (7) Discard disposable cover after each treatment and when soiled.
  (8) Cuddle or feed infant during treatment as per routine.

TABLE 45-2
Complications of Phototherapy

| Problem | |
Clinically Relevant	Suggested Intervention
Skin changes increased pigmentation erythema, or rash burns	Reposition to allow even tanning. Avoid topical therapy. Prevent plastic diapers or plastic wrap from direct contact.
Diarrhea, loose stools	Increase fluid intake.[27]
Dehydration	Increase free water.[28]
Hyperthermia	Shield servocontrol thermometer from light. Keep free air flow in incubator. Decrease distance from light unit.
Bronze baby syndrome	Stop phototherapy.[29]
Hemolysis of red cells	Shield blood during transfusion.[30,31]
Spuriously low bilirubin level	Turn off phototherapy during lab phlebotomy.
Change in photosensitive medication: nitroprusside, amphotericin, vitamin injectables	Shield solutions from light.
Staff discomfort with blue or green bulbs	Hang yellow plastic to filter light. Replace blue with white or gold bulb.
Difficulty assessing cyanosis	Use oximetry and monitoring if infant at particular risk. Turn lights off periodically for exam.
Separation from parents	Encourage parental visitation and assistance in care.[32] Consider alternative technique.

Theoretical or Clinically Minor	
Retinal damage from light exposure	Keep eyes effectively covered.[33,34]
DNA damage	Use gonadal shield if desired.[20,21]
Hypocalcemia in premature infants	Monitor serum calcium.[35]

TABLE 45-2
(continued)

Theoretical or Clinically Minor	
Transient drop in LH values[36]	No intervention needed.
Depressed plasma riboflavin[37]	No intervention needed.
Depressed free tryptophan levels[38]	No intervention needed.

G. COMPLICATIONS

See Table 45-2.

References

1. COSTARINO AT, ENNEVER JF, BAUMGART S, ET AL: Bilirubin photoisomerization in premature neonates under low- and high-dose phototherapy. Pediatrics 75:519, 1985
2. ONISHI S, ISOBE K, ITOH S, ET AL: Metabolism of bilirubin and its photoisomers in newborn infants during phototherapy. J Biochem 100:789, 1986
3. BROWN AK, KIM MH, WU PY, BRYLA DA: Efficacy of phototherapy in prevention and management of neonatal hyperbilirubinemia. Pediatrics (suppl) 75:393, 1985
4. SCHEIDT PC, BRYLA DA, NELSON KB, ET AL: Phototherapy for neonatal hyperbilirubinemia: Six year followup of the NICHD clinical trial. Pediatrics 85:455, 1990
5. HINDERLITER SA: Hyperbilirubinemia. In Gomella TL (ed): Neonatology, Basic Management, On-Call Problems, Diseases, Drugs '88/89. Norwalk, CT. Appleton Lange, 1988, p 232
6. TAN KL: The pattern of bilirubin response to phototherapy for neonatal hyperbilirubinemia. Pediatr Res 16:670, 1982
7. ALLEN FH JR, DIAMOND LK: Erythroblastosis Fetalis: Including Exchange Transfusion Technique. Boston, Little, Brown, 1957, p 57
8. OSBORN LM, LENARSKY C, OAKES RC, REIFF MI: Phototherapy in full-term infants with hemolytic disease secondary to ABO incompatibility. Pediatrics 74:371, 1984

9. Osborn LM, Bolus R: Breast feeding and jaundice in the first week of life. J Fam Pract 20:475, 1985

10. Rubaltelli FF, Jori G, Reddi E: Bronze baby syndrome: A new porphyrin-related disorder. Pediatr Res 17:327, 1983

11. Onishi S, Itoh S, Isobe K, et al: Mechanism of development of bronze baby syndrome in neonates treated with phototherapy. Pediatrics 69:273, 1982

12. Balistreri WF: Neonatal Cholestasis: Lessons from the past, issues for the future. Seminar in Liver Disease (Foreword) 7(2), 1987

13. Brown AK, McDonagh AF: Phototherapy for neonatal hyperbilirubinemia: Efficacy, mechanism and toxicity. In Barness LA (ed): Advances in Pediatrics, Vol 27. Chicago, Year Book Medical Publishers, 1980, p 341

14. Fort FL, Gold J: Phototoxicity of tin protoporphyrin, tin mesoporphyrin, and tin dilododeuteroporphyrin under neonatal phototherapy conditions. Pediatrics 84:1031, 1989

15. Tan KL: Efficacy of fluorescent daylight, blue, and green lamps in the management of nonhemolytic hyperbilirubinemia. J Pediatr 114:132, 1989

16. Amato M, Inaebnit D: Clinical usefulness of high intensity green light phototherapy in the treatment of neonatal jaundice. Eur J Pediatr 150:274, 1991

17. Warshaw JB, Ggagliardi J, Patel A: A comparison of fluorescent and nonfluorescent light sources for phototherapy. Pediatrics 65(4):795, 1980

18. Karsdon J, Schothorst AA, Ruys JH, Berger HM: Plastic blankets and heat shields decrease transmission of phototherapy light. Acta Paediatr Scand 75:555, 1986

19. Hay W: Physiology of oygenation and its relation to pulse oximetry in neonates. J Perinatol 7(4):309, 1987

20. Rosenstein BS, Ducore JM: Induction of DNA strand breaks in normal human fibroblasts exposed to monochromatic ultraviolet and visible wavelengths in the 240–546 nm range. Photochem Photobiol 38:51, 1983

21. Ting CC, Rogers MJ: Mutagenicity and toxicity of visible fluorescent light to cultured mammalian cells. Nature 266:724, 1977

22. Eggert LD, Pollary RA, Folland DS, Jung AL: Home phototherapy treatment of neonatal jaundice. Pediatrics 76:579, 1985

23. Committee on Fetus and Newborn, American Academy of Pediatrics 76:136, 1985

24. Gale R, Dranitzki Z, Dollberg S, Stevenson D: A randomized, controlled application of the Wallaby phototherapy system compared with standard phototherapy. J Perinatol 10(3):239, 1990

25. Wallaby phototherapy system: Instruction manual. Allentown, PA, Fiberoptic Medical Products, Inc.

26. BiliBlanket phototherapy light: Operation, maintenance, and service manual. Columbia, MD, Ohmeda, 1990

27. Curtis MD, Guandalini S, Fasano A, et al: Diarrhoea in jaundiced neonates treated with phototherapy: Role of intestinal secretion. Arch Dis Child 64:1161, 1989

28. Oh W, Karecki H: Phototherapy and insensible water loss in the newborn infant. Am J Dis Child 124:230, 1972

29. Kopelman AE, Brown RS, Odell GB: The "bronze" baby syndrome: A complication of phototherapy. J Pediatr 81:466, 1972

30. Opitz JC, Baldauf MC, Kessler DL, Meyer JA: Hemolysis of blood in intravenous tubing caused by heat. J Pediatr 112:111, 1988

31. Tozzi E, Tozzi-Ciancarelli MG, DiGiulio A, et al: In vitro and in vivo effects of erythrocyte phototherapy on newborns. Biol Neonate 56:204, 1989

32. Telzrow RW, Snyder DM, Tronick E, et al: The behavior of jaundiced infants undergoing phototherapy. Dev Med Child Neurol 22:317, 1980

33. Moseley MJ, Fielder AR: Phototherapy: An ocular hazard revisited. Arch Dis Child 63:886, 1988

34. Dobson V, Cowett RM, Riggs LA: Long-term effect of phototherapy on visual function. J Pediatr 86:555, 1975

35. Ramagnoli C, Polidori G, Cataldi L, et al: Phototherapy-induced hypocalcemia. J Pediatr 94:815, 1979

36. Lemaitre B, Toubas PL, Guillot M, et al: Changes in serum gonadotropin concentrations in premature babies submitted to phototherapy. Biol Neonate 32:113, 1977

37. Gromisch DS, Rafael L, Cole HS, Cooperman JM: Light (phototherapy)-induced riboflavin deficiency in the neonate. J Pediatr 90:118, 1977

38. Zammarchi E, LaRosa S, Pierro U, et al: Free tryptophan decrease in jaundiced newborn infants during phototherapy. Biol Neonate 55:224, 1989

46 Intraosseous Infusions

Mary E. Revenis

A. INDICATIONS

1. Emergency intravenous access when other venous access is not readily available. See Table 46-1 for types of fluids that have been infused.[1-3]

B. CONTRAINDICATIONS[3-5]

1. Bone without cortical integrity (fracture, previous penetration): extravasation of infusate
2. Sternal site: potential damage to heart and lungs[6]
3. Overlying soft tissue infection
4. Osteogenesis imperfecta
5. Obliterative diseases of marrow such as osteopetrosis

C. EQUIPMENT

Sterile

1. Surgical gloves
2. Cup with antiseptic solution
3. Gauze squares
4. Aperture drape
5. 1% lidocaine in 1-ml syringe with 25-gauge needle
6. Needle, in order of preference[1-3,7-9]
   a. Bone marrow (18 gauge) (stylet and adjustable depth indicator preferred)
   b. Short spinal needle with stylet (18 or 20 gauge)
   c. Short hypodermic needle (18 or 20 gauge)
   d. Butterfly needle (16–19 gauge)
7. 5-ml syringe on a three-way stopcock
8. Syringes with saline flush solution
9. Intravenous infusion set and intravenous fluid

Unsterile

1. Small sand bag or rolled towel to aid in stabilizing limb
2. Tape
3. Arm board
4. Disposable plastic cup (optional)

D. PRECAUTIONS

1. Limit use to emergency vascular access only when peripheral or central venous access are not available.
2. Avoid inserting needle into infected skin or subcutaneous tissue.
3. Stabilize limb with counter pressure directly opposite proposed site of penetration to avoid bone fracture.
4. Limit needle size to decrease chance of fracture of bone.

TABLE 46-1

Types of Intraosseous Infusates Reported in the Literature[18,19,22,27,37]

---

1. Fluids[24,27,28,37]
   a. Normal saline
   b. Crystalloid solutions
   c. Glucose (dilute if possible when using D50)[18,19,29]
   d. Ringer's lactate[22]
2. Blood and blood products[27,28,37]
3. Medications
   a. Anesthetic agents[28]
   b. Antibiotics
   c. Atropine[22,31]
   d. Calcium gluconate
   e. Dexamethasone[22]
   f. Diazepam
   g. Diazoxide,[22] Phenytoin[36]
   h. Dobutamine[34]
   i. Dopamine[29,34,35]
   j. Ephedrine[32,33]
   k. Epinephrine[32,33]
   l. Heparin[22]
   m. Insulin[31]
   n. Isoproterenol[35]
   o. Lidocaine
   p. Morphine[31]
   q. Sodium bicarbonate (dilute if possible)[19,30]
4. Contrast material[17,24]

---

5. Administer drugs in the usual doses for intravenous administration, but when possible, dilute hypertonic or strongly alkaline solutions prior to infusion to lessen possible danger of bone marrow damage.[2]
6. Discontinue intraosseous infusion as soon as alternate venous access is established to lessen risk of osteomyelitis.

E. TECHNIQUE

Proximal tibia[1-3,8,10,11] (Fig. 46-1)

1. Position patient supine.
2. Place sand bag or towel roll behind knee.
3. Clean proximal tibia with antiseptic solution.
4. Put on sterile gloves.
5. Apply aperture drape.
6. If appropriate, inject lidocaine into skin, soft tissue, and periosteum.[12]
7. Determine penetration depth on needle: rarely more than 1 cm in infants.
   a. For needle with adjustable depth indicator, adjust sheath to allow desired penetration.
   b. For needle without an adjustable depth indicator, hold the needle in the dominant hand with blunt end supported by the palm and the index finger approximately 1 cm from the bevel of the needle to avoid pushing it past this mark.
8. Palpate tibial tuberosity with index finger.
9. Insert needle on the flat antero-medial surface of the tibia, 1 to 2 cm below the tibial tuberosity.
10. Direct needle at an angle of 10 to 15 degrees toward the foot to avoid the growth plate.
11. Support bone directly behind insertion site to reduce bone fracture.

12. Advance needle, using firm pressure with a twisting motion until there is a sudden, slight decrease in resistance, indicating puncture of the cortex.
13. Do not advance the needle beyond cortical puncture.
14. Remove the stylet.
15. Confirm the position of the needle in the marrow cavity.
   a. Needle should stand without support.
   b. Securely attach a 5-ml syringe and attempt to aspirate blood or marrow. Aspiration is not always successful when using an 18- or 20-gauge needle.

   If aspirated, the bone marrow can be analyzed for blood chemistry values, partial pressure of arterial carbon dioxide, pH, hemoglobin level,[13-15] type and crossmatch, or culture.[13,15]

   c. Attach syringe of saline flush solution and infuse 2 to 3 ml slowly while palpating the tissue adjacent to the insertion site to detect extravasation. There should be only mild resistance to fluid infusion.
16. If marrow cannot be aspirated and significant resistance to fluid infusion is met
   a. The hollow bore needle may be obstructed by small bone plugs.
      (1) Reintroduce the stylet, or
      (2) Introduce a smaller gauge needle through the original needle.
      (3) Attach syringe of saline flush and flush 2 to 3 ml of fluid.
   b. The bevel of the needle may not have penetrated the cortex.

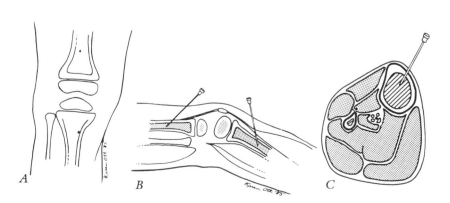

FIG. 46-1
A, anterior view. *B*, sagittal section. *C*, cross-section through tibia. (Reproduced with permission from Hodge D: Intraosseous infusions: A review. Pediatr Emerg Care 1(4):215, 1985).

(1) Redetermine estimated depth needed.
(2) Advance
(3) Flush with saline.

  c. The bevel of the needle may be lodged against the opposite cortex.

(1) Withdraw needle slightly.
(2) Flush with saline.

17. Observe the site for extravasation of fluid indicating

  a. The placement is too superficial, or

  b. The bone has been penetrated completely.

  c. If extravasation occurs, withdraw needle and select a different bone.

18. When needle position is confirmed

  a. Attach syringe and infuse medications or fluid directly into the needle. Clear medications with saline flush.

  b. For continuous infusion, attach a standard intravenous infusion set with an infusion pump to the intraosseous needle and administer at the same rate as for IV infusion.[2]

19. Secure intraosseous needle and maintain a clean infusion site while the needle is in place.

  a. Tape the flanges of the needle to the skin to prevent dislodgement.

  b. If desired, cover the exposed end of the needle with a disposable cup, taping the cover down.

Caution: this may make visualization of any subcutaneous infiltration difficult.

20. Secure intravenous tubing with tape to the leg.
21. Secure the leg to armboard.
22. Obtain x-ray to confirm position of needle and to rule out fracture.
23. Discontinue intraosseous infusion as soon as alternate intravenous access is achieved.

  a. Remove needle.

  b. Apply a sterile dressing over the puncture site.

  c. Apply pressure to the dressing for 5 minutes.

Distal tibia[2,9] (Fig. 46-2)

1. Position patient in supine.
2. Prepare site and needle as for proximal tibia, above.
3. Insert needle in the medial surface of the distal tibia just proximal to the medial malleolus.
4. Direct needle cephalad away from the joint space.
5. Proceed as for proximal tibia, above.

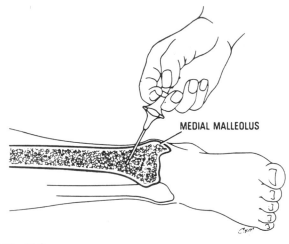

MEDIAL MALLEOLUS

FIG. 46-2
Intraosseous infusion into the distal tibia. (Reproduced with permission from Spivey WH: Intraosseous infusions. J Pediatr 111(5):639, 1987).

Distal femur[1,3,8,10] (Fig. 46-1)

1. Position patient supine.
2. Place sand bag or towel roll behind knee.
3. Prepare site and needle as for proximal tibia, above.
4. Insert needle 1 to 3 cm above the external condyles in the anterior midline.
5. Direct needle cephalad at a slight angle of 10 to 15 degrees.
6. Proceed as for proximal tibia, above.

F. COMPLICATIONS

1. Fracture of bone[21]
2. Complete penetration of bone[22]
3. Osteomyelitis[16,19,20,23,24]
4. Periostitis[18,19]
5. Subcutaneous abscess
6. Cellulitis
7. Sepsis
8. Extravasation of fluid from the puncture site
9. Subperiosteal or subcutaneous infiltration or hematoma
10. Subcutaneous sloughing
11. Death (reported only with sternal bone site)[20]
12. Theoretical (as yet unreported)

  a. Embolization of bone fragments or fat[25,26]

  b. Damage to bone marrow[18]

  c. Damage to growth plate

References

1. FISER D: Intraosseous infusion. N Engl J Med 322:1579, 1990

2. SPIVEY W: Intraosseous infusions. J Pediatr 111:639, 1987

3. HODGE D: Intraosseous infusions: review. Pediatr Emerg Care 1:215, 1985

4. MANLEY L, HALEY K, DICK M: Intraosseous infusion: Rapid vascular access for critically ill or injured infants and children. J Emer Nurs 14:63, 1988

5. MINER WF, CORNELI HM, BOLTE RG, ET AL: Prehospital use of intraosseous infusion by paramedics. Pediatr Emerg Care 5:5, 1989

6. TURKEL H: Deaths following sternal puncture. JAMA 156:992, 1954

7. ROGERS SN, BENUMOF JL: Intraosseous infusions. In Roberts JR Hedges JR (eds.): Clinical Procedures in Emergency Medicine. Philadelphia, WB Saunders, 1985, p 339

8. Infusions. In Hughes W, Buescher E (eds): Pediatric Procedures, 2nd Ed. Philadelphia, WB Saunders, 1980, p 117

9. ISERSON K, CRISS E: Intraosseous infusions: A usable technique. Am J Emerg Med 4:540, 1986

10. BROENNLE AM, GEWITZ MH, HANDLER SD, ET AL: Illustrated techniques of pediatric emergency procedures. In Fleisher G, Ludwig S (eds): Textbook of Pediatric Emergency Medicine, 2nd Ed. Baltimore, Williams and Wilkins, 1988, p 1246

11. PARRISH G, TURKEWITZ D, SKIENDZIELEWSKI J: Intraosseous infusions in the emergency department. Am J Emerg Med 4:59, 1986

12. MOFENSON HC, TASCONE A, CARACCIO TR: Guidelines for intraosseous infusions. J Emerg Med 6:143, 1988

13. BALDWIN ST, JOHNSON C: Intraosseous infusion: A technique whose time has returned. Ala Med 56:29, 1987

14. BRINKMAN K, REGA P, GUINNESS M: A comparative study of intraosseous, intravenous and intra arterial pH changes during hypoventilation in dogs (abstr). Ann Emerg Med 16:510, 1987

15. ORLOWSKI JP, POREMBKA DT, GALLAGHER JM, VAN-LENTE F: The bone marrow as a source of laboratory studies. Ann Emerg Med 18:1348, 1989

16. ROSETTI V, THOMPSON B, MILLER J, ET AL: Intraosseous infusion: An alternative route of pediatric intravascular access. Ann Emerg Med 14:885, 1985

17. QUILLIGAN JJ JR, TURKEL H: Bone marrow infusion and its complications. Am J Dis Child 71:457, 1946

18. WALLDEN TM, LENNART W: On injuries of bone and bone marrow after intraosseous injections: An experimental investigation. Acta Chir Scand 96:152, 1947

19. HEINILD S, SONDERGAARD J, TUDVAD F: Bone marrow infusions in childhood: Experiences from a thousand infusions. J Pediatr 30:400, 1947

20. TOCANTINS LM, O'NEILL JF: Complications of intraosseous therapy. Ann Surg 122:266, 1945

21. LA FLECHE F, SLEPIN M, VARGAS J, MILZMAN D: Iatrogenic bilateral tibial fractures after intraosseous infusion attempts in a 3-month-old infant. Ann Emerg Med 18:1099, 1989

22. VALDES MM: Intraosseous administration in emergencies. Lancet 1:1235, 1977

23. PAPPER EM: The bone marrow route for injecting fluids and drugs into the general circulation. Anesthesiology 3:307, 1942

24. TOCANTINS LM: Rapid absorption of substances injected into the bone marrow. Proc Soc Exp Biol Med 45:292, 1940

25. WILE UJ, SCHAMBERG IL: Pulmonary fat embolism following infusions via bone marrow. J Invest Dermatol 5:173, 1942

26. Pediatric Forum. Emergency bone marrow infusions. Am J Dis Child 139:438, 1985

27. TOCANTINS LM, O'NEILL JF, JONES HW: Infusions of blood and other fluids via the bone marrow: Application in pediatrics. JAMA 117:1229, 1941

28. BAILEY H: Bone marrow as a site for the reception of infusions, transfusion, and anesthetic agents. Br Med J (Clin Res) 2:181, 1944

29. NEISII SR, MACON MG, MOORE JW, GRAEBER GM: Intraosseous infusion of hypertonic glucose and dopamine. Am J Dis Child 142:878, 1988

30. SPIVEY WH: Comparison of intraosseous, central and peripheral routes of sodium bicarbonate administration during CPR in pigs. Ann Emerg Med 14:1135, 1985

31. MACHT DI: Absorption of drugs through the bone marrow. Proc Soc Exp Biol Med 47:299, 1941

32. MACHT DI: Studies on intraosseous injection of epinepherine. Am J Physiol 138:269, 1943

33. SHOOR PM, BERRYNILL RE, BENUMOF JL: Intraosseous infusion: Pressure-flow relationship and pharmacokinetics. J Trauma 19:772, 1979

34. BERG R: Emergency infusion of catecholamines into bone marrow. Am J Dis Child 138:810, 1984

35. BILELLO JF, O'HAIR KC, KIRBY WC, MOORE JW: Intraosseous infusion of dobutamine and isoproterenol. Am J Dis Child 145:165, 1991

36. WALSH-KELLY C, BERENS R, GLAESER P, LOSEK J: Intraosseous infusion of phenytoin. Am J Emerg Med 4:523, 1986

37. TOCANTINS LM, O'NEILL JF: Infusions of blood and other fluids into the circulation via the bone marrow. Proc Soc Exp Biol Med 45:782, 1940

47 Tapping Ventricular Reservoirs

Mary Ann Fletcher
Dennis L. Johnson

A reservoir (Fig. 47-1) may be inserted prior to permanent ventricular catheter drainage in obstructive hydrocephalus when

1. Intermittent lumbar punctures fail to drain ventricles effectively
2. Infant's condition precludes insertion of ventriculoperitoneal shunt
   a. Sepsis or bacteremia
   b. Abdominal pathology
      (1) Necrotizing enterocolitis
      (2) Peritonitis
      (3) Recent or anticipated bowel surgery
   c. Severe life-threatening systemic disease

A. INDICATIONS

1. Clinical symptoms of increased intracranial pressure
   a. Apnea, bradycardia
   b. Poor feeding
   c. Somnolence
   d. Hypotonia
2. Ultrasonographic evidence of progressive ventriculomegaly

B. CONTRAINDICATIONS

1. Low circulating blood volume
2. Cellulitis or abrasion over reservoir site
3. Sunken fontanelle

C. EQUIPMENT

1. Povidone iodine surgical scrub and prep solution
2. Scalp-vein needle: 25 gauge
3. Standard infant lumbar puncture set or
4. Sterile gauze sponges 4×4 and
5. Clamp to hold sponges
6. 1 to 3 10-ml syringes
7. Aperture drape

D. PRECAUTIONS

1. Maintain strict asepsis.
2. Monitor and correct serum electrolytes every other day if more than 10 ml removed daily.
3. Be prepared to provide rapid fluid replacement should infant not tolerate large volumes removed. Replace fluid removed with intravenous normal saline.
4. If skin breakdown occurs, select insertion site away from broken area.
5. Do not use local anesthetic.
6. Do not place IVs on same side of scalp.

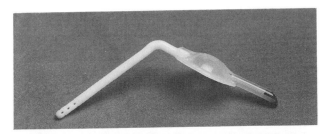

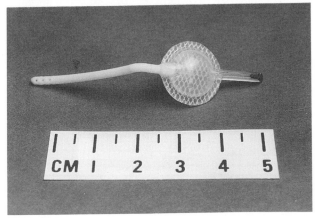

FIG. 47-1
McComb reservoir. Ventricular access device—side and front views.

E. TECHNIQUE

1. Restrain recumbent infant with head in neutral position in anticipation of a 20- to 25-minute procedure.
2. Clip any long hair that interferes with the surgical area but do not shave operative area.
3. Wearing sterile gloves, scrub with surgical scrub over the reservoir and a surrounding circle of skin with a radius of 4 cm.
   a. Continue for full 10 minutes.
   b. Use light but firm contact.
4. Dry area by blotting with gauze pads.
5. Paint with povidone iodine solution and allow to dry.
6. Position aperture drape to maintain patient visibility.
7. Insert scalp-vein needle through skin just into reservoir bladder.
   a. Select an insertion site different from the one most recently used.
   b. Angle needle at 30 to 45 degrees from the skin.
   c. Avoid puncturing the bottom of reservoir.
8. Aspirate fluid into syringe at a rate of 1 to 3 ml/min over 10 minutes.
9. Limit total volume of cerebrospinal fluid (CSF) aspirated at each tapping to no more than 30 ml.

   The initial puncture should not exceed 10 ml in volume and can be increased on sequential taps at a rate of not more than 5 ml/day.

10. Sample CSF for culture, cell count, glucose, and protein every 3 days.

    If fluid is dark because it still contains old blood, only culture results will be meaningful. Culture dark fluid every 3 days.

11. Remove needle and hold firm pressure for 2 minutes or until CSF leakage from skin stops.
12. Increase daily fluid intake to compensate for volume removed.
13. Repeat taps at intervals dictated by clinical response.

   a. Repeat usually once a day but as often as twice daily.
   b. Aim to remove a daily volume sufficient
      (1) To prevent progressive ventriculomegaly and
      (2) To maintain growth of the head circumference at less than 1 cm per week.

Clinically, a "sufficient volume" is defined as the amount aspirated that causes the fontanelle to become very concave and the cranial bones to overlap at the sutures. If a sufficient volume is taken, the fontanelle should be full 24 hours later and the cranial bones touching but not split apart. When the cranial bones are still overlapping the next day and the fontanelle remains slack, the interval for tapping should be lengthened to every other day. If there is no buildup of fluid between intervals, the taps may eventually be stopped without need for a shunt.

   c. Follow response with cranial ultrasonography.
   d. Continue until infant weighs 2 kg and is a suitable candidate for surgery.

Reservoirs are seldom removed even if they are no longer needed.

F. COMPLICATIONS

1. Local skin breakdown[1]
2. Intravascular fluid depletion
3. Hypoproteinemia
4. Hyponatremia[1]
5. Wound or reservoir infection
6. CSF leak from puncture site
7. Obstruction of ventricular catheter
8. Ventriculitis

References

1. LEONHARDT A, STEINER HH, LINDERKAMP O: Management of posthaemorrhagic hydrocephalus with a subcutaneous ventricular catheter reservoir in premature infants. Arch Dis Child 64(1 Spec No):24, 1989

48 Cryotherapy for Retinopathy of Prematurity

Aileen T. Kelly
Kathleen M. Cronin

A. CLASSIFICATION OF RETINOPATHY OF PREMATURITY[1] (FIG. 48-1)

1. Location
   Zone I—Circle whose center is the optic disc, and whose radius is twice the distance from the optic disc to the center of the macula
   Zone II—The area peripheral to Zone I, and defined by a circle centered on the optic disc. The radius of this circle extends to the nasal ora serrata.
   Zone III—The crescent of retina anterior to Zone II
2. Extent of Disease
   The retina is divided into segments, each subtending a 30-degree angle and called a "clock hour." A description of the extent of retinopathy specifies the number of clock hours involved.
3. Staging the Disease (Color Figs. 48-1 to 48-3 at the front of this book)
   Stage 1—Demarcation line: A flat white line that lies in the plane of the retina, separating avascular retina anteriorly from vascular retina posteriorly.
   Stage 2—Ridge: Elevated mass of pink fibrovascular tissue extending up out of the plane of the retina.
   Stage 3—Ridge with extraretinal fibrovascular proliferation: Fibrovascular tissue forms and leaves the plane of the retina. It may cause the posterior border of the ridge to appear ragged, or be seen extending into the vitreous perpendicular to the plane of the retina (Color Fig. 48-1).
   Stage 4—Retinal detachment: This may be caused by either an effusion or by traction.
   "Plus" disease —Dilatation and tortuosity of vessels in the posterior pole (Color Fig. 48-2)
   "Threshold ROP"—5 contiguous or 8 cumulative clock hours of Stage 3 ROP in Zones I or II along with plus disease (Color Fig. 48-3)
   Other features that may be seen in advanced ROP include iris vascular engorgement and pupillary rigidity.

B. SCREENING FOR RETINOPATHY OF PREMATURITY

1. Direct ophthalmoscopy—Dilated and tortuous vessels in Zone 1 (plus disease) may be seen with a direct ophthalmoscope. In rapidly progressive disease, neonatologists may detect plus disease prior to routine eye exam by ophthalmologist. This allows early referral for advanced cases.
2. Indirect ophthalmoscopy—Referral to an ophthalmologist for evaluation at 5 to 6 weeks for premature infants of birth weight $\leq$ 1500 gm and 8 to 10 weeks for prematures of birth weight $\geq$ 1500 gm.[5]

C. INDICATIONS FOR CRYOTHERAPY

Threshold retinopathy of prematurity (ROP)[2-4]

D. CONTRAINDICATIONS

1. Cicatricial ROP advanced beyond threshold (e.g., retinal detachment or large vitreous hemorrhage obscuring retina)[4,6]
2. Instability of medical condition sufficient to make the stress of cryotherapy inadvisable
3. Lethal medical illness

E. PERSONNEL AND EQUIPMENT[2,7]

Personnel
1. Ophthalmologist
   a. Administers topical and subconjunctival anesthetic
   b. Performs the cryotherapy
   c. Watches for and treats (as necessary) any ocular

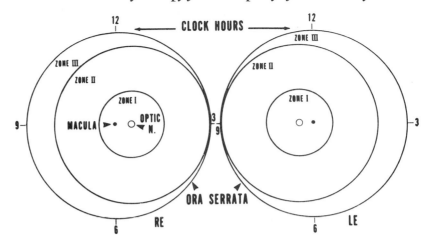

FIG. 48-1
Scheme of retina of right eye (RE) and left eye (LE) showing zone borders and clock hours employed to describe location and extent of retinopathy of prematurity. (The Committee for Classification of Retinopathy of Prematurity: An international classifiction of retinopathy of prematurity. Arch Ophthalmol 102:1130, 1984. Reprinted with permission).

complications that may arise during and after the procedure

2. Neonatology fellow, attending physician, or pediatric anesthesiologist
   a. Administers systemic anesthetic agents
   b. Observes patient for and treats any systemic complications that develop during or after cryotherapy
   c. Provides information to the ophthalmologist regarding the patient's overall condition throughout the procedure
3. Assistant to the ophthalmologist
   a. Helps with the cryotherapy instruments and unit
   b. Records the stage of ROP at the time of the exam, and the number of freezes performed by the ophthalmologist
4. Neonatal nurse
   a. Immobilizes the patient
   b. Monitors the patient's airway

Equipment
1. Cardiorespiratory, blood pressure, and O_2 saturation or transcutaneous O_2 monitors
2. Appropriate respiratory support (ventilator, laryngoscope and ET tubes, face mask, Ambu bag, suction and oxygen source)
3. Supply of emergency medications (atropine, epinephrine, bicarbonate, calcium, phenobarbital)

   Precalculation of weight-appropriate doses is helpful.

4. 1% xylocaine without epinephrine
5. Topical ocular anesthetic (e.g., Ophthaine)

6. Cycloplegic and mydriatic eye drops: Cyclomydril® (cyclopentolate hydrochloride 0.2% and phenylephrine hydrochloride 1%) or 0.5% cyclopentolate and 1 to 2.5% phenylephrine
7. 2-ml syringe with 27-gauge needle
8. Sterile gloves
9. Sterile drapes and towels
10. Straight needle holder
11. 6-0 plain suture
12. Betadine swabs
13. Cotton-tipped applicators
14. Balanced salt solution
15. Neonatal eyelid speculum (Fig. 48-2)
16. Flynn scleral depressor (Fig. 48-2)

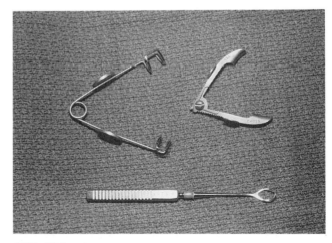

FIG. 48-2
Lid speculae, Flynn depressor.

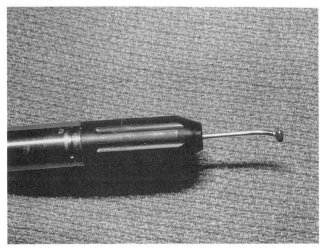

FIG. 48-3
Baby hammerhead cryoprobe handpiece.

17. Pediatric retinal cryoprobe (Fig. 48-3) and cryotherapy unit
18. Smooth and toothed forceps
19. Indirect ophthalmoscope with 28 or 30, and 20 diopter lenses

F. PRECAUTIONS (TABLE 48-1)

1. Check nitrous oxide tank on cryotherapy unit to be sure it is full.
2. Treat the more advanced eye first if both eyes have threshold ROP. Consider treating the second eye 2 to 3 days later.

> It is less stressful for the patient to have one eye treated at a time. In addition, upon examining the treated eye following cryotherapy, serious complications may be found that may alter the plan to treat the second eye.

3. Discontinue feedings at least 4 hours before the procedure, or empty the stomach with an orogastric tube.
4. Establish IV access for infusions of medications and maintenance of IV fluids.
5. Observe transcutaneous O_2 or O_2 saturation monitor carefully, and adjust administered oxygen appropriately to avoid hypoxemia.
6. If necessary, correct electrolyte imbalances.
7. Avoid using more than 1% phenylephrine if there is a history of hypertension.

8. Wipe off any excess liquid spilling onto the skin after instillation of eyedrops, to avoid transcutaneous absorption (skin vessel blanching occurs with phenylephrine).[8]

G. TECHNIQUE[7,8]

1. General preparation
   a. Instill eyedrops (per orders from ophthalmologist) into both eyes at 2 and 1 hours prior to procedure.
      (1) Two hours prior to surgery—0.25% scopolamine
      (2) One hour prior to surgery—1 to 2.5% phenylephrine
      (3) At the time of surgery (if pupils are not fully dilated)—Cyclomydril® or 0.5% cyclopentolate and 1 to 2.5% phenylephrine
   b. Transport patient to surgical suite or designated procedure room in the nursery.

   > A special room is recommended, to provide a sterile environment, privacy, and an area suitable for the personnel and equipment required.

   c. Ensure monitors are attached and functioning.
2. Immobilize infant.
3. Administer anesthesia (local or general).

   > If local anesthesia is to be used, a combination of topical (Ophthaine), infiltrative (subconjunctival xylocaine), and systemic analgesic/sedative (IV morphine) medications are administered.

4. Retract lids.
5. Perform indirect ophthalmoscopy to confirm stage of ROP.
6. Applications are made with the probe to the avascular retina through conjunctiva, causing whitening of retina. Freezing is then stopped immediately, allowing the area to thaw. Each cryoapplication takes 2 to 3 seconds.

   > The area frozen extends beyond the diameter of the cryoprobe tip. An attempt is made to perform the cryotherapy in a contiguous fashion. While avoiding overlap between frozen areas, there are often skipped areas. These may need to be retreated in 1 week if the ROP is not regressing.

7. Make a row of applications at the ora serrata, followed by more posterior applications, covering the

TABLE 48-1

Complications During Cryotherapy[2,4,8,9]

Problem	Treatment
I: Systemic	
Bradycardia	Interrupt cryotherapy to relieve pressure on orbit.
	Reassess airway, ventilation, and oxygen delivery.
	Atropine 0.1 mg IV
Hypoxia/cyanosis	Evaluate airway.
	Administer supplemental oxygen.
Apnea	Evaluate airway.
	Gentle stimulation.
	Administer supplemental oxygen.
	Hand ventilate with Ambu bag and face mask.
Tachycardia	Assess pain control (give additional analgesia).
	Monitor blood pressure and perfusion closely.
Hypertension	Assess pain control.
	If moderate, observe
	If severe, consider hydralazine 0.1 mg/kg IV
Arrhythmia	Manage as appropriate for particular arrhythmia.
Seizure (etiology is uncertain, but may be anticholinergic effect in susceptible patients)	Supportive care
	Phenobarbital
II: Ocular	
Conjunctival/subconjunctival hematoma	Close follow up
Conjunctival laceration	Apply antibiotic ointment to area 3 times a day for 3 days
Retinal/preretinal/vitreous hemorrhage	Close follow up
	If obscuring treatment zone, interrupt cryotherapy until it clears enough to continue (2–7 days)
Retinal necrosis from overfreezing	Close follow up
Closure of central retinal artery	Usually transient
	Increase interval between freezes.
Freezing to area outside target zone	Close follow up
Possible complications: eye muscle injury, damage to optic nerve or wall of orbit, perforation of globe	Close follow up and management as indicated (Surgical repair is required for a perforated globe.)

avascular retina, extending back as far as the anterior edge of the fibrovascular ridge.

By beginning cryoapplications anteriorly and then moving posteriorly, the intraocular pressure decreases, therefore often allowing treatment of the entire avascular zone without incising the conjunctiva.[9]

8. Have an assistant count and record the number of applications.
9. Withdraw the cryoprobe from the fornices at intervals to avoid elevated intraocular pressure.

I. POSTOPERATIVE CARE[7]

1. Instill eyedrops in treated eye: 0.25% scopolamine hydrobromide (continue through 5th postoperative day).
2. Apply antibiotic ointment to treated eye (Polysporin, Bacitracin).

   Continue this twice daily for 3 days if the conjunctiva was opened.

3. Examine eye 24 hours after surgery for external signs of complications (Table 48-2).

TABLE 48-2
Postoperative Complications

Problem	Treatment
I: Systemic	
Apnea	Cardiorespiratory monitors for 48–72 hours postoperative
Increased oxygen requirement	Oxygen saturation or transcutaneous oxygen monitor
II: Ocular	
Swelling of eyelid	Observe
	If patient cannot open eye after 24 hours, patch the untreated eye to prevent amblyopia.
Infection	Antibiotic ointment to eye (postoperative)
	Continue antibiotic ointment three times a day for 3 days if conjunctiva was opened.
Vitreous hemorrhage	Close follow up
Anterior chamber hemorrhage	Close follow up
	Monitoring of intraocular pressure and treatment as indicated

4. Apply an occlusive patch to untreated eye to prevent amblyopia if treated eye is swollen shut beyond 24 hours.
5. Monitor patient with a cardiorespiratory monitor for 24 to 72 hours.
6. Perform a dilated retinal exam 1 week after procedure.
7. Consider retreating skipped areas if plus disease persists at 1 week after treatment.[2]
8. Be aware that 22 to 31% of eyes with Stage III ROP and plus disease develop retinal folds or detach-

ments, or retrolental tissue obscuring the posterior pole, despite cryotherapy.[2,3,6]

If a retinal detachment occurs, appropriate surgical intervention by a retina–vitreous specialist is recommended.

References

1. The Committee for Classification of Retinopathy of Prematurity: An international classification of retinopathy of prematurity. Arch Ophthalmol 102:1130, 1984
2. Cryotherapy for Retinopathy of Prematurity Cooperative Group: Multicenter trial of cryotherapy for retinopathy of prematurity: Three-month outcome. Arch Ophthalmol 108:195, 1990
3. TOPILOW HW, ACKERMAN AL: Cryotherapy for Stage 3+ retinopathy of prematurity: Visual and anatomic results. Ophthalmic Surg 20:864, 1989
4. BEN SIRA I, NISSENKORN I, KREMER I: Retinopathy of prematurity. Surv Ophthalmol 33:1, 1988
5. REISNER SH, AMIR J, ET AL: Retinopathy of prematurity: Incidence and treatment. Arch Dis Child 60:698, 1985
6. TOPILOW HW, ACKERMAN AL, WANG FM, STROME RR: Successful treatment of advanced retinopathy of prematurity. Ophthal Surg 19:781, 1988
7. Multicenter Trial of Cryotherapy for Retinopathy of Prematurity Cooperative Group. Manual of Procedures. Springfield, VA, National Technical Information Service, US Department of Commerce, 1985. PB 88-163530
8. Physician's Desk Reference (PDR) for Ophthalmology, 19th Ed. Oradell, NJ, Medical Economics Company Inc., 1990, p 2329
9. TOPILOW HW, ACKERMAN AL, WANG FM: The treatment of advanced retinopathy of prematurity by cryotherapy and scleral buckling surgery. Ophthalmology 92:379, 1985

49 Peritoneal Dialysis and Continuous Arteriovenous Hemofiltration[1-4]

Kathleen A. Marinelli
Majid Rasoulpour

Acute Peritoneal Dialysis[1-4]

For most newborns, peritoneal dialysis (PD) is preferred over hemodialysis (HD), continuous arteriovenous hemofiltration (CAVH), and continuous arteriovenous hemodiafiltration (CAVHD) because

1. The access in PD is technically easier
2. The clearance is superior to CAVH
3. Rapid shifts of fluid and fall of plasma osmolality are less likely than with HD.

Because the peritoneal surface area/kg body weight is relatively larger in newborns and children than in adults, it usually allows adequate clearance and removal of excess fluid.[5]

A. INDICATIONS

1. Renal failure when conservative management has failed to adequately control the following conditions[6]
   a. Hypervolemia
   b. Hyperkalemia
   c. Hyponatremia
   d. Acidosis
   e. Hyperphosphatemia
   f. Azotemia
2. Inherited disorders of organic and amino acid metabolism when hemodialysis is unavailable or contraindicated[7,8]

B. EQUIPMENT (FIGS. 49-1 TO 49-3)

1. Masks, sterile drapes, gowns, and gloves
2. Cotton-tipped skin cleanser, povidone iodine
3. 1% xylocaine without epinephrine
4. 3-ml syringe with 25-gauge needle
5. Intravenous cutdown tray with No. 11 surgical blade
6. Waterproof tape
7. 22-gauge angiocath
8. A temporary catheter such as an infant size Trocath* or a 14-gauge angiocath. Other temporary catheters are also available.
9. Dialysis solution (1.5, 2.5, or 4.25%). Other concentrations can be made by manual mixing of standard solutions.
10. Heparin
11. Blood/fluid warmer†
12. 2 Inpersol Administration Sets‡
13. Blood/fluid warming set§
14. Y set‖
15. Plastic tubing connector.¶ This should be sterilized.
16. Urimeter (urine collection device)

*Trocath Peritoneal Dialysis Catheter. Kendall McGaw Laboratories. Sabana Grande, Puerto Rico 00747
†American Pharmaseal Company. Valencia, CA 91355-8900
‡Inpersol System 1 Extended Life Administration Set B. Abbott Laboratories. North Chicago, IL 60064
§DWC-100 Blood/Fluid Warming Set. American Pharmaseal Company. Valencia, CA 91355-8900
‖Y Check Set—Luer Lock with Injection Site. Medlon, Inc., 3325 N Glenoaks, Burbank, CA 91504
¶Plastic Tubing Connector. Pharmaseal. Ooa Alta, Puerto Rico 00758

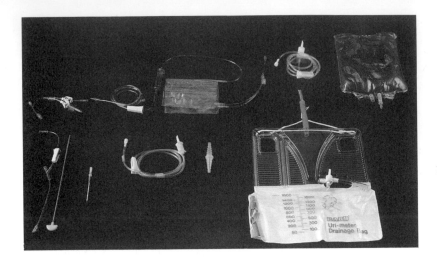

FIG. 49-1
Top row, right to left: Dialysis solution, Inpersol Administration Set, blood/fluid warming set, Y set. Bottom row, left to right: Trocath connector, Trocath, 14-gauge angiocath, Inpersol Administration Set, plastic tubing connector, urimeter.

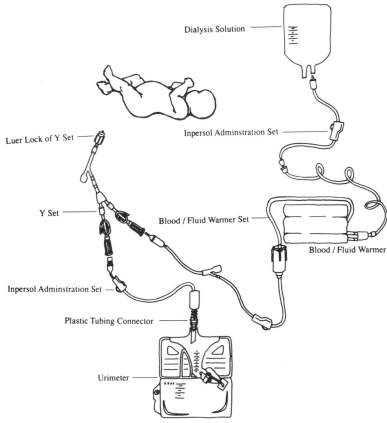

FIG. 49-3
Peritoneal dialysis circuit.

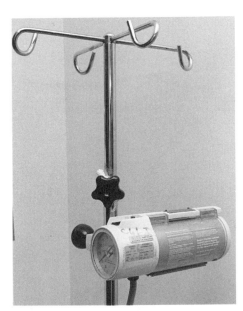

FIG. 49-2
Blood/fluid warmer assembled on an intravenous administration pole.

C. PRE-PROCEDURE CARE

1. Obtain informed consent.
2. Check body weight and abdominal girth.
3. Check for infection at the insertion site.
4. Decompress the stomach.
5. Catheterize the bladder.
6. Place pre-weighed diaper under the patient.

Before assembly of system, wash hands and wear a mask. All connections should be made using sterile technique.# Universal precautions should be observed (Chap. 4). Keep all tubing clamped. See Figure 49-3 for connections.

7. Add 500 units of heparin to each 1 liter of the dialysis solution. Start with 1.5% dialysate.
8. Spike the Inpersol Administration Set into the dialysate.
9. Install the blood/fluid warming set into the blood/fluid warmer.
10. Remove protector from the female luer of blood/fluid warming set and attach to the luer lock of Inpersol Administration Set.
11. Remove protector from the male luer of blood/fluid warming set and attach to one of the 2 female luer locks of the Y set as illustrated.
12. Attach the other female luer of the Y set to the luer lock of the 2nd Inpersol Administration Set.
13. Cut off the long connecting tubing of the urimeter using sterile technique.
14. Spike the 2nd Inpersol Administration Set into a sterile plastic tubing connector. Spike the other end of the plastic tubing connector into the stump of connecting tubing of the urimeter. Secure the connections with waterproof tape. Secure the urimeter to the bedside, as low as possible.
15. Remove protector from the Y set luer lock.
16. Unclamp the inflow line and prime with the dialysis solution. Clamp inflow line and replace protector on the Y set luer lock.

D. PROCEDURE

An alternative technique to percutaneous catheter placement is surgical insertion of a flexible Tenckhoff

#Inpersol-CAPD System 1 Prep Kit. Abbott Laboratories, North Chicago, IL 60064

catheter. This procedure can be performed in the NICU and under local anesthesia. The catheter is tunneled from the peritoneum to an exit site on the skin. For short-term dialysis a Trocath or an angiocath is satisfactory.

1. Monitor vital signs.
2. Restrain infant in supine position.
3. Scrub.
4. Prepare the skin of the abdomen (Chap. 4).
5. Drape to expose the insertion site.

The best insertion site depends on the preference of the physician, presence of postoperative wounds, abdominal wall infection, and organomegaly. A location one-third the distance from the umbilicus to the symphysis pubis in the midline or a site lateral to the rectus sheath in either of the lower quadrants are preferred.

6. Infuse approximately 0.5 ml of xylocaine around the insertion point.
7. Select either a 14-gauge angiocath or a Trocath as the temporary dialysis catheter. We suggest Trocath or temporary catheters other than angiocath because dialysis by an angiocath may not be efficient. An alternative method is to use 2 angiocaths, one each for inflow and outflow (omit Y set).
8. If you elected to use a 14-gauge angiocath
    a. Insert the angiocath at the insertion point.
    b. Remove the stylet.
    c. Connect the Y set to the angiocath.
    d. Proceed to #10.
9. If you elected to use a Trocath
    a. Insert a 22-gauge angiocath at the insertion point. This is used to prime the abdominal cavity with dialysis solution.
    b. Remove the stylet.
    c. Connect the Y set to the angiocath.
    d. Unclamp the inflow line.
    e. Allow 30 ml/kg of dialysis solution to run into peritoneal cavity.
    f. Clamp the inflow line.
    g. Disconnect the Y set from the angiocath.
    h. Remove the angiocath.
    i. Make a small stab wound at the insertion site, but not through the peritoneum
    j. Insert Trocath. Use gentle, steady pressure with a twisting motion until a "give" is felt as the peritoneum is perforated.

k. Remove trocar.

l. Advance catheter toward pelvic gutter until a slight resistance is felt.

m. Cut catheter to leave a short stump.

n. Connect the special rubber connector (included in Trocath package) to the stump.

o. Unclamp the Trocath set. Allow the peritoneal fluid to prime the Trocath set. Clamp the set.

p. Connect the male luer of the Trocath set to the luer lock of the Y set.

q. Unclamp the outflow line and drain the peritoneal fluid until it slows down. Clamp the outflow line.

10. Test patency of the entire system.

a. Unclamp the inflow line.

b. Allow approximately 30 ml of dialysis solution to enter peritoneal cavity by gravity.

c. Clamp inflow line.

d. Unclamp outflow line.

e. Repeat the above four steps several times.

This procedure usually results in a positive fluid balance (the volume drained less than the volume infused). This retention is acceptable.

11. If inflow and outflow occur readily, secure the catheter with purse-string suture and tape.

E. MANAGEMENT

1. Establish a cycle time. This is usually about 60 minutes and consists of a fill by gravity, dwell time of 45 minutes, and drain by gravity.

2. Establish a dialysis volume per pass. Starting volume is usually 20 to 30 ml/kg.

3. Clamp the outflow line.

4. Unclamp the inflow line.

5. Allow the dialysate to flow in as quickly as possible, while carefully observing the vital signs.

6. Clamp the inflow line.

7. Allow the fluid to dwell.

8. Unclamp the outflow when dwell time completed.

9. Allow 5 to 10 minutes for drain.

10. Clamp the outflow line.

11. Repeat the cycle.

12. Increase the volume by 5 ml/kg/cycle slowly. Maximum volume 40 ml/kg if tolerated, attained over 12 to 24 hours.

13. Continue 500 units of heparin/liter, until dialysate effluent is clear.

14. Add 3 mEq/L of K if serum K is at or below 4 mEq/L.

F. MONITORING

1. Maintain hourly PD flow sheet.

a. Volume in

b. Volume out

c. Net/hr $(+/-)$

d. Net over the course of dialysis $(+/-)$

e. Intakes (enteral, parenteral)

f. Outputs (urine, gastric, insensible water loss, etc.)

2. Establish a desired fluid balance. Proceed gently if negative balance is required. Reassess the state of hydration frequently.

3. Measure serum glucose and potassium every 4 hours for the 1st 24 hours or until stable, then twice a day. Obtain other serum electrolytes twice daily. Check BUN, serum creatinine, serum calcium, serum phosphorus, and serum magnesium once a day.

4. Obtain cell count, gram stain, and culture of peritoneal effluent every 12 hours.

5. Recognize that some drug dosages may need adjustment.[9-11] (See Appendix D.)

G. COMPLICATIONS

See Table 49-1.

Continuous Arteriovenous Hemofiltration in Newborns

Continuous arteriovenous hemofiltration (CAVH) is an extracorporeal technique for removing plasma water and its disolved solutes of <50,000 Daltons, over an extended period of time. Using an arterial access line of the largest possible diameter and a venous access line, blood enters the extracorporeal circuit (arterial tubing, hemofilter, and venous tubing) by way of the arterial line and returns to the patient by way of the venous line (Figs. 49-4 and 49-5). The arteriovenous pressure gradient usually generates an adequate pressure, allowing the blood to flow through the circuit. Addition of a blood pump may be necessary if the flow is inadequate.

TABLE 49-1

Complications of Peritoneal Dialysis

Problem	What to Do
Perforation of bladder, bowel, or major vessels	• Surgical consultation
Puncture site bleeding	• Apply pressure gently. Purse-string suture
Blood-stained dialysis maintained after several cycles	• Check hematocrit frequently. Continue heparin. R/O major vessel bleeding
Leakage from exit site	• Reduce dwell volume until leakage stops.
Extravasation of dialysate into the anterior abdominal wall	• Replace with a new catheter.
More than 10% of solution retained in each of several consecutive cycles (outflow obstruction)	• Reposition the infant gently. Reposition the catheter by rotation and slight retraction. *Do not advance.* Remove if unchanged. Replace with a new catheter.
Two-way obstruction	• Irrigate catheter with small amount of dialysate or saline aseptically. Reposition. Remove if unchanged.
Dislodgement of catheter	• Replace with a new catheter.
Hydrothorax	• Reposition the infant, head and chest above the level of the abdomen. Decrease dwell volume.
Hyperglycemia	• Avoid high concentrations of dialysate unless outflow is inadequate. Low dose of insulin if needed
Lactic acidosis	• Use bicarbonate dialysate.*
Hyponatremia	• Reduce fluid intake. Aim to increase the outflow if secondary to fluid overload.
Hypernatremia	• Increase fluid intake if 2° to excessive ultrafiltrate.
Exit site infection	• Systemic antibiotics Excision of exit site PRN
Peritonitis	• Several rapid flushing exchanges Cephalothin 250 mg/L of dialysate plus gentamycin 8 mg/L For fungal peritonitis, systemic therapy is needed and the catheter should be removed.
Removal of therapeutic drugs	• See Appendix D

*1.5% bicarbonate dialysis solution: 140 mEq/L of Na, 110 mEq/L of Cl, 30 mEq/L of HCO_3, 15 gm glucose, add sterile water to 1000 ml

As blood flows through the extracorporeal device, plasma water and dissolved solutes are filtered out (ultrafiltered) through the pores of the hemofilter. We use a hollow fiber hemofilter, which is composed of many fine capillaries of highly water-permeable membranes located within a cylindric case. The filtered-off fluid (ultrafiltrate) is drained out by way of an exit incorporated on the surface of the hemofilter. The ultrafiltrate is collected inside a calibrated collecting bag. The fluid removed has all the characteristics of an ultrafiltrate of plasma water. The sodium, potassium, phosphorus, urea, and creatinine concentrations of the fluid are very similar to those of plasma; chloride and bicarbonate concentrations are slightly higher and calcium concentration is about 60% of plasma. It is free of protein, but contains aminoacids and water-soluble vitamins.

The volume of ultrafiltrate (ultrafiltration rate) depends upon the pressure gradient across the capillary

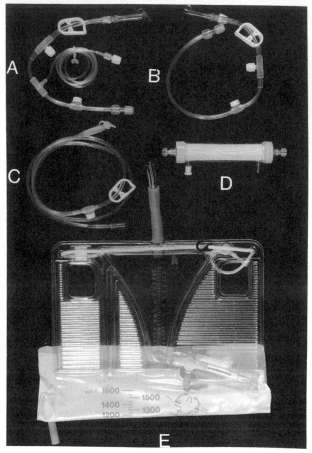

FIG. 49-4
Hemofilter kit and urimeter: (*A*) arterial tubing, (*B*) venous tubing, (*C*) ultrafiltrate tubing, (*D*) hemofilter, (*E*) urimeter.

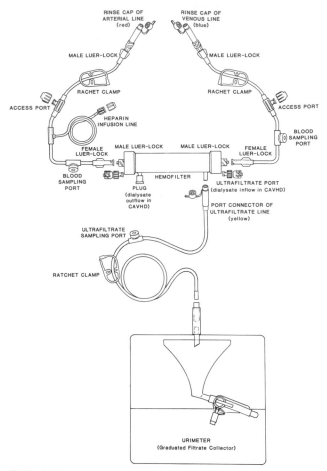

FIG. 49-5
A continuous arteriovenous hemofiltration circuit.

membranes of the hemofilter. Systemic arterial blood pressure exerts a positive effect on the ultrafiltration rate, whereas plasma oncotic pressure exerts a negative effect. By virtue of creating suction on the hemofilter, the height of the tubing which links the exit and collecting bag exerts a positive effect on the ultrafiltration rate (suction mmHg = height cm × 0.74). Continuous anticoagulation is usually necessary.

A. INDICATIONS[12,14-21]

1. Hypervolemia resistant to diuretics
2. Parenteral nutrition in patients requiring fluid restriction
3. Alternative therapy to hemodialysis or peritoneal dialysis

B. CONTRAINDICATIONS

Severe hypotension

C. EQUIPMENT (SEE FIGS. 49-4 AND 49-5)

1. Catheters for vascular access (Largest possible diameter is recommended. CAVH catheters are preferred.)[22]

2. Hemofilter kit.*

   Circuit volumes of Minifilter and Minifilter Plus are 12 ml and 21 ml respectively.

3. Collecting bag (a urimeter or equivalent)
4. One liter bag of 0.9% NaCl with 5,000 units of heparin/liter for priming hemofilter kit (priming with 2 liters is optional)
5. One 500-ml bag of 0.9% NaCl with 5,000 units of heparin/500 ml, for continuous anticoagulation
6. An activated clotting time (ACT) machine (optional)
7. One 250-ml bag of 0.9% NaCl with 25 mg of protamine sulfate/250 ml, for regional heparinization (optional)
8. One 500-ml bag of Ringer's solution as replacement fluid. It is advisable to modify the replacement fluid according to the patient's needs. Total parenteral nutrition (TPN) fluid or a modified saline solution with calcium (approximately 2.4 mEq/L), Mg (approx. 1.4 mEq/L), dextrose, and lactate or acetate (approx. 30 mEq/L) as the buffering anion is suggested.
9. Three infusion pumps (one each for heparin, protamine sulfate, and replacement fluid).
10. One sterile basin with >500 ml capacity.
11. Masks, sterile gowns, gloves and drapes, IV tubing, and two rubber-shod Kelly clamps.

D. TECHNIQUE[14-16,19,20,23]

Preprocedural Care

1. Obtain informed consent.
2. Obtain baseline CBC; serum sodium, potassium, chloride, bicarbonate, calcium, phosphorus, magnesium, glucose, and creatinine; BUN; total plasma protein, plasma albumin, PTT, and ACT (if available).
3. Obtain arterial and venous access by accepted methods. (Arterial access is obtained by way of femoral, brachial, or umbilical artery; venous access by way of femoral, jugular, or umbilical vein.)
4. Have replacement fluid available.

---

*Minifilter Plus or Minifilter (Amicon, Amicon Division, WR Grace & Co., 72 Cherry Hill Drive, Beverly MA 01915-1065)

Procedure

Note: Strict aseptic technique and universal precautions must be used (Chap. 4). Wear mask, sterile gown, gloves, and goggles.

1. Prime the hemofilter.
   a. Place a sterile drape on a flat surface to form a sterile field.
   b. Place unpacked hemofilter kit on the sterile field.
   c. Attach IV tubing to the one liter bag of heparinized saline (priming solution).
   d. Connect the arterial (color coded red) and venous (color coded blue) tubings to the arterial and venous ends of the hemofilter. (The arterial tubing should be connected to the port farthest from the ultrafiltrate exit.) Close the ratchet clamps.
   e. Connect the ultrafiltrate tubing (color coded yellow) to the exit that is near to the venous end. Close the ratchet clamp. (Secure the cap of the other exit that is near to the arterial end.)
   f. Place a three-way stopcock on the access ports of the arterial and venous tubing. Remove the red cap of the arterial tubing. Connect the IV tubing of priming solution to the arterial tubing.
   g. Place the Kelly clamp (provided), or a rubber-shod Kelly clamp, on the arterial tubing between the heparin infusion line and the filter.
   h. Open the ratchet clamp on the arterial tubing and prime the heparin infusion line by removing the cap and allowing some of the priming solution to drip into the sterile basin. Clamp the IV tubing of priming solution and replace the cap of the heparin infusion line.
   i. Open the Kelly clamp.
   j. Remove the blue cap of the venous tubing. While holding the end of the venous tubing over the basin, open the ratchet clamp. Position the hemofilter vertically, with the venous end up. Allow approximately 500 ml of priming solution to flow through the arterial tubing, hemofilter, and venous tubing. Close the ratchet clamp of the venous tubing.
   k. Unclamp the ratchet clamp of the ultrafiltrate tubing. While holding hemofilter horizontally with the ultrafiltrate exit facing up, allow the

priming solution to remove all the air (approx. 200 ml of priming solution is adequate). Close the ratchet clamp of ultrafiltrate tubing.

l. Unclamp the venous tubing again and let most of the remaining priming solution flow through the arterial tubing, hemofilter, and venous tubing. Remove air bubbles. *Clamp all the tubes tightly with the ratchet clamps before priming solution bag is empty.*

m. Disconnect the IV tubing from the arterial tubing.

n. Close the red and blue caps.

2. Connect the arterial and venous tubings to the patient's arterial and venous access lines, by accepted methods. Secure the luer lock connections tightly.

3. Connect the ultrafiltrate tubing to the collecting bag.

4. Proceed to systemic anticoagulation unless contraindicated, e.g., by bleeding disorders. Wait for several minutes. Start continuous infusion of heparin.

> Several minutes before the circuit is opened, a loading dose of 20–40 U/kg of heparin is suggested. For continuous infusion, approximately 10 U/kg/hr of heparin is required. PTT is usually kept 1.5–2 times normal. If ACT is used, it is usually kept 40–80% above baseline. For regional heparinization[13] to neutralize heparin's systemic effect, 1 mg of protamine sulfate is administered, via the venous tubing, for each 100 units of heparin. (Caution: Protamine may cause hypotension or anaphylactoid reaction.)

5. Unclamp the ratchet clamps of arterial and venous tubing.

6. Keep the hemofilter level with the heart. Make sure blood lines are not kinked.

7. Keep the collecting bag below the level of the hemofilter (usually by 50–100 cm). This height can be adjusted based on the desired volume of ultrafiltrate.

8. Unclamp the ultrafiltrate line.

9. Start replacement fluid as needed.*

> This is usually administered via the access port of venous tubing (postdilution mode). Administering the replacement fluid via the arterial access port (predilution mode) may increase solute

---

*Replacement fluid ml/hr = output (ultrafiltrate, urine, etc.)/hr + IWL/hr − intakes/hr − net desired fluid loss/hr.

clearance and ultrafiltration rate, and it may also reduce the dose of heparin required. If predilution mode is chosen, some of the replacement fluid will be filtered via the hemofilter.

E. REPLACEMENT OF THE HEMOFILTER

The extracorporeal system is replaced if the ultrafiltration rate is very low or the ultrafiltrate appears pink or red (Table 49-2).

Equipment

1. Two syringes of normal saline for flushing

2. Masks, sterile gowns, gloves, and drapes

3. Two rubber-shod Kelly clamps

4. Hemofilter kit

5. One liter bag of 0.9% NaCl with 5,000 units of heparin/liter for priming the new hemofilter kit (priming with two liters of solution is optional).

6. One sterile basin with >500-ml capacity

7. IV tubing

Procedure

Note: Strict aseptic technique and universal precautions should be used. Wear mask, sterile gown, gloves, and goggles.

1. Prime a new hemofilter kit. (See Procedure D.)

2. Place sterile drape(s) under arterial and venous access catheters.

3. Soak the arterial and venous access catheter connections to the arterial and venous tubings with povidone iodine solution for 5 minutes.

4. Clamp the arterial and venous access catheters with rubber-shod Kelly clamps.

5. Clamp the ratchet clamps of arterial, venous, and ultrafiltrate tubing.

6. Disconnect the arterial tubing from the arterial access catheter.

7. Attach saline flush to the arterial catheter. Draw back the plunger to remove clots, if any. Maintain the patency of the arterial access catheter.

8. Disconnect the venous tubing from the venous access catheter.

9. Attach saline flush to the venous catheter. Draw back the plunger to remove clots, if any. Maintain the patency of the venous access catheter.

TABLE 49-2

Complications of Continuous Arteriovenous Hemofiltration

Problem	What to Do
Decreased ultrafiltration rate without systemic hypotension	• Check if any of the extracorporeal lines are kinked. Find out whether the collecting bag has been displaced to a higher position. Consider replacing the circuit if clotting seems to have occurred (see Section E).
Filters clot quickly while cardiac output and access lines appear free of clot.	• Check whether the anticoagulation is adequate. Find out if ultrafiltration rate has been excessive. Consider administering the replacement fluid by predilution mode when hemofilter kit is replaced (see D, Procedure 9).
Extracorporeal system has been disconnected OR ultrafiltrate is pink/blood tinged because of ruptured membranes of hemofilter.	• Clamp the access lines with the rubber-shod Kelly clamps. Close the ratchet clamps of hemofilter kit. Disconnect the access lines from arterial and venous tubing of the hemofilter kit, if connected, one at a time. Attach saline flushes to the access lines. Draw the plungers to remove clots, if any. Maintain the patency of access lines by accepted methods. Connect a new hemofilter (see Section E).
Blood tubing filled with clear fluid because of clotting of arterial or venous line	• Clamp the access lines with the rubber-shod Kelly clamps. Close the ratchet clamps of hemofilter kit. Disconnect the access lines from all the tubing one at a time. Attach saline flush to the access lines. Draw the plungers to remove clots. If clots are removed but the hemofilter kit needs replacement, maintain the patency of access lines by accepted methods. Connect a new filter (see Section E).
Hypotension	• Close the ratchet clamp of the ultrafiltrate line. Infuse fluids, if required, either via the arterial access port or through a conventional line.

10. Connect the arterial and venous tubing to the arterial and venous access lines. Secure the luer lock connections tightly.
11. Connect the ultrafiltrate tubing to the collecting bag.
12. Proceed to systemic anticoagulation, if necessary (See Procedure D4.)
13. Follow Procedures D5–9.
14. Discard the used CAVH extracorporeal circuit.

F. DISCONTINUATION OF CAVH

Equipment
1. Two syringes of normal saline for flushing
2. Two syringes of heparinized saline for flushing (0.5 U heparin/ml of normal saline)
3. Two luer lock injection caps for arterial and venous access lines
4. IV solutions and infusion pumps, if the access lines are to be used immediately for IV infusion
5. Masks, goggles, sterile gown, gloves, and drapes
6. Two rubber-shod Kelly clamps

Procedure
Note: Strict aseptic technique and universal precautions must be used. Wear mask, sterile gloves, and goggles.

1. Place sterile drape(s) under the patient's arterial and venous access catheters.
2. Soak the arterial and venous access catheter connections to the arterial and venous tubing with povidone iodine solution for 5 minutes.

3. Close the ratchet clamps of arterial and ultrafiltrate tubing.
4. Clamp the arterial access catheter with a rubber shod Kelly clamp.
5. Disconnect the arterial tubing from the access catheter.
6. Attach saline flush to the access catheter. Draw back the plunger to remove clots, if any. Cap the catheter with a luer lock injection cap. Flush with heparinized saline.
7. Clamp the venous access catheter with a rubber-shod Kelly clamp.
8. Clamp the ratchet clamp of the venous tubing.
9. Disconnect the venous tubing from the access catheter.
10. Attach saline flush to the venous access catheter. Draw back the plunger to remove clots, if any. Cap the catheter with a luer lock injection cap. Flush with heparinized saline.
11. Discard CAVH extracorporeal circuit.

G. MONITORING

1. Maintain hourly CAVH flow sheet. Include all sources of the fluid intake and output, including insensible water loss (IWL).
2. Establish a desired fluid balance. Keep the ultrafiltration rate at a moderate level. Besides hypotension, an aggressive ultrafiltration leads to marked hemoconcentration at the venous end of the hemofilter, reducing its performance. Check ultrafiltration rate frequently at the initiation of CAVH, and whenever any adjustment of the ultrafiltration rate is in progress.
3. Measure clotting studies (PTT or ACT) hourly until no further adjustment is required, then every 4 to 8 hours unless the rate of heparin infusion is changed.

> Patients at risk of bleeding may undergo the procedure without heparin. If there is no risk of bleeding, keep PTT at 1.5 to 2 times the normal value or follow the ACT protocol of your institution. At the initiation of CAVH, a blood sample for baseline PTT or ACT should be drawn from the arterial access line only. All the other samples are drawn from the venous access line to determine the coagulation status of the blood passing through the hemofilter.

4. Measure serum electrolytes and glucose every 2 hours until stable, then every 6 to 12 hours. Check the CBC, serum calcium, phosphorus, magnesium, creatinine, and BUN once daily. Serum electrolytes, creatinine, and BUN can be measured on the ultrafiltrate sample rather than a blood sample.
5. Drug removal is very limited, and replacement is usually unnecessary.[2] If replacement is required Supplemental dose = (desired drug level − arterial level) × volume of distribution × body weight (kg)
6. Inspect the insertion sites of the vascular access lines daily for signs of infection.

H. COMPLICATIONS

See Table 49-2.

References

1. BLATZ S, PAES B, STEELE B: Peritoneal dialysis in the neonate. Neonatal Network 8:41, 1990
2. STAPLETON FB, JONES DP, GREEN RS: Acute renal failure in neonates: Incidence, etiology and outcome. Pediatr Nephrol 1:314, 1987
3. MEEKS ACG, SIMS DG: Treatment of renal failure in neonates. Arch Dis Child 63:1372, 1988
4. MATTHEWS DE, WEST KW, RESCORLA FJ, ET AL: Peritoneal dialysis in the first 60 days of life. J Pediatr Surg 25:110, 1990
5. ESPERANCA MJ, COLLINS DL: Peritoneal dialysis efficiency relation to body weight. J Pediatr Surg 1:162, 1966
6. ANAND SK: Acute renal failure in the neonate. Pediatr Clin North Am 29:791, 1982
7. BATSHAW ML, BRUSILOW SW: Treatment of hyperammonemic coma caused by inborn errors of urea synthesis. J Pediatr 97:893, 1980
8. GARTNER L, LEUPOLD D, POHLANDT F, BARTMAN P: Peritoneal dialysis in the treatment of metabolic crises caused by inherited disorders of organic and amino acid metabolism. Acta Paediatr Scand 78:706, 1989
9. TROMPETER RS: A review of drug prescribing in children with end-stage renal failure. Pediatr Nephrol 1:183, 1987
10. AANDGIL A, SRIVASTAVA RN: Drug prescribing in children with renal failure. Indian Pediatr 26:693, 1989
11. BENNETT WM, BLYTH WB: Use of drugs in patients with renal failure. In Schrier RW, Gottschalk CW (eds): Disease of the Kidney, 4th Ed. Boston, Little, Brown Co., 1988, p 3437

12. Giusti RJ, Kurtin P: Extended hemofiltration in a neonate: A case report and a review of the literature. Am J Perinatol 4:198, 1987

13. Golper TA, Wedel SK, Kaplan AA, et al: Drug removal during continuous arteriovenous hemofiltration: Theory and clinical observations. Int J Artif Organs 8:307, 1985

14. Golper TA: Continuous arteriovenous hemofiltration in acute renal failure. Am J Kidney Dis 6:373, 1985

15. Kaplan AA, Longnecker RE, Folkert VW, et al: Continuous arterio-venous hemofiltration: A report of six months experience. Ann Intern Med 100:358, 1984

16. Kiely MA: Continuous arteriovenous hemofiltration. Critical Care Nurse, 4:39, 1984

17. Lieberman KV: Continuous arteriovenous hemofiltration on children. Pediatr Nephrol 1:330, 1987

18. Lieberman KV, Nardi L, Bosch JP: Treatment of acute renal failure in an infant using continuous arteriovenous hemofiltration. J Pediatr 106:646, 1985

19. Ronco C, Brendolan A, Bragantini L, et al: Treatment of acute renal failure in the newborn by continuous arteriovenous hemofiltration. Trans Am Soc Artif Intern Organs 31:634, 1985

20. Suddaby EC, Bell SB, Murphy KJ: Continuous hemofiltration in infants and children. Pediatr Nurs 16:79, 1990

21. Zobel G, Ring E, Muller W: Continuous arteriovenous hemofiltration in premature infants. Crit Care Med 17:534, 1989

22. Jenkins RD, Kuhn RJ, Funk JE: Clinical implications of catheter variability on neonatal continuous arteriovenous hemofiltration. Trans Am Soc Artif Intern Organs 11:108, 1988

23. Merrill RH: The technique of slow continuous ultrafiltration. J Crit Illness 6:289, 1991

24. Kaplan AA, Petrillo R: Regional heparinization for continuous arteriovenous hemofiltration (CAVH). Trans Am Soc Artif Intern Organs 33:1, 1987

50 Conjunctival Scraping

Marilea Kay Miller
Mhairi G. MacDonald

A. INDICATIONS

To obtain specimen for cytologic and other testing (Table 50-1) to determine the cause of conjunctivitis.[1-8]

1. Most useful in active phase of disease
2. Permits detailed study of cells, inclusion bodies, and cell response
3. Tool for detecting intracellular bacteria

B. RELATIVE CONTRAINDICATIONS

When conjunctival swab will provide an adequate sample. However, although samples collected by conjunctival swabbing may be satisfactory for culture[6] the flourescein-labeled monoclonal antibody test for chlamydia (Syva Micro Trak®*), which directly detects chlamydial elementary bodies, requires a specimen containing at least 10 columnar epithelial cells.[7,8] Conjunctival scraping will more reliably provide an adequate sample.

C. EQUIPMENT

(Select appropriate equipment for proposed study.)

1. Sterile, cotton-tipped applicators
2. Appropriate culture media, for example
   a. Bacteria
      (1) Trypticase soy broth
      (2) Blood agar plate
      (3) Chocolate agar plate—*Haemophilus influenzae, Neisseria gonorrhoeae*
   b. Virus-holding medium
   c. Chlamydia culture transport medium (sucrose-phosphate)
   d. Sabouraud's agar with preservative if fungal conjunctivitis suspected.

3. Suitable topical anesthetic (e.g., proparacaine hydrochloride [Ophthaine]) (optional)
4. Sterile 5% glucose
5. Metal/plastic-shafted Ca alginate swabs
6. Presterile aluminum or platinum spatula or nasopharyngeal (NP) swab[†]

   a. Flexible wire portion of NP swab is bent into a small, smooth loop before unwrapping.[9]
   b. Use of wooden instruments may introduce artifact/inhibit growth.[10]

7. Glass microscope slides, frosted at one end for labeling
8. Pencil for labeling slides
9. Stains
   a. Gram's stain
   b. Giemsa stain
10. Absolute alcohol in slide-staining rack
11. Light microscope with oil-emersion lens
12. Syva Micro Trak® chlamydia trachomatis specimen collection kit

   If kit is not used, the following is required:

   a. Microscope slides with 8-mm wells (methanol-resistant paint required)
   b. Cyto brush
   c. Dacron swab
   d. Methanol fixative
   e. Container for slide transport to laboratory

D. PRECAUTIONS

1. Always consider gonococcal conjunctivitis in differential diagnosis. Take cultures from oro/nasopharynx, anus, and vagina, because concomitant infection at these sites is common.[11] (In the case of conjunctival samples positive for chlamydia, repeat

---

*Syva Company, Palo Alto, CA 94303

†For example, Kimura Platinum E-109 Spatula, STORTZ Instrument Company, St. Louis, MO 63101

TABLE 50-1
Analysis of Conjunctival Scrapings

Test	Organism(s) Identified	Finding
Gram's stain	Neisseria gonorrhea	Gram-negative diplococci
Giemsma stain	Chlamydia trachomatis	Intraepithelial intracytoplasmic inclusions
Papanicolaou stain	Herpes simplex virus	Multinucleate giant cells and inclusion-bearing cells
Direct antigen detection techniques		
Immunofluorescent indicator system	Chlamydia trachomatis	
Immunosorbent assay (ELISA)	Chlamydia trachomatis Herpes simplex virus	
Flourescein-labeled monoclonal antibodies (Syva MicroTrak®)	Chlamydia trachomatis	Extracellular elementary bodies
Indirect fluorescence	Herpes simplex virus	
Culture		
Specific Media		
Thayer-Martin	Neisseria gonorrhea	
Aerobic	Gram-positive and gram-negative bacteria	
Anaerobic	Anaerobic bacteria	
Viral transport	Herpes simplex virus	
Chlamydia culture	Chlamydia trachomatis	

nasopharyngeal cultures in 4 to 6 weeks are advisable to detect infants at risk for nonbacterial pneumonia.)

2. Avoid use of cotton-tipped applicator to obtain sample.
  a. Insufficient sample obtained/wooden shaft (see C6 above)
  b. Sample contaminated with strands from tip
3. Recognize that diphtheroids, *Staphylococcus albus,* and *Micrococcus* are normal conjunctival flora.[9]
4. Keep spatula blade flat against tarsal conjunctiva at all times to avoid corneal injury.
5. Use separate sterile spatula (or NP swab) for each eye.

E. METHOD FOR EVERTING EYELIDS

Upper Lid (Fig. 50-1)

1. Grasp lashes and border of lid between thumb and index finger of nondominant hand.
2. Draw lid downward and away from eyeball.
3. Indent upper lid, with handle of cotton-tipped ap-

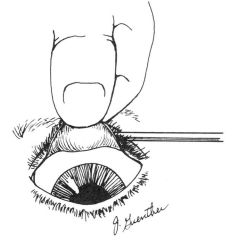

FIG. 50-1
Everting the upper eyelid.

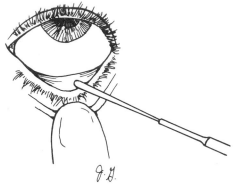

FIG. 50-2
Using Kimura platinum spatula to take scraping from lower eyelid.

plicator held in dominant hand, and pull lid back and upward over applicator.

4. Remove applicator and hold lid in place with non-dominant hand by gently pressing border of lid against superior orbital margin.

Lower Lid

1. Place index finger of nondominant hand on margin of lower lid.
2. Pull downward, as in Figure 50-2.

F. PROCEDURE[1,9,12,13]

1. Obtain cultures from each eye prior to conjunctival scraping.
   a. Moisten Ca alginate swabs with 5% glucose or liquid culture medium.
   b. Evert eyelid, as in E.
   c. Gently apply alginate swab to bulbar and palpebral conjunctiva of upper and lower fornices of eye.
   d. Apply swab directly to culture media.
   e. Label cultures.
   f. Incubate cultures immediately at 37°C.
2. Instill topical anesthetic, with lids everted, or into medial canthus of eye, with head tilted to that side (optional).
3. Scrape upper or lower tarsal conjunctiva.
   a. Evert eyelid as described in E.
   b. Swab off excess discharge.
   c. Take scraping approximately 2 mm from lid margin (see Fig. 50-2).

Epithelium at lid margins is naturally keratinized and may be mistakenly considered pathologic.

   d. Pass spatula (or NP swab) two to three times in same direction (not back and forth) firmly but avoiding bleeding.
4. Spread specimen from spatula onto clean glass slide.

   Specimen for culture may be inoculated directly into transport medium.

   a. Remove excess fluid from specimen by tapping spatula on edge of slide.
   b. Place spatula flat on slide, and pass back and forth over 3- to 5-mm area until cohesive material appears.
   c. Spread evenly and gently to avoid maceration or clumping of cells.
5. Fix smears as required for proposed tests.
   a. Remove slides and allow to air dry.
   b. Label slides with patients' name, prior to staining with Gram's stain (bacteriologic examination) or Giemsa stain (cytologic examination) examination under oil-emersion objective of light, microscope, or other examination.

G. INTERPRETATION OF CONJUNCTIVAL CYTOLOGY

1. Cellular reactions
   a. Polymorphonuclear reaction
      (1) Bacterial infections
      (2) Chlamydial infection and trachoma
      (3) Monilial keratitis
      (4) Erythema multiforme
      (5) Very severe viral infection
   b. Mononuclear reaction—viral infections
   c. Eosinophilia and basophilia—allergic states
   d. Plasma cells—chlamydial infection
2. Intraepithelial cell inclusions[3,5,6,12]
   a. Chlamydial infection
      (1) Acidophilic inclusions in cytoplasm, capping epithelial cell nuclei (See Color Fig. 50-1 at the beginning of this book.)
      (2) Basophilic "initial bodies" in cytoplasm (See Color Fig. 50-2 at beginning of book.)
   b. Viral infection
      Giant, multinucleated, epithelial cells may be seen (e.g., herpetic keratoconjunctivitis).

3. Keratinization of conjunctival epithelial cells
   a. Always pathologic, except at lid margins
   b. Seen in
      (1) Vitamin-A deficiency
      (2) Exposure
      (3) Cicatrization (e.g., chronic chlamydia infection)

H. COMPLICATIONS

1. Conjunctival bleeding[12]
2. Injury to cornea
3. Transfer of infection from infected to noninfected eye
4. Occular irritation, pain, photophobia, lacrimation, tarsal swelling, conjunctival hyperemia, inflammation, discharge[6]

References

1. Aronson S, Elliott J: Diagnostic principles. In Aronson S, Elliott J (eds): Ocular Inflammation. St. Louis, CV Mosby, 1972, p 68
2. Dawson C: Therapy of diseases caused by Chlamydia organisms. Int Ophthalmol Clin 13:93, 1973
3. Foster R: Ophthalmia neonatorum. In Duane T (ed): Clinical Ophthalmology, Vol 4. Hagerstown, MD, Harper & Row, 1976, p 5
4. Kimura S, Thygeson P: The cytology of external ocular disease. Am J Ophthalmol 39:137, 1955
5. Vastine D: Infections of the ocular adnexa and cornea. In Peyman G, Saunders D, Goldberg M (eds): Principles and Practice of Ophthalmology. Philadelphia, WB Saunders, 1980, p 288
6. Darougar S, Jones BR: Conjunctival swabbing for the isolation of TRIC agent (*Chlamydia*). Br J Ophthalmol 55:585, 1971
7. Uyeda CT, Welborn P, Ellison-Birang N, et al: Rapid diagnosis of chlamydial infections with the Micro-Trak® Direct Test. J Clin Microbiol 20:948, 1984
8. Rapoza PA, Quinn TC, Keissling LA, et al: Assessment of neonatal conjunctivitis with a direct immunoflourescent monoclonal autobody strain for *Chlamydia*. JAMA 255:3369, 1986
9. Marks MI, Welch DF: Diagnosis of bacterial infections of the newborn infant. Clin Perinatol 8:548, 1981
10. Hammerschlag MR: Chlamydial infections. Pediatr Rev 3:77, 1981
11. Cattin BW: Nutritional profiles of *Neisseria gonorrhoeae*, *Neisseria meningitides* and *Neisseria lactamica* in chemically defined media and the use of growth requirements for gonococcal typing. J Infect Dis 128:178, 1973
12. Furigiuele F: Disorders of the conjunctiva. In Harley R (ed): Pediatric Ophthalmology. Philadelphia, WB Saunders, 1975, p 261
13. Goscienski P: Inclusion conjunctivitis in the modern infant. J Pediatr 77:19, 1970

Appendix A

Chapter 5

TABLE A1
Elimination Half-lives of the Opioids

Opioid	Relative dose	$T_{1/2}\beta$ Neonate	$T_{1/2}\beta$ Child
Morphine	0.1 mg	6.8 hr	2.2 hr
Fentanyl	1–5 μg	250 min	208 min
Sufentanil	0.2–1 μg	737 min	140 min
Alfentanil	5–25 μg	525 min	84 min

From: Arnold JH, Anand KJS. Anesthesia and analgesia in the neonate. *In* Avery GB, Fletcher MA, MacDonald MG (eds.). Neonatology—Pathophysiology and Management of the Newborn. Fourth Edition. Philadelphia, PA, J.B. Lippincott, 1993. Reprinted with permission.

TABLE A2
Recommended Dosages and Oral/Parenteral Ratios for Opioids

Drug	Routes of Administration	Parenteral Dosage (mg/kg)	Frequency	Oral/Parenteral Ratio	Frequency
Morphine	IM, IV SQ, PO, PR Neuraxial*	0.05–0.2	q 1–2 hr IV q 2–4 hr IM/SQ	3–6	q 4–6 hr‡ q 8–12 hr§
Meperidine	IM, IV, SQ, PO	0.5–1.5	q 1–2 hr IV q 2–4 hr IM/SQ	4	q 4–6 hr
Codeine	IM, IV, SQ, PO	0.5–1.0	q 2–4 hr	1.5–2	q 4–6 hr
Hydromorphone	IM, IV, SQ, PO, PR	0.02–0.04	q 2–4 hr	2–4	q 4–6 hr PO q 6–8 hr PR
Methadone	IM, IV, SQ, PO	0.05–0.2	q 12–24 hr	2	q 24 hr
Fentanyl	IM, IV, TM/TD† Neuraxial*	0.001–0.005	q 1–2 hr	—	

IM = intramuscular, IV = intravenous, SQ = subcutaneous, PO = by mouth, PR = per rectum, TM/TD = transmucosal/transdermal, q = every.

*Neuraxial (epidural, subarachnoid) administration can be performed only by qualified and experienced anesthesiologists.

†TM/TD preparations have not been standardized for use in term or preterm neonates.

‡Pertains to regular oral preparations (e.g., MSIR®, Roxanal®, tablets and oral solutions).

§Pertains to slow release oral or rectal preparations (e.g., MS Contin®, Duramorph®, Roxanol SR®).

From Arnold JH, Anand KJS: Anaesthesia and analgesia in the neonate. In Avery GB, Fletcher MA, MacDonald MG (eds.): Neonatology: Pathophysiology and Management of the Newborn, Fourth Edition. Philadelphia, JB Lippincott, 1993.

TABLE A3

Recommended Dosages for Non-steroidal Anti-inflammatory Drugs

Drug	Dosage (mg/kg)	Routes of Administration	Frequency
Acetaminophen	10–20	PO, PR	q 4–6 hr
Aspirin	10–15	PO	q 4 hr
Choline-magnesium trisalicylate	10–15	PO	q 6–8 hr
Ibuprofen	5–15	PO, PR	q 6–8 hr
Naprosyn	5–7	PO	q 8–12 hr
Tolectin	5–7	PO	q 8–12 hr
Ketorolac tromethamine	0.3–0.6	PO, IM, IV	q 6–8 hr

PO = by mouth, PR = per rectum, IM = intramuscular, IV = intravenous, q = every.

From Arnold JH, Anand KJS: Anaesthesia and analgesia in the neonate. In Avery GB, Fletcher MA, MacDonald MG (eds): Neonatology: Pathophysiology and Management of the Newborn, Fourth Edition. Philadelphia, JB Lippincott, 1993. Reprinted with permission.

Appendix B

Chapter 28

TABLE B1

Basic, All-purpose Instrument Tray

Sponge forceps (2–3)
  a. Straight or curved
  b. Serrated 7″
Medicine glass (1)
  a. For antiseptic solutions
  b. 1 oz
Surgical drapes (1–3)
  a. Single use: transparent, adhesive or
  b. Multiple use
    (1) Fenestrated (circumcision)
    (2) Fan-folded towels
Knife handle (1) or disposable scalpel
Scissors (1–2)
  a. Fine or delicate scissors
  b. Straight or slightly curved
  c. Sharp/sharp (1) and
  d. Sharp/blunt (1)
  e. 4–5½″
Dressing forceps without teeth (3–4)
  a. Eye or delicate
  b. Half curved (2) and
  c. Straight (1–2)
  d. 5½″
Tissue forceps with teeth, 1 × 2 (1–2)
  a. Thumb or iris
  b. 5½″
Ring-handled tissue forceps 5 × 6 (1)
  a. Allis or Babcock design
  b. 6″
Hemostatic forceps, ring handled (2–3)
  a. Fine or mosquito
  b. Straight and curved
  c. 5″ or 5½″
Vein retractor with small-width blades (1)
Probe with eye, 5½″ (1)
Needle holder (1)

Numbers in parentheses are suggested quantities. Descriptors are given for ordering but are subject to individual preference. Disposable, single-use, or plastic instruments from commercially prepared trays are not suitable for all procedures.

TABLE B2
Selected Sutures Appropriate for Common Neonatal Procedures

Types	Raw Material	Tissue Use	Advantages	Disadvantages
Absorbable				
Chromic gut	Mammalian collagen with chromium salt to delay absorption	Subcutaneous (Use plain gut for mucosa)	Retains strength for up to 90 days Versatile Can be used in presence of infection Requires only square knot tie	Moderate tissue reaction (3+) Tends to fray when tied Faster absorption the smaller the caliber
Vicryl® or Dexon®	Synthetic Copolymers	Subcutaneous Fascia	Mild tissue reaction (2+) Low infectivity rate For absorbable suture or ligature Maintains knots	Cannot be used for approximation under stress 60% strength at 2 weeks Safety in cardiovascular tissue not established Requires flat and square ties with extra throws
Nonabsorbable				
Silk	Braided protein filament from silk worm	Skin Fascia	Best knot holding Easiest to use Strong for size Gone after 1–2 years	High infectivity rate High tissue reaction (4+)
Nylon	Polyamide polymer Mono or braided filament	Monofilament: skin closure and plastic surgery Braided: any tissue	Inert Least tissue reaction (0–1+) Lowest infectivity Very strong for size	Poor knot-holding, requires at least 6 ties Not as easy to handle
Polypropylene Prolene®	Polymer of propylene Monofilament	Skin Pull-out subcuticular	Inert Low tissue reaction (0–1+) Low infectivity Very strong for size Holds knot better than nylon Easier to tie	Remains encapsulated Completely nonabsorbable
Mersilene® Dacron	Polyester polyethylene terephthalate	Skin	Easy to use Low infectivity rate Holds knot well Good overall suture	Mild reactivity (2+)
Skin closure tape	Reinforced nylon filaments to back or porous paper tape	Skin superficial laceration or when subcuticular suture also used	Easy to place and remove Quick to apply No skin reactivity Least scarring No anesthetic required	Will not stick to wet or oily skin (Wipe skin with alcohol first) Will not hold if wound is widely separated or under tension Cannot evert wound edges

Appendix C

Chapter 40

TABLE C1
Blood Products

Product	Available Volume	Shelf Life	Advantages	Disadvantages	Comments
I. Whole Blood A. Whole Blood Unit Hct = 40%	450 ± 45 ml + 63 ml CPD	1. CPA-1 = 35 days 2. CPD = 21 days 3. Heparin = 48 hours	1. Provides volume 2. RBC mass 3. Provides some coagulation factors	1. WBCs and platelets relatively nonfunctional unless fresh and unrefrigerated 2. Exposure to WBCs and platelet antigens 3. Risk of infectious disease transmission 4. Storage lesion defects (K^+, NH_3) tx in plasma faction	1. Use for exchange tx 2. Use for rapid, acute blood loss 3. Must be ABO identical
B. Quad Pack Collection Hct = 40%	450 ± 45 ml + 63 ml CPD	1. CPDA-1 = 35 days 2. CPD = 21 days 3. Usually used by 5 days	1. Allows multiple tx to one infant 2. Allows tx to multiple infants from one unit 3. Volume of each quad adjustable 4. Can be made into PRBCs	1. May outdate in small neonatal unit 2. Some wastage expected	1. Best collection device for active neonatal unit 2. Can use quad pieces for older patients after 5 days 3. Potential for small-volume collection by decreasing anticoagulant volume with ratio of 14 : 100 of anticoagulant : blood
C. Modified Pack Collection Hct = 40%	450 ± 45 ml + 63 ml CPD	1. CPDA-1 = 35 days 2. CPD = 21 days	1. Same as quad 2. Use of small-volume collection a. Allows repeated donations b. Allows donations from lower-weight persons	Not always practical to rebleed donor	See I,B,3, above

			Advantages	Disadvantages	Comments
D. Walking Donor Hct as in donor	Variable volume; drawn in heparin	No shelf life	1. Allows rebleeding of donor 2. Low cost 3. Freshest product 4. No storage lesion defects 5. Maintenance of Ca^{++} and pH	1. Loss of blood-bank control 2. Inadequate screening for infectious diseases 3. Risk of contamination in collection 4. Potential anticoagulation of recipient if high heparin : blood ratio	Disadvantages outweigh advantages when good blood banking is available Not a licensed product in USA
II. Reconstituted Whole Blood Hct variable by formula	Variable should not exceed 450 ± 45 ml	24 hours	1. Allows preparation of group-O cells with low titers of A and B antibody 2. Allows preparation of whole blood from stored RBCs (packed, frozen, or rejuvenated)	Time for preparation, especially with frozen products	1. Use for exchange tx of A, B, or AB infant 2. Provides replacement equivalent of fresh whole blood 3. Use following formula for reconstitution: $$\text{Volume plasma to add} = \text{Volume PRBCs} \times \left[\frac{\text{Hct PRBCs}}{\text{Hct desired}} - 1\right]$$
III. Autologous Fetal Blood Hct ≅ 50%–60%	50 ml or less (heparin)	<4 hours	1. Potential immediate availability in delivery room 2. Same infectious disease risk as mother 3. No foreign antigens 4. No storage lesion defects	1. Risk of bacterial contamination 2. Microaggregation 3. Difficult to obtain correct heparin : blood ratio (2–3 units/1 ml blood) 4. Requires anticipatory preparation for best procedural control	1. Use microaggregate or 3rd-generation leukocyte removal filter 2. Follow infant for coagulation defect and bacteremia 3. Properly prepared banked blood generally a better choice when time permits

(continued)

Product	Available Volume	Shelf Life	Advantages	Disadvantages	Comments
IV. Red-Cell Products					
A. Packed Red Blood Cells (PRBCs) Hct 70%–90+%	250 ml or variable from quad pack	1. CPDA-1 = 35 days 2. CPD = 21 days 3. Additive solutions = 42 days	1. Readily available 2. Easy to prepare	1. Presence of foreign antigens (platelet, WBC, and plasma) 2. Accentuated storage lesion defects if unit at end of shelf life	1. Principal use in replacement of iatrogenic blood loss 2. Must be ABO compatible
B. Sedimented Red Blood Cells Hct 65%	As above	As above	Does not require centrifugation	1. Hct may not be as high as desired 2. Contains more plasma	As above
C. Leukocyte-poor Red Blood Cells Hct variable (~70%) 1. Buffy-coat poor	As above	As above	Centrifugation with removal of 65%–90% PMNs	Time required for preparation	
2. Washed red blood cells	As above	24 hours	1. Removes 90% PMNs (70% total WBCs) 2. Removes platelets, K⁺, anticoagulants 3. Reduces transmission of CMV, other virus 4. Allows use of older blood 5. Hct adjustable 6. Less viscosity 7. Reduces alloimmunization to HLA and WBC antigens	1. Time required for preparation 2. More expensive than buffy-coat poor 3. Expires 24 hours after washing	1. Can wash pieces of quad pack 2. Can combine with fresh, frozen plasma for exchange transfusions
D. Deglycerolized Red Blood Cells	1. 250 ml in 0.9% NaCl with 2% Dextrose 2. Variable (see comments)	24 hours after thawing and washing	1. Excellent maintenance of 2,3-DPG and ATP 2. Removes 90% PMNs; >80% WBCs 3. Allows storage of rare types of blood or autologous blood	1. Higher cost than other preparations 2. Not universally available 3. Expires 24 hours after washing	If frozen in aliquots can thaw and wash as needed for a given infant

Product	Volume	Storage	Advantages	Disadvantages	Comments
E. Rejuvenated Red Blood Cells	1. Variable 2. See comments	Unknown	4. Same advantages as washed RBCs, above. Revitalizes older and outdated red blood cells	1. Experimental 2. Anticipated higher cost	1. Unlikely to be used in neonates 2. Rejuvenating solutions contain inosine, pyruvate, phosphate, high glucose
V. Plasma Products A. Fresh, Frozen Plasma or Single Donor Plasma	250 ml or 90 ml in Pedipack	1. 1 year, frozen (−18°C) 2. 24 hours, thawed	1. Available for general coagulation disorders 2. Generally available	1. 20 to 45 minutes thawing time 2. Must be transfused within 24 hours after thawing	1. Use blood filter 2. Must be ABO-group compatible
B. Albumin 5%	250 ml or 500 ml	3 years, at room temp	1. Heat treated to reduce risk of infectious diseases 2. Requires no crossmatch 3. Increases plasma oncotic pressure	Expense	1. Requires no filter 2. Na = 110 mEq/liter 3. Cl = 50 mEq/liter
C. Albumin 25%	20 ml, 50 ml, and 100 ml	3 years, at room temp	1. Requires no crossmatch 2. Provides increased oncotic pressure with low volume 3. Mobilizes extravascular fluid accumulation 4. Increased protein binding sites (bilirubin)	1. Expense 2. Short-lived response	1. Requires no filter 2. Na = 140 mEq/liter 3. Cl = 120 mEq/liter
D. Plasma–Protein Fraction	250 ml, 500 ml	5 years, at room temp	See albumin 5%	1. Contains globulin as well as albumin 2. Vasoactive peptides may cause hypotension	Not recommended for use in neonates
E. Cryoprecipitate	10 ml	1 year, frozen at −18°C	1. Treatment of deficiency of Factor VIII, Factor IX, and of von Willebrand's disease*	Must be used within 6 hours of thawing	1. Use blood filter 2. Should be ABO compatible

(*continued*)

Appendix C (Continued)

Product	Available Volume	Shelf Life	Advantages	Disadvantages	Comments
			2. Provides fibrinogen in higher concentration than FFP		
VI. Platelet Products A. Platelet Concentrate (random donor)	1. 45 ml–75 ml 2. 25 ml after concentration	3 to 5 days, depending on type of bag used	Approximately 5.5 × 10^10 platelets per bag	Contains some WBCs, few RBCs, and plasma	1. Use platelet administration set 2. Best transfused by gravity drip 3. Use immediately from blood bank 4. Should be ABO compatible 5. Store at 20–24°C with gentle agitation
B. Single-donor Pheresis	300 ml	1 to 5 days depending on technique used	1. 3 × 10^11 platelets per bag 2. Allows selection of HLA & PLA 1 compatible donor 3. Repeated pheresis possible	1. Requires special order 2. Large volume, unless concentrated 3. May have high WBC count	1. Complete transfusion within 3 hours after removal from blood bank 2. Store at 20–24°C with gentle agitation 3. Used for bleeding owing to thrombocytopenia in presence of antiplatelet, or anti-HLA antibodies

Key: *ATP*, adenosine triphosphate; *CMV*, cytomegalovirus; *CPD*, citrate phosphate dextrose; *CPDA-1*, citrate phosphate dextrose and adenine; *2,3-DPG*, diphosphoglycerate; *Hct*, hemocrit; *PMN*, polymorphonuclear leukocytes; *PRBC*, packed red blood cell; *RBC*, red blood cell; *tx*, transfusion; *WBC*, white blood cell

*Proven hemophilia A or B requires specific factor concentrates for major bleeding and surgery.

Appendix D

Chapter 49

TABLE D1
Drugs Requiring Adjustment in Severe Renal Failure

Drug	Method	Adjustment	Elimination by PD
Acetaminophen	i	q 8 hr	no
Acyclovir	i	q 48 hr	no
Allopurinol	i	q 12–24 hr	
	d	50%	
Amikacin	i	q 24 hr	yes
	d	20–30%	
Amoxicillin	i	q 12–16 hr	no
Amphotericin B	i	q 24–36 hr	no
Ampicillin	i	q 12–16 hr	no
Bumetanide		unchanged	
Captopril	d	50%	
Carbamazepine	d	75%	
Carbenicillin	i	q 24–48 hr	no
Cefaclor	d	33%	yes
Cefamandole	i	q 8 hr	no
Cefazole	i	q 24–48 hr	no
Cefotaxime	i	q 12–24 hr	no
Cefoxitin	i	q 24–48 hr	no
Ceftazidime	i	q 24–48 hr	no
Ceftriaxone		unchanged	no
Cefuroxime	i	q 48–72 hr	yes
Cephalexin	i	q 6–12 hr	no
Cephalothin	i	q 8–12 hr	yes
Chloral hydrate		Avoid	
Chloramphenicol		unchanged	no
Cimetidine	d	50%	no
Clavulanic acid	d	50–75%	no
Clindamycin		unchanged	no
Dexamethasone		unchanged	
Diazepam		unchanged	
Diazoxide		unchanged	yes
Dicloxacillin		unchanged	no
Digitoxin	d	50–75%	no
Digoxin	i	q 48 hr	no
	d	10–25%	no
Diphenhydramine	i	q 9–12 hr	
Erythromycin		unchanged	no
Ethambutol	i	q 48 hr	Yes
	d	unchanged	Yes

(continued)

TABLE D1   (*Continued*)

Drug	Method	Adjustment	Elimination by PD
Fentanyl		30–50%	
Flucytosine	i	q 24–48 hr	Yes
	d	20–30%	
Furosemide		unchanged	
Gentamicin	i	q 24 hr	Yes
	d	20–30%	
Heparin		unchanged	no
Hydrocortisone		unchanged	
Hydralazine	i	q 8–16 hr	no
Indomethacin		unchanged	
Insulin (Reg)	d	50%	
Isoniazid		unchanged	Yes
Kanamycin	i	q 24 hr	Yes
	d	20–30%	
Ketoconazole		unchanged	no
Labetalol		unchanged	
Lidocaine		unchanged	
Lorazepam	d	50%	
Meperidine		unchanged	
Metoprolol		unchanged	
Metronidazole	i	q 12–24 hr	no
Morphine		unchanged	no
Nafcillin		unchanged	
Naloxone		unchanged	no
Oxacillin		unchanged	
Penicillin G	i	q 12–16 hr	no
	d	25–50%	
Pentobarbital		unchanged	
Phenobarbital	i	12–16 hr	yes
Phenytoin		unchanged	
Prednisone		unchanged	
Propranolol		unchanged	
Rifampin		unchanged	no
Secobarbital		unchanged	no
Sodium nitroprusside		unchanged	
Theophylline		unchanged	yes
Thiazide		avoid	
Ticarcillin	i	q 24–48 hr	yes
Tobramycin	i	q 24 hr	yes
	d	20–30%	
Trimethoprim-sulfamethoxazole	i	24 hr	no
Valproic acid		unchanged	no
Vancomycin	i	q 24 hr	no
Verapamil	d	50–75%	

Renal failure alters the clearance of most drugs to a degree that is inversely proportional to the glomerular filtration rate. Drugs that are entirely cleared by the liver are administered without renal adjustment. Dose is adjusted by either administering a percentage of normal dose (d) or by increasing the interval (i) between the doses by hours.[9-11] The normal loading dose can be administered for virtually all drugs. Unlike hemodialysis, peritoneal dialysis usually has no significant effect on the clearance of most drugs. However, a supplemental dose is sometimes required. Blood levels of drug, if available, are the best guide.

Index